HOME REMEDIES: WHAT WORKS

HOME REMEDIES: WHAT WORKS

* *

THOUSANDS OF AMERICANS REVEAL THEIR FAVORITE HOME–TESTED CURES FOR EVERYDAY HEALTH PROBLEMS

* *

GALE MALESKEY, BRIAN KAUFMAN
and the editors of *PREVENTION* Magazine Health Books

Rodale Press, Emmaus, Pennsylvania

Copyright ©1995 by Rodale Press, Inc.

All rights reserved. No part of this publication may be reproduced or transmitted in any form or by any means, electronic or mechanical, including photocopying, recording or any other information storage and retrieval system, without the written permission of the publisher.

Prevention is a registered trademark of Rodale Press, Inc.

Printed in the United States of America on acid-free ∞, recycled paper ♻

Library of Congress Cataloging-in-Publication Data

Maleskey, Gale
     Home remedies: what works: thousands of Americans reveal their favorite, home-tested cures for everyday health problems / by Gale Maleskey, Brian Kaufman and the editors of Prevention Magazine.
     p.   cm.
     Includes index.
     ISBN 0–87596–233–5   hardcover
     ISBN 0–87596–407–9   paperback
     1. Medicine, Popular.   I. Kaufman, Brian, 1961–
II. Prevention (Emmaus, Pa.)   III. Title.
RC81.M218   1995
615.8'8—dc20   94–30876

Distributed in the book trade by St. Martin's Press

     4 6 8 10 9 7 5   hardcover

 2 4 6 8 10 9 7 5 3 1 paperback

─── OUR PURPOSE ───

*"We inspire and enable people to improve
their lives and the world around them."*

Thomas Platts-Mills, M.D., Ph.D. Professor of medicine and head of the Division of Allergy and Clinical Immunology at the University of Virginia Medical Center in Charlottesville

David P. Rose, M.D., Ph.D, D.Sc. Chief of the Division of Nutrition and Endocrinology at Naylor Dana Institute, part of the American Health Foundation in Valhalla, New York

William B. Ruderman, M.D. Chairperson of the Department of Gastroenterology at Cleveland Clinic Florida in Fort Lauderdale

Yvonne S. Thornton, M.D. Professor of clinical obstetrics and gynecology at Columbia University College of Physicians and Surgeons in New York City and director of the Perinatal Diagnostic Testing Center at Morristown Memorial Hospital in Morristown, New Jersey

Lila A. Wallis, M.D. Clinical professor of medicine and director of "Update Your Medicine," a continuing medical education program for physicians, at Cornell University Medical College in New York City

Andrew T. Weil, M.D. Associate director of the Division of Social Perspectives in Medicine at the University of Arizona College of Medicine in Tucson

Contents

CONTENTS

CONTENTS

CONTENTS

CONTENTS

CONTENTS

CONTENTS

CONTENTS

CONTENTS

CONTENTS

CONTENTS

CONTENTS

CONTENTS

CONTENTS

Introduction

Question: How does a home remedy get to be a *favorite* home remedy?

Answer: It works.

It happens something like this: You hurt. You try a home remedy you heard about. The pain goes away. Next time you hurt, you know just what to grab. When you find a way to deal with any one of life's common health problems, you use that trusted remedy again and again. And you undoubtedly tell your friends about it when they have that same problem to deal with.

That's what this book is about—people sharing their *best* home remedies, the stuff that really gets the job done.

A little more than a year ago, the editors at *Prevention* Magazine Health Books decided to tap into people power—the vast underground reserve of healing wisdom that exists across America. We figured there must be a lot of people who might be willing to share their favorite remedies in a major way . . . in a book. And were we ever right!

Working with Princeton Research Survey Associates, headquartered in New Jersey, we sent out a survey questionnaire to thousands of people across the country asking them to tell us about the home remedies that work for them. Then we sat back and waited. Within days, thousands of letters came pouring in, containing thousands and thousands of home remedies.

What a treasure we had in our hands. Remedies for hundreds of common health problems. Remedies that have been passed down for generations. Remedies from Europe, Asia, Latin America, the Caribbean, from American Indians. Remedies gathered from friends, trusted doctors, the corner pharmacist and from grandmothers and elderly family members.

And, what's really interesting, most of these remedies came packaged with a great story. One of my personal favorites is a headache cure from Margaret, a 74-year-old resident of La Puente, California. Margaret says to banish the pain, you simply soak raw potato slices in vinegar, then tuck them snugly into a headband. Frankly, our first reaction when we read that letter was to laugh. *Sure, Margaret, you really think I'm going to fall for that one and walk around with potatoes on my head?*

So, what were we going to do with Margaret's remedy? After all, she took the trouble to write the letter. It sounded way-out and wacky, but perhaps she was sincere. . . . So we called up a doctor who's an expert on headaches. (*You* try asking a doctor about something this bizarre; it's not easy.) The doctor didn't laugh. On the contrary, he assured us that this remedy would undoubtedly work for many people because of the clever combination of cold and pressure from the potato disks. Oh.

With this kind of verification coming from doctors, we learned quickly to view *all* the simple remedies that were sent to us with respect. But what were we going to do with all those wonderful letters containing all that outlandish advice? (Dab mouthwash on your head to cure dandruff, rub a backyard weed on yourself to cancel out poison ivy, stick your fingers in your ears to banish hiccups and so forth.)

It was obvious right from the start that this was not going to be your typical health book. And what we had to do soon became obvious as well.

We wanted to make sure that our readers were getting the best remedies available for each condition. So, in addition to the survey, we put a request in *Prevention* magazine asking for remedies. More letters rolled in.

We were touched by how much care went into all these letters. The people who wrote to us put such love into their stories. Think about it. Who has the time to write a letter these days? The people who wrote to us were sending healing information to perfect strangers. We decided that the best thing we could do, whenever possible, was to let folks tell about their remedies in their own words.

So, authors Gale Maleskey and Brian Kaufman spent the good part of a year calling people who had written us. They asked about where the remedies came from and for all the details on how they work. For a whole year they talked to the friendliest, warmest, most helpful people in the country.

We also knew that we couldn't just pass these remedies on to you without verifying them. Rodale Books takes its commitment to safety seriously. So we ran all the remedies by medical experts asking them two important questions: Does this really work? Is it safe? We had to eliminate a few remedies for safety reasons, but we were happy to do that.

INTRODUCTION

What you're holding in your hands represents the generous healing gifts of thousands of Americans, verified by top medical authorities. These remedies are safe, effective, home-grown and home-tested. And they work.

Alice Feinstein
Editor

Acne

Tactics for Smoother Skin

Compared with the war against life-threatening diseases, the battle over blemishes may seem about as important to your health as a coup d'état in a banana republic. Unless you're one of the walking wounded. Unless you bear the scars of the struggle. Unless you've got a bright red pimple on your nose the size of an American Legion hall.

The hostilities start when sebaceous glands beneath your skin pump oil through your pores to keep your skin from drying. Unfortunately, sometimes oil and dead cells are produced faster than they can exit from a pore, creating a solidified plug called a whitehead or blackhead. (A closed-off pore produces a whitehead. If the pore stays open, the top surface of the plug can darken, becoming a blackhead.)

If a whitehead ruptures the wall of a pore, invading bacteria can jump in and cause what's known as a pimple. And before you know it, those dreaded bumps are busting out all over.

But it's possible to fight back. Our army of survey takers have been on the front lines of acne eradication, and they've got some victories to report.

SO, BE AN EGGHEAD

Susan, a former cosmetologist, reaches no further than her refrigerator for her favorite blemish buster. The 42-year-old Grafton, West Virginia, resident recalls that when she was going to beautician's school, the students gave each other facials made with egg whites. "They were just great for the complexion. The egg white just seemed to draw the oil from my face," she says.

When a bump threatens today, Susan still wastes little time before cracking an egg. After removing makeup or grime with soap or a cleansing lotion, Susan breaks an egg, separating the yolk from the white as you would when baking a cake. She then dips her finger or a cotton swab into the egg white and applies it to her blemish.

"If I use this technique when a blemish is just beginning, usually by the next morning it's a lot better," she says.

Susan's egg remedy may be everything it's cracked up to be—and more, says James Fulton, M.D., a dermatologist in private practice in Newport Beach, California. "Egg white is a mild astringent—meaning it can help tighten skin—and probably contains some anti-inflammatory proteins," he says. "So it's not surprising that this remedy should have some benefit."

A SUPER BOWL OF OATMEAL PROVES ITS POWER

Here's a story that should make oatmeal lovers smile. It seems that Wilma, 44, of Lebanon, Missouri, had a son who was suffering from severe acne. After visiting a dermatologist, the young man was prescribed Retin A, a powerful and often successful acne treatment. Within a week, however, his skin was raw from an apparent allergic reaction, and he stopped using the medication.

At her grandmother's suggestion, Wilma mixed up a bowl of oatmeal. After letting the cereal cool, she spread it on her son's face, covered it with a clean, damp washcloth, left it there for 15 minutes and then washed it off. Wilma repeated this procedure each day for a week.

To her and her son's amazement, by the end of two weeks his acne had vanished. "Oatmeal seemed to help him—and it's cheap!" says Wilma. "Now, when he gets a flare-up, he just reapplies it for a day or two until the problem is gone."

In fact, for centuries women have believed that oatmeal has a unique ability to keep complexions clear—and with good reason, says Dr. Fulton. "Oatmeal is a natural astringent that also contains beneficial proteins," he says.

VINEGAR: A LITTLE DAB DOES HER

When Arlene was a teen, Gloria Swanson was wowing moviegoers with her great looks and smooth skin. So it's no surprise that the legendary star's acne-ending tactics inspired Arlene to develop her own cleansing plan.

While reading one afternoon, Arlene learned that Ms. Swanson used nothing but pure lemon juice on her skin. "At the time I didn't have any lemons. But I remember thinking, 'Vinegar has acid in it like lemon juice, so why wouldn't that work just as well?' "

After soaking a cotton ball in apple cider vinegar, Arlene dabbed some on her face and waited for the reviews to come rolling in.

She gave her remedy four stars. "It really stung when I put it on, but in a day or so it worked beautifully," says the 62-year-old church organist from Columbia Station, Ohio. "It seemed to dry up the blemishes right away."

As it turns out, Arlene's improvisation also gets critical raves for technical excellence. "Both lemon and vinegar *do* contain acids that can help flush out the pores. And either is great as an acne wash," says Dr. Fulton.

HOPE FROM SOAP

When Cindy's son was suffering from an infection on his hands, a pharmacist told her about Fels-Naptha soap. The product not only worked well for his hands, it took care of the whole family's blemishes. They haven't used another product for daily facial cleansing since. "I have no idea what makes it work, but we wouldn't use anything else," says Cindy.

Fels-Naptha works well but is an "aggressive" soap that's probably best for very oily skin, says Dr. Fulton. If you have dry, sensitive skin, he suggests washing with old-fashioned soaps like Sweetheart, which contain natural ingredients that he says are less irritating to the skin.

THEY ZAP 'EM WITH ZINC

About 10 percent of our survey takers zero in on what they believe are the acne-fighting effects of zinc. For Sandi of Chillicothe, Illinois, and her teen-age daughter with a troubled complexion, zinc was literally their last resort.

"At age 14 or 15, skin problems can be just earth-shattering," says Sandi. "But when we went to dermatologists, they gave my daughter things that just irritated her skin more."

Finally, Sandi read that some adolescents' acne might be linked to zinc deficiency. That was enough for her—she promptly bought some zinc supplements and suggested that her daughter take them.

Within a few months, Sandi noticed fewer blemishes on her daughter's face. But there was something else: "Her skin almost glowed. It was as if her skin chemistry changed," says this satisfied mom. Her daughter continued taking zinc for about a year and had no further skin problems, Sandi reports.

Zinc enthusiasts like Sandi may be onto something. "The theory is controversial, but using zinc seems to cut down on inflammation, and that reduces scarring," says Dr. Fulton.

EDITOR'S NOTE: Before adding zinc supplements to your diet to fight acne, consult your doctor. Among other findings, researchers have discovered that taking high doses of zinc may interfere with the way your body absorbs other minerals. According to experts, you shouldn't take more than 15 milligrams a day without medical supervision.

SHE BLAMES FATTY FOODS

With three teens in the house, Marie was on full acne alert during her tour of duty as a housewife in Potlatch, Idaho. And while the family *did* enjoy some success with over-the-counter acne preparations, she says it was their all-out war against dietary fat that sealed the victory.

"Eating high-fat foods like chocolate, pork, beef, potato chips and nuts really seemed to cause eruptions in my kids—as quickly as the very next day," says the 57-year-old school librarian.

The notion that certain foods—candy, milk, and fried or greasy foods, for example—cause skin problems has a wide following among the general public. But scientific studies detailing a direct diet/acne link are rare. Even so, it's wise to avoid a particular food if you break out after eating it, says Michael Ramsey, M.D., a Wharton, Texas, dermatologist and a clinical instructor of dermatology at Baylor College of Medicine in Houston.

One proven culprit in food is the mineral iodine. Because iodine-rich foods like clams, crabs and other shellfish have been associated with acne, it's best not to eat these in large quantities if you are susceptible to blemishes, notes Dr. Ramsey.

THE CASE OF THE DIRTY PILLOWCASE

As a nutritionist in McKinleyville, California, Kathie believes that what you put in your mouth can have an effect on your face. But she has discovered something else as well: It's important to rest your face on a fresh and clean pillowcase.

"While I was representing a line of skin care products, the company provided us with a questionnaire for our customers," says Kathie. "One of the questions was: Do you change your pillowcase at least once a week? At first, I thought it was an odd question. But after I researched the subject, I found out that it's really important."

Kathie says she learned tiny flakes of dead skin are constantly falling off your face—even while you sleep. Meanwhile, your sebaceous glands continue producing oil, which also attracts dirt. And all that material has nowhere to go but onto your pillowcase and sheets, she says.

"So each night you spend eight hours rubbing your face in the accumulation of dead skin cells, oil and dirt," says Kathie. "By the end of the week, that's not very pleasant—or good for your skin."

Kathie says she invariably receives several not-so-subtle reminders when she forgets to change her bed linen at least once a week. "No doubt about it. I start having a few more blackheads and a pimple here or there."

Dermatologists say nearly anything that touches your face—even a telephone receiver or your fingers—has the potential to block pores, causing blemishes. And if you go to bed wearing greasy hair care products or makeup, you run an even greater risk of acne for that same reason.

Age Spots

Ways to Make 'Em Fade

They may look cute splashed across the nose of a six-year-old, but when brown-colored spots start to dot the backs of your hands or dapple your brow...well, let's just say they're a lot cuter on a freckle-faced kid.

Age spots, also called liver spots, are areas of increased skin pigmentation caused both by aging and too much sun. Usually they look like dark, smooth freckles, but sometimes they are slightly raised. They are generally harmless enough, although any skin discoloration that starts to increase in size or to change color or texture should be checked by a doctor.

Although our survey participants don't seem particularly concerned about age spots, a small percentage of people suggested a number of ways to make them fade away.

GRATEFUL FOR LEMON AID

"Using a cotton-tip applicator, I dab fresh lemon juice on the spots at least twice a day," says Millie, a retired school teacher in Tucson, Arizona. She says this remedy really works for her, provided it's combined with a second important ingredient: patience. "It takes a month or two before I see results."

Millie also applies sunscreen over the lemon juice, and continues to use the sunscreen after the spots have faded. "If I don't protect my skin from the sun, those spots come back before I know it," she says.

The secret of lemon juice's success could be its mild acidity. The citric acid it contains is just strong enough to safely peel off the skin's upper layer, says Jerome Z. Litt, M.D., a Cleveland dermatologist and author of *Your Skin: From Acne to Zits*. That peeling action can remove or lighten some age spots, he says. Citric acid is also the active ingredient in some cosmetic bleaches sold to lighten freckles and nails.

HER MOM WASHED IN BUTTERMILK

Long before there was Avon or Mary Kay, there was buttermilk. Beth of Elberton, Georgia, recalls that, at the end of a long day outdoors, her mother would wash her hands in buttermilk she'd made herself. "It was a treatment passed down by the women in my family, and my mother said it did work to fade age spots," Beth recalls.

Long used as a skin cleanser and beauty treatment, buttermilk contains lactic acid, an ingredient also found in some cosmetics.

Splashed on, then lightly blotted, buttermilk coats the skin with a slightly acidic mantle. As with lemon juice, this may cause some gentle peeling of upper skin layers that helps fade superficial age spots.

ALOE HELPS IN THE SUN BELT

"Since I have retired to the South, I am outside a lot, and my hands and face are exposed to a lot of sunlight," reports Martha, of Bayonet Point, Florida. "Both my friends and I use aloe vera gel, often straight from the plant, to fade age spots on our hands and faces." It takes about a month of applying the gel once or twice a day to see results, Martha says.

Aloe vera gel is another beauty treatment that seems to have withstood the test of time. This clear liquid is pressed from the thick, fleshy leaves of the aloe vera plant. In laboratory studies, fresh aloe vera gel has been found to promote the growth of normal skin cells. Commercial products containing "stabilized" aloe vera gel, however, did not have this beneficial effect. So if you're going to try aloe, the fresh material may be your best bet.

SUNSCREEN: A WISE PRECAUTION

"I don't think I'm old enough to have age spots, but I do tend to develop some large brown patches on the back of my hands if I'm out in the sun a lot," reports Marie, 38, of Denver. Both gardening and biking expose the tops of her hands to plenty of direct sunlight. "I noticed these spots fade during the winter, when I'm outdoors less often. So I started using a sunscreen with a protection factor of 30 during the summer months. This is the second summer I've used it, and my hands look much better now." To avoid having a greasy grip, she wipes the palms of her hands with a paper towel after applying the lotion.

It's no surprise that slathering on sunscreen should help prevent age spots or make them fade. After all, it's the sun's skin-damaging rays that help cause age spots in the first place. In fact, doctors say that, regardless of what remedy you use to fade age spots, you should top it off with a coat of sunscreen with a sun protection factor (SPF) of at least 15.

A LINK WITH ZINC?

"On a friend's recommendation, I started taking a zinc supplement every day," says Etta, 79, of Lowell, Arkansas. She says that soon afterward, the age spots on her hands and arms began to fade, and eventually they disappeared.

Just a coincidence? Perhaps not. In fact, one type of skin spot—actually a small bruise that some people might mistake for age spots—can result from zinc deficiency, doctors at England's East Birmingham Hospital reported. They found that 20 people with purplish brown spots called senile purpura had lower zinc levels than 20 others whose skin was free of spots.

"This condition does respond to zinc replacement," says Alexander Zemtsov, M.D., associate professor of dermatology at Texas Tech University in Lubbock. While senile purpura and age spots are not quite the same, zinc is generally known to be involved in tissue repair and wound healing. Whether or not it could actually help fade true age spots has not been studied, Dr. Zemtsov says.

EDITOR'S NOTE: Large amounts of zinc can hinder your body's absorption of other minerals. So experts recommend that you don't take more than 15 milligrams a day without medical supervision.

HERBAL CONCOCTION IS HER CURE

"For occasional age spots, I use gotu kola, an ancient Chinese herb, sold in health food stores," says Grace, 70, a Tucson, Arizona, woman who says she's been studying herbs for 20 years. She mixes about ⅛ teaspoon of powdered gotu kola into a cup of herbal tea or else adds it to plain hot water along with ⅛ teaspoon of ginseng and a pinch of cayenne.

"I'll drink this if I notice age spots appearing on my hands. For me, it clears the spots in two to three days," she says.

In some parts of the world—India, especially—gotu kola is taken by people who believe it promotes longevity. Long-lived elephants have been observed feeding extensively on the leaves of this creeping plant. Whatever its antiaging properties, however, the herb does contain an ingredient that apparently stimulates wound healing, according to Varro E. Tyler, Ph.D., a professor of pharmacognosy in the School of Pharmacy and Pharmacal Sciences at Purdue University in West Lafayette, Indiana, and author of *The Honest Herbal.*

EDITOR'S NOTE: Gotu kola's effectiveness and safety have yet to be scientifically proven, Dr. Tyler says. For that reason, it's best used under medical supervision. Like drugs, herbs often contain active ingredients that can have unwanted side effects. For instance, in large doses, gotu kola acts as a sedative.

Anal Fissures

Mending the Tears

Let's face it: Anal fissures are a pain in the butt! But as our survey takers have discovered, these small tears in the skin around the anus are preventable. Among the best approaches: mending bad bowel habits. They also say they've learned how to soothe the pain. Here's how they do it.

V IS FOR VASELINE

Vaseline, that all-purpose petroleum jelly, prevailed in our survey as both the preferred preventive and the main treatment for painful anal fissures.

In Mary's case, the best defense against an anal fissure is a good offense—and to her that means plenty of Vaseline. "If you've ever had one of these, all you need is something hard to pass through there, and it will reopen if you haven't taken precautions," says the 51-year-old Doylestown, Pennsylvania, housewife.

Using a piece of toilet tissue, Mary says she liberally applies Vaseline to the area just before a bowel movement. If her fissure reopens and bleeding occurs, Mary says she also applies some cortisone cream to speed healing.

"I used to just put up with it, but this is far preferable," she says. "It works for me."

Frank, 48, from Indiana, also says he "coats the entire area" with Vaseline. Mary, 78, says she gently massages sore fissures with Vaseline or "any oily based ointment."

All three are on their way to a full recovery, says Lester Rosen, M.D., associate clinical professor at Hahnemann University School of Medicine in Philadelphia and a board member of the American Society of Colon and Rectal Surgeons. "Any lubricant or cream over the short term, which would facilitate easier passage of the bowel movement, would probably help heal most superficial cracks or acute fissures," says Dr. Rosen.

EDITOR'S NOTE: Be careful using cortisone creams for any length of time. "More than three or four weeks of topical steroid preparations can actually thin the lining of the skin, so when the tear heals, it's actually weaker than it should be, setting you up for more superficial tears," Dr. Rosen says.

SHE COMBATS CONSTIPATION

It's just common sense to Viola, but she says drinking lots of water helps keep her from getting constipated and, as a result, from getting fissures. "When I worked, I used to keep a glass of ice water on my desk all the time," says the 75-year-old Amarillo, Texas, resident. "They say you're supposed to have about eight glasses a day. I couldn't drink that many, but I try to have at least five."

In another fissure-fighting move, Mary says she eats lots of fruit and bran products to keep her bowels moving easily.

If you don't take daily, practical steps to maintain regularity, you could end up with much more than just pain, says Dr. Rosen. "When you strain or have severe bouts of diarrhea, the little superficial cracks can go deep into the muscle, setting up a spasm that prevents the rectum from stretching," he says. "Unfortunately, when this kind of fissure opens up, it really can't be treated effectively with anything other than surgery."

And just how much water and fiber do you need to keep the surgeon at bay? Dr. Rosen recommends between six and eight glasses of water and 15 to 35 grams of fiber a day. "We tell people to balance their diet with a certain amount of fiber, like fruit or vegetables. A good bran cereal has about 8 to 10 grams of fiber. And sometimes people enjoy a psyllium preparation (a key in-gredient in many natural laxatives) which will give them a hefty dose of fiber. Depending on the cereal you choose, that puts you about a fraction of the way there." (If you're not currently eating this much fiber, Dr. Rosen recommends upping your intake gradually to avoid problems with gas and bloating.)

Because most fruits and vegetables contain about 1.5 to 2 grams of fiber, eating four or five servings of these, in addition to your psyllium-cereal regi-men, should provide all the fiber you need to keep your bowels healthy.

Also try avoiding dairy products for a time if you're constipated. Milk, cheese and ice cream can block your bowels, says Dr. Rosen. Spicy foods can also cause problems, he says, so avoid them until your regularity returns.

SHE OPTS FOR ALOE VERA

Normally, Joan saves her beloved aloe vera for treating sunburn. But when several over-the-counter remedies failed to heal her painful anal fissures, she decided to give the plant a new challenge. "I know aloe vera is good for sunburns and rashes and things like that because I use it all the time," says the 56-year-old San Jose, California, day care center director. "So I thought, why not experiment with this?"

Snipping a leaf from an aloe vera plant in her garden, Joan squeezed out the aloe and applied it liberally with a cotton swab or her finger twice a day for about two weeks. "It worked out great," she says. "It was so soothing, and it healed the fissure nicely."

And when she needs more gel than her aloe plant can give, Joan says she buys a gallon jug at her local health-food store.

Medical researchers have found that aloe gel speeds the healing of surgical wounds, burns, pressure sores and frostbite. And in addition to containing salicylates, the same anti-inflammatory painkiller found in aspirin, aloe vera also may inhibit the histamine reactions that cause itching and irritation.

SHE LIKES A GOOD SOAK

The fissure-fighting choice of one 70-year-old woman: the ever-popular sitz bath. For the uninitiated, a sitz bath is sitting in three or four inches of warm bath water with your knees raised. "I take a hot sitz bath after bowel movements," the woman reports.

"Probably one of the greatest things to relieve rectal pain is the warm, not hot, sitz bath," says Dr. Rosen. "It's fairly well known that the moist heat can also relax the anal sphincter muscles, which can help subside spasm."

EDITOR'S NOTE: *If your fissures or bleeding continue for any length of time, see your doctor. "If you were to have one hard bowel movement and feel a tear and you bleed and it stops, then it's not a big issue; but certainly persistent bleeding should get attention, just as if you were bleeding from any other part of your body," says Dr. Rosen.*

Arthritis

Help for the Pain and Stiffness

Perhaps because so many people have at least a touch of arthritis, it seems that just about everyone knows of a home remedy for this painful condition. The people who answered our survey told us of dozens of arthritis self-care treatments they favored—from alfalfa tea to stretching exercises to zinc supplements.

Several survey participants have developed their own home-care programs combining nutrition, exercise, heat, massage, rest and other methods to keep arthritis pain at bay. "I tried lots of things, and over time, I figured out what worked for me," explains a 76-year-old Minneapolis grandmother who's had mild arthritis in her knees for more than 20 years. Her response typifies the group's spirit of trial-and-error learning and persistence.

Some people say they need to limit their use of arthritis drugs as much as possible because those drugs have so many side effects. So they're using home remedies rather than relying on medication. And many of those remedies—hot baths and exercise, for instance—are actually recommended by their own doctors.

But many of the remedies we heard about—especially those involving vitamins, minerals or herbs—are not often recommended by doctors. In fact, several people told us their doctors laughed, got angry or expressed disbelief when they learned a patient was using vitamins, minerals or an herbal preparation specifically to help their arthritis.

"I don't bother to tell a doctor that I take vitamins A, B, C, E, calcium, garlic, and herbal teas—that way I don't have to watch his pained expression," says a 76-year-old Missouri woman. Even without the doctor's approval, she feels confident that there are benefits to her own remedies—and she continues to use them.

Someone who has rheumatoid arthritis—the serious inflammatory form of the disease—experiences many flare-ups and remissions, so it's dif-

11

ficult to evaluate whether the remedy is helping or whether the arthritis is just following its natural course. Osteoarthritis is the more common "wear-and-tear" type of arthritis: It may progress intermittently, and sometimes even reverse itself, so it's hard to tell whether the remedies are working or the condition has just been put on hold for a while. Top that off with the fact that even experts have no idea what causes the occasional sponta-neous remission in rheumatoid arthritis, or why some people with os-teoarthritis do so much better than others, and you can understand why there are so many remedies and so much debate over which remedies work and which don't. That debate isn't likely to be resolved any time soon.

With that in mind, here are the best of the home remedies we heard about from the people who use them.

EXERCISE KEEPS THEM MOBILE

"Keep moving!" a Princeton, New Jersey, grandmother admonishes. Many others follow that advice, too. In fact, 26 percent of those who replied to this survey question say they walk, swim, stretch, cross-country ski or bike on a regular basis to keep their joints flexible, their muscles strong, their energy flowing and their emotions on an even keel.

"Five days a week, I walk for ten minutes, bike for ten minutes and work out to a stretching tape for ten minutes," reports Joyce, a Warren, Texas, woman who has Sjögren's syndrome, a disorder in the rheumatoid arthritis category characterized by dry eyes and mouth, along with joint and muscle pain. "Exercise helps to keep up my energy, and it's one of my main forms of stress release."

"I'm creaky, and it hurts sometimes, but I do those exercises!" adds Marge, a registered nurse in San Antonio, Texas, who has arthritis "just about everywhere." She does a series of stretches for her back and also spends time on a stair climber, exercise bike and rowing machine. "I may not like it when I start out, but by the time I'm done, I feel wonderful. And if I don't exercise, in about three days I feel terrible," she says. "The body was meant to be in motion!"

"My physical therapists really stress exercise. I don't dare not do it!" says Janice, 75, of Wilbraham, Massachusetts. She swims for a half-hour two or three times a week in a balmy Olympic-sized indoor pool. "I'm not a great swimmer. I can only do the side stroke, and so that's what I do." Swimming has helped ease the arthritis pain in her hips and knees, she says.

In fact, studies show that staying active is one of the most important things people with arthritis can do. Too much rest ultimately makes arthritis symptoms worse, not better. It makes joints stiffen up and become even more painful. It weakens muscles, depletes stamina and erodes people's ability to do even simple things for themselves, which can lead to dependence, fear and depression.

Researchers have found that both walking and water aerobics programs are well tolerated by most people with osteoarthritis or rheumatoid arthritis. These activities improve stamina while reducing joint pain.

HEAT SEEKERS FIND RELIEF

Almost instinctively, many survey participants seek out sources of heat to keep their joints warm and comfortable. Whether it's a heating pad, hot water bottle, steaming dishwater, balmy beach, goose down sleeping bag or pile-lined sweatsuit, about 80 percent of those who use heat say it works wonders.

"If my fingers and wrists hurt, I'll offer to do the evening dishes," says Mary, 48, of Baltimore. Of course, it helps that her husband is always ready to oblige her by letting her do the dishes!

"I use the whirlpool at the YMCA," says Linda, 53, a teacher in Boston. "After I've been in the pool for a few minutes and I'm warmed up, I do range-of-motion exercises that help to keep my joints flexible. The buoyancy and warmth provided by the water really make these exercises easier for me to do."

"When I'm trying to fall asleep, I'll use a heating pad on my back or wherever I hurt most," says Joyce, of Texas. "It eases the pain enough so that I can sleep."

EDITOR'S NOTE: As a safety matter, you shouldn't fall asleep when you're using a turned-on heating pad. If you're planning to use a heating pad at bedtime, invest in a timer that will automatically switch off the pad after several minutes. Better yet, use a hot water bottle wrapped in a cloth, which will cool down on its own.

VITAMINS AND MINERALS TOP THE LIST

Most people in our survey told us they take a variety of vitamins and minerals to relieve their arthritis pain. Those who suggested individual supplements were most likely to list vitamin C or calcium. Vitamins B_6 and E, zinc, magnesium, beta-carotene and a number of other nutritional supplements were also mentioned.

"My pain really and truthfully is gone. I just wish other people with arthritis could have my success," says Evalee, 56, who with her husband manages a soybean and corn farm in Mount Pleasant, Iowa. She attributes her recovery to a combination of nutrients: calcium and magnesium, vitamins A and D, vitamins C (300 milligrams a day) and E (200 international units, or IU, daily), along with beta-carotene and the B-complex vitamins. It took her a few years to settle on that combination. She chose some of the nutrients as a result of reading about nutrition and started taking others when her husband went on a diet and was given supplements. Her own doctor gives no credit to vitamins.

"I couldn't tell you exactly which vitamin or mineral is providing the benefits," she says. "I think it's all of them together. I had terrible pain in my wrists, fingers, thumb and one elbow, but in the three years I have been taking these vitamins, my pain has gone. This summer, I spent three long days pulling weeds. It was hard, hard work, and believe me, there was a time when my elbow and wrists would have been sore and tender for weeks after that kind of hard use. But this time I had no pain at all."

Herman, 84, a retired engineer in Freehold, New Jersey, credits vitamins C and E, calcium, magnesium and zinc, along with other nutrients, for the fact that he has been able to cut back on the amount of aspirin he needs to take for the arthritis in his hips. Herman does other things as well—he walks every day and avoids certain foods.

"It's hard to tell for sure which things are working, but I seem to be doing better in general, so I must be doing something right," he says. Herman, too, does not discuss his at-home arthritis treatments with his doctor. "We do not see eye-to-eye on this," he admits.

Kathy, a 47-year-old government worker in Annapolis, Maryland, read about vitamin E relieving osteoarthritis pain and decided to try it for herself. "I have osteoarthritis in both knees as a result of high school gymnastics injuries, and they were getting to be quite painful," she says. "I took vitamin E for a couple of months before I noticed that it really was working. Mainly, I have less morning stiffness and pain."

Some people discover what they consider to be a nutritional link to arthritis purely by accident. "I started to eat better and take vitamins simply because I didn't have the energy I wanted," explains Lynn, a 47-year-old Denver cashier. "I was surprised—and delighted—when the pain I sometimes had in my back, hips and shoulders slowly improved. Now, I can be as active as I want, with practically no pain."

Lynn takes a multivitamin and mineral supplement, along with extra calcium and magnesium, and vitamins C and E. "Plus, I bought a juicer and started to drink carrot juice a few times a week. I rely on that as a source of extra beta-carotene and potassium." She made her dietary changes as a result of reading about nutrition and visiting a health spa.

Research on the use of vitamins and minerals for arthritis has produced mixed results. No single nutrient seems to stand out as having a significant impact on either rheumatoid arthritis or osteoarthritis. Several, however, may play a supporting role in helping to prevent joint deterioration or reduce inflammation. For instance, calcium, selenium and vitamin C are known to be involved in the formation of bone, cartilage and connective tissue and in the formation of biochemicals that have anti-inflammatory properties in the body.

Inflammation tends to deplete the body's stores of vitamin C, and some arthritis drugs interfere with vitamin C metabolism and excretion. For these reasons, some doctors recommend higher-than-normal doses of vitamin C for their patients with rheumatoid arthritis.

People with arthritis may be lacking in other nutrients as well. A study by Finnish researchers showed reduced blood levels of vitamins A and E, along with zinc, in people with rheumatoid arthritis. All three of these nutrients play a role in building immunity and may help to control inflammation in the body.

Vitamin E was found helpful in relieving pain from osteoarthritis in a study by Israeli researchers. More than half of the 32 patients taking 600 IU of vitamin E a day for ten days experienced marked relief of pain.

EDITOR'S NOTE: If you have arthritis and want to try nutritional therapy, it's best to seek the guidance of a doctor or other health professional knowledgeable in nutrition.

THEY GET TRIED AND TRUE HELP FROM THE DRUGSTORE

A fair number of people said they also use over-the-counter products like aspirin, ibuprofen, Ben-Gay or Mineral Ice to ease their arthritis pain. "I exercise and use hot baths, but I'll also take aspirin if and when I need it," explains Carolyn, an elementary school teacher in White Plains, New York. She's found that enteric-coated aspirin is easiest on her stomach.

"I rub Ben-Gay on my hands and wrists when they get sore," says Martha, 69, of Providence, Rhode Island. She finds this ritual especially soothing to perform at night, before she goes to bed, while watching television. "I massage my hands, and they get warm and loosened up," she explains. "They're not so stiff in the morning after I do this."

SHE'S CONVINCED COPPER BRACELETS WORK

An old and apparently discredited arthritis remedy—the copper bracelet—was suggested by two people. One woman described how the bracelet provided significant benefits, both to her and her sister.

"I had been in agony for months from the arthritis in my wrists and especially in my right leg. My sister too has arthritis in her wrists and legs," says Florence, of Morris, New York. "We read about the copper bracelets in a book and decided to try them. We bought four bracelets and put them on our wrists. The pain died down in our wrists almost instantly, and my leg quieted down a bit. But then the pain in my leg got worse. My doctor took X-rays and said I had acute arthritis.

"My sister, just kidding one night, said, 'It's too bad you can't put a bracelet around your ankle.' So I thought, why not? I pulled the bracelet open far enough so I could put it around my ankle, and I pulled a sock up over it to help keep it on. It worked so well that now we both wear copper bracelets around our ankles, too. I feel it's like a miracle. I can stand longer now—I don't feel as if I am going to fall. And I am taking fewer painkilling pills."

Her health care provider, a nurse practitioner, laughed when he saw the sisters wearing copper anklets, Florence says. "But he's not laughing now," she says.

EDITOR'S NOTE: The official word from the medical establishment is that copper bracelets are just plain silly. If you do decide to wear a copper bracelet, medical experts warn: Don't count on that as your only arthritis remedy. It's important to keep up other treatments that have been proven effective.

SPECIAL DIETS EASE SYMPTOMS

Traditionally, medical experts have denied any link between rheumatoid arthritis flare-ups and food. But several of our survey participants disagree. They've learned to be picky eaters—and apparently it's been to their benefit, at least as far as their arthritis symptoms go.

"I've pretty much eliminated red meat, dairy products, sugar, nightshade plants (including peppers and tomatoes) and food preservatives," says Joyce of Warren, Texas. "I am so sensitive that if I eat red meat, my hands start to swell up within ten minutes or so." She has replaced these foods with vegetables, fruits, legumes, nuts and seeds.

It's not easy to stay on this sort of diet, she admits. "But when you suffer like I do, and doctors can't help, you just do the best you can."

Several arthritis sufferers say they noted flare-ups connected to refined sugar. "Because I am overweight, I don't usually eat sugar. But I noticed that after weekends when we'd had company and I'd eaten sugar, my knees would swell up for a few days," says Ruby, 65, of Mahtomedi, Minnesota. "If I stay away from sugar, I have a lot less pain."

A few people say citrus fruits aggravate their symptoms. Others say coffee or cola seems to precipitate a flare-up.

A variety of studies suggest that, for a small number of sensitive people, certain foods may provoke a kind of allergic inflammatory reaction in joint tissue—in much the same way that a particular food might cause other people to break out in hives. Eliminating suspect foods from the diet sometimes helps. For instance, one study found that a strictly vegetarian diet—no meat, eggs or dairy products—improved the symptoms of some people who are susceptible to rheumatoid arthritis.

EDITOR'S NOTE: Doctors caution that if you steer away from more than one or two foods, or if you avoid foods that are a major source of a particular nutrient— such as calcium-rich dairy products—you should make sure you are getting the nutrients you need from other sources, including supplements if necessary.

THEY SAY NO TO TOMATOES

Most people who say foods aggravate their rheumatoid arthritis find that simply eliminating one food, or a group of related foods, seems to do the trick. Tops on their avoid-at-all-costs list are tomatoes, followed by other vegetables in the nightshade family: potatoes, eggplant, peppers (red and green bell peppers, chili peppers and paprika—but not black pepper) and tobacco.

In fact, the members of this botanical family contain a known toxin, solanine, which has been associated with joint inflammation in animals that resembles rheumatoid arthritis. However, most doctors believe there isn't enough solanine in any of these foods to do much harm. So they discount the nightshades–arthritis connection.

But that connection is real, some of our survey participants contend. For example, Ray, a 48-year-old business consultant from Landing, New Jersey, considers himself lucky to have made the connection between the arthritis developing in his knees and his frequent forays to a Mexican restaurant near his house.

"I was eating spicy salsa two or three times a week, and I noticed that the next day my knees would be aching and swollen," he says. "It took me a while to see the link, but I decided to avoid the salsa. I did, and within a week my knees were back to normal. I tried eating the salsa again, and the pain and swelling returned. So I'm convinced this food had something to do with it."

Julia, a Huntsville, Alabama, gardener, claims she grows the best tomatoes around. But she finds that her fingers swell up whenever she eats them. "I eat them anyway," she says. "I don't mind a little discomfort."

GREEN GROW THE OLD-TIME REMEDIES

It sounds like rabbit food, but some people say that alfalfa in the form of tablets or tea eases their arthritis pain. And others say products made with barley grass work for them.

"I take five alfalfa tablets in the morning and five at night, and it does seem to make a difference," says Helen, of Hendrum, Minnesota. She has osteoarthritis in her knees.

"I've tried alfalfa tea, and I find that if I use it regularly, it takes the edge off my pain," says Claudia, of Hopewell, New Jersey. "This remedy was recommended to me years ago by a chiropractor, who said it may help to reduce inflammation." She has arthritis in one injured knee and one wrist, along with back pain.

Alfalfa is one of those old-fashioned, hard-to-prove-it-works remedies. Arthritis sufferers have recommended it again and again as a treatment, but their recommendations are not backed up by scientific evidence.

Both alfalfa and barley grass are said to contain vitamins and minerals which may account for some of their alleged benefits. Both also are a rich source of chlorophyll, the pigment that makes plants green. Some people have claimed that chlorophyll has anti-inflammatory properties, but those properties have yet to be proven in the laboratory.

FISH OIL HELPS A FEW

A few people report that they take fish oil capsules to ease their rheumatoid arthritis pain. "I find fish oil very helpful for my arthritis, especially the morning stiffness and joint pain," says Mickey, 58, of Searcy, Arkansas. A night admissions clerk at a local hospital, she has had rheumatoid arthritis in her knees, shoulders and hands since she was in her twenties.

"I usually take one capsule a day, and it keeps me from getting too bad. If I do start having trouble, I'll up the dosage a little bit, to two or three capsules a day, for a while."

She notes that she can't expect to get overnight relief from taking fish oil. "I have to take it every day for a least a week or ten days before it begins to work," she says. For immediate relief, she relies on ibuprofen.

Another person notes that "fish oil has not cured my arthritis, but the attacks are less severe and of shorter duration."

Researchers think that fish oil may interfere with the inflammation process in arthritis, possibly preventing flare-ups and slowing the progress of the disease. In several studies, people taking fish oil had fewer arthritis symptoms related to inflammation—pain, morning stiffness and fatigue—

than other people taking olive oil (considered a neutral agent).

Some people prefer to get their fish oil directly from the fish. A woman from Lookout Mountain, Tennessee, says, "After years of taking various medications for arthritis pain, I have been able to control the flare-ups for the last five years by eating three cans of sardines a week."

Experts say there may be benefits in adopting a diet lower in total fat, while eating more fatty fish such as mackerel, tuna, salmon, sardines and bluefish. But along with that, arthritis sufferers should probably stay away from polyunsaturated fats like those found in vegetable oils and margarine.

EDITOR'S NOTE: One person mentioned the use of cod liver oil for arthritis. This old-time remedy may have some of the same inflammation-taming effects as fish oil. But unlike fish oil, cod liver oil contains large amounts of vitamin A (one brand has 10,000 IU of vitamin A per dose, about twice the recommended Daily Value) along with a hefty amount of vitamin D. Large amounts of vitamins A and D can be toxic. So don't take more than a teaspoon a day without medical supervision.

THEY SIDE WITH CIDER VINEGAR

Several people say they use apple cider vinegar as a remedy for arthritis. Most drink it. However, one person, Bill, of Yuba City, California, sits in it. He says he relieves his arthritis pain by soaking in a hot bath that contains a cup of apple cider vinegar and a cup of Epsom salts.

"I actually do believe apple cider vinegar helps me," says Franceline, of West Branch, Minnesota, who adds that she gets aggravated by the costs of arthritis medicines. When the arthritis in her hands acts up, she sips a glass of hot water containing two parts honey to one part apple cider vinegar. "I don't measure the amounts I put in. I just eyeball it." And the result may not be everyone's cup of tea. "It's an acquired taste," she admits.

Doctors say there is no scientific evidence suggesting that apple cider vinegar can relieve any form of arthritis. At present, it must be considered a folk remedy in search of medical validation.

Asthma

Airway Openers That Help in a Pinch

Theodore Roosevelt. President, adventurer, asthma sufferer. But home remedy expert? You bet your Bull Moose! He of the bully pulpit and the walrus mustache used to swill tea to help fight his asthma.

Of course, asthma treatment has improved markedly since Teddy was riding rough over the American body politic. No matter what pulls your asthmatic trigger today—cold air, dust mites, exercise, pet dander, smoke, even springtime—when your airways are swollen and inflamed, doctors say there's usually no better medicine than your inhaler.

A puff or two later, the medication from this handy device has begun to do its job: The spasms have slowed, the mucus begins clearing and oxygen is rushing through your windpipe again.

The participants in our survey who take doctor-prescribed medicine are grateful for it. But they also claim they've found some home remedies that—used in a pinch—are worthy of presidential acclaim.

THEY'RE STEAMED UP OVER THIS REMEDY

Several people proclaim their success at fighting asthma with steam.

Dolly, 79, of Martinez, California, says she didn't say hello to asthma until she turned 71. But when the symptoms developed, she was prepared.

"Mother had used steam for her asthma," she says. "And as a child I also used to inhale steam when my nose was clogged by a cold and I had difficulty breathing."

So Dolly started using the remedy again with good results. After filling a teapot with water, she brings it to a boil and removes it from the stove. Carefully holding a towel over both her head and the pot to trap the steam, she then breathes deeply.

"It usually takes about five minutes for my airways to clear," she says. "But depending on how congested I am, I might repeat the treatment again within a half-hour."

For even greater asthma-clearing punch, Dolly sometimes adds a drop of eucalyptus oil (available at health-food stores) to the water before boiling. "Then when I breathe in the steam, I can feel it all the way down into my chest," she says.

A number of other people with asthma told us they use a steam treatment by turning on a hot shower and sitting in the bathroom for 10 to 15 minutes.

Using steam power against asthma is anything but hot air, according to Gary N. Gross, M.D., a clinical associate professor of internal medicine at the University of Texas Health Science Center at Dallas Southwestern Medical School and the author of several articles on coping with asthma.

"One of the problems with asthma is that it creates thick mucus secretions, and this mucus has a tendency to stick to the airways. But the steam can thin out these secretions," says Dr. Gross. "The other potential benefit of steam is that it may also clear secretions out of sinus passages. We now know that asthma can be worse if someone has a sinus infection."

According to Dr. Gross, any kind of steam treatment is fine—including the boiling-water-on-the-stove and the steam-filled bathroom. "You don't need expensive steam machines, steam rooms and other fancy equipment," he says.

SYMPTOMS ARE VAPORIZED

Mary, a 51-year-old housewife from Doylestown, Pennsylvania, opts for a different kind of vapor strategy in her bid to stop asthma. Before going to sleep, she clicks on the vaporizer in her bedroom, pumping much-needed moisture into the air.

"Low indoor humidity seems to be enough to bring on my asthma," says Mary. "But since I've been using the vaporizer for about a year, I've been feeling much better."

Another report of a vapor-related remedy for asthma came to us from Linda, a 40-year-old secretary in Columbus, Ohio. It seems that Minnie, her pet hamster, became sick late one evening. After diagnosing Minnie with bronchitis, the veterinarian told Linda to heat up some Vicks VapoRub in a small pan on the stove and give Minnie a whiff.

Linda did just what the doctor ordered, and Minnie made a marvelous recovery. And that made Linda wonder: "If this works for a hamster, what would it do for my asthma?"

EDITOR'S NOTE: Right idea, wrong product, according to Jim Schwartz, a spokesman for Procter & Gamble, the makers of Vicks products. "The only safe way to get the benefit of VapoRub aromatics is to use our other product, VapoSteam, in a hot steam vaporizer. It contains the same aromatic ingredients as VapoRub, but is designed for use in a hot steam vaporizer."

According to Schwartz, VapoRub should only be rubbed on the chest and throat—and it should never be heated on the stove or in a microwave oven.

THE CASE FOR CAFFEINE

A retired registered nurse, Fern isn't afraid to try a new, but logical-sounding treatment when she hears about one. The 63-year-old Berrien Springs, Michigan, resident learned there was some scientific evidence that the caffeine in coffee could help exertional asthma—the kind that is brought on by certain kinds of exercise.

"My asthma is triggered by things like shoveling snow, sweeping the walk, even walking," she says. "If I'm not careful, I'll work for a while and not notice how hard I'm going, and then I'll pay for it the next hour—wheezing and coughing."

That's where Fern's occasional cup of coffee comes in. "I don't really like the taste of coffee, but if I take my first sip even before my breathing becomes too labored, it really seems to help."

In fact, nearly 25 percent of people suffering from asthma who responded to our survey felt that a cup of joe gives their symptoms a healthy jolt. And a review of studies sponsored by the National Heart, Lung and Blood Institute seems to back up their findings. Researchers discovered that asthmatic adults who are regular coffee drinkers suffer a third fewer symptoms than non–coffee drinkers.

The research did not determine for certain whether caffeine ingestion produces any long-term beneficial effects for people who have asthma. However, it appears that coffee may possibly help reduce the frequency of asthmatic symptoms.

EDITOR'S NOTE: The bottom line: Caffeine is a chemical that opens breathing tubes, say medical researchers. Just don't make a habit of substituting caffeine-containing beverages like tea, coffee or cola for your medicine. That's not an effective way of controlling symptoms over the long term, doctors warn.

VITAMIN C GETS AN A IN ARIZONA

Each year, when mittens and jackets made their appearance in Des Arc, Arizona, asthma was sure to follow for Kathern's son. Playing in the chilly air would start him wheezing. That is, until Kathern read that vitamin C seems to help some asthma sufferers.

"I started keeping vitamin C–rich orange juice on hand for him to drink," she says. "Since he likes it, he drank about a gallon a week."

The next time snowflakes fell, instead of sucking wind, her son performed like he was auditioning for the Ice Capades, says Kathern. "He went outside and played for at least two hours without having an asthma attack," she says. And the improvement continued.

Asthma sufferers may have good reason to warm up to vitamin C. Several studies show modest improvements in lung capacity following increased intake of the nutrient. A few researchers speculate that vitamin C may help reduce exercise-induced bronchial constriction and spasms. Several other studies suggest that a vitamin B_6 deficiency may also be linked to asthma.

"I don't think all the answers are in yet on vitamins and asthma. But if you find vitamins are beneficial for you, taking them is a reasonable thing to do," says Dr. Gross. Just make sure to tell your doctor what you're taking and how much, he says.

EDITOR'S NOTE: Two other nutritional supplements that allegedly fight asthma—bee pollen and brewer's yeast—should be avoided because they contain known allergens that could possibly make some people's asthma worse, says Dr. Gross.

FOOD TRIGGERS ARE NO FISH STORY

A spry 74-year-old, Patricia, of Sun City, Arizona, had only one health complaint—periodic, early morning chest pain associated with her asthma. After reading that food allergies can trigger both asthma and related pain, she decided to start keeping a food diary.

"I had never been a great fish lover, but I noticed that the day before my last attack I had eaten a tuna salad sandwich for lunch and fresh trout for dinner. From that point on, I decided to avoid all fish and have not had a recurrence of the pain since."

Eating—or even smelling—foods that an individual is sensitive to can trigger an asthma attack. "Some of the most common foods that trigger asthma are milk, eggs, nuts and seafood," says allergist John Carlston, M.D., associate professor of medicine at Eastern Virginia Medical School in Norfolk.

The problem with seafood is its high histamine content. When people who are allergic eat a food high in histamine, it can trigger an asthmatic reaction felt as chest discomfort or breathing difficulty, says Gary Guarka, M.D., an immunologist at St. Elizabeth's Hospital in Boston. "Deep-water fish, including trout, tuna, bluefish, salmon and swordfish, are the most concentrated food sources of histamine," he says. "Distributed throughout their flesh, it acts as a natural antifreeze to prevent the fish from freezing to death in the cold water."

People with asthma should also consider steering clear of sulfites (used as a food preservative) and monosodium glutamate, or MSG (a flavor enhancer). One woman with asthma told us that after eating pepper steak containing MSG at a Chinese restaurant, she thought she was going to die. Only a quick cup of coffee prevented her from gagging, she says.

While sulfites have been proven to cause serious problems for some asthma sufferers, the evidence for MSG's involvement is less convincing, says Dr. Gross. If you believe you've had a reaction to either, however, you should probably avoid them, he says. Sulfites are commonly found in beer, wine and dried foods. MSG is often added to sauces, soups and many other prepared foods—especially Chinese foods—so read labels carefully.

WAGING WAR AGAINST DUST

Grounding airborne allergens before they take off is Mary's favorite tactic for beating asthma.

"We use cheesecloth over our heating vents to reduce the amount of dust getting through," says the Columbus, Ohio, woman. "And we also use it on our vacuum cleaner, taping triple-thickness cheesecloth over the exhaust airflow. This cuts down so much on dust in the home that it's no longer necessary for me to wear a mask when I clean."

Studies have shown that vacuum cleaners can kick up two to ten times the amount of allergens (like pollen, mold, dust mites, animal dander and insect fragments) normally floating around the house. And that extra onslaught can persist for up to an hour after you finish vacuuming.

EDITOR'S NOTE: To pass safety tests, vacuum cleaners have to be able to operate with one layer of cheesecloth over the vent without danger of fire. But using two or more layers may be unsafe, experts caution.

Mary would be better off selecting any one of a number of filtering bags or exhaust filters for vacuum cleaners now sold in stores. "You can eliminate the potential for problems by using one of these special filters," says Dr. Gross.

Some brands of filter bags are available at stores where vacuum cleaners are sold. Or you can call 1-800-422-DUST to get more information about special allergy-control products.

MAKING HAY: THE BENEFITS OF HORSING AROUND

With not one but two teenage sons suffering from exertional asthma, Lori, of Oak Brook, Illinois, was afraid that they would have to cut way back on sports activities and general horsing around.

But by using their metered-dose inhalers, and following the regimen prescribed by their doctor, the boys get the precise amount of medication needed to prevent asthma attacks. They have stayed healthy and extremely active, excelling in both baseball and basketball, says the 47-year-old housewife.

"They've been able to lead normal lives," she says. "Before they exercise, they use their inhalers. And they keep them nearby just in case they need to use them when they're competing. We feel that prevention is much better than treatment."

For those who can tolerate it, engaging in some type of aerobic exercise three times a week is good for a variety of reasons, says Dr. Gross. "It can reduce the frequency of asthma attacks and give you a way to monitor how you're doing," he says. "It also helps move the mucus around so you can cough it up."

THEY RELAX AND BREATHE EASY

Several people say they took the easy way out of an asthma attack by learning relaxation techniques and controlled breathing.

Nancy didn't have far to go to pick up her relaxation tips: She learned them from her roommate, Pat.

When she's at home and feels an attack coming on, the Tempe, Arizona, resident will use her inhaler and then lie down in a dark, quiet room. She finds that counting backwards helps her to relax. Or she just "talks herself" into relaxing for a few moments.

But can a few quiet moments yield big asthma-beating benefits? You better believe it, says Dr. Gross.

"When you're short of breath, there's a natural tendency to try to breathe faster to get more air," he says. "But faster breathing requires more energy and effort at a time when you're already under stress, making the problem even worse."

On the other hand, slowing their breathing rate can make some asthmatics feel better almost immediately, he says. One technique: controlled breathing. While lying on your back, first fill your belly with air, then allow your chest to expand and fill. Exhale, and repeat. To practice (and make sure you're doing the techniques properly), rest your right hand on your stomach and your left hand on your chest. Your right hand should rise before the left one does, says Dr. Gross.

Listening to soothing music, even self-hypnosis, have all been used effectively against asthma, he says. "All these things have some potential benefit, but it's like telling someone that they won't get hurt as much if they can keep from getting tense when they're involved in an automobile accident. It's hard to relax when you feel like you're struggling for breath—but it can be done."

SHE TOOK THE PLUNGE

Painting at poolside in the summer heat, Estella felt herself becoming more susceptible to a pollen-provoked asthma attack with every brush stroke.

But as she felt the symptoms coming on, the 56-year-old Dagsboro, Delaware, resident remembered reading that, in an emergency, jumping into a swimming pool could ward off a severe asthma attack.

With her breathing now labored—and hardly waiting to put down her paintbrush—Estella took the plunge, clothing and all. For her, the result was well worth the inconvenience of getting soaked. "In less than five minutes I had calmed right down and was able to breathe much better," she says.

EDITOR'S NOTE: If a sudden, overpowering run-in with pollen should cause an asthma attack, experts say there's a chance even your inhaler won't help you in time. Hopping in a pool or dousing yourself with a hose really can help by banishing pollen quickly; but for safety's sake, make sure there is someone nearby.

MULLEIN DID THE TRICK

When her 84-year-old mother wouldn't stop complaining about her asthma symptoms, Beth, of Athens, Georgia, took a trip to her local herb store in search of a cure.

The store owner said many of his customers with asthma breathe the smoke of mullein leaves to relieve their condition. He urged her to find some in her backyard and to give the remedy a try.

Although Beth's mother breathed easier after inhaling the smoke of the mullein leaves, she refused to try it again. "I don't think she felt comfortable about smoking it," Beth says.

In fact, tincture of mullein is available in some health-food stores. And it can be taken orally for chest congestion and bronchial coughs, according to Andrew Weil, M.D., associate director of the Division of Social Perspectives in Medicine at the University of Arizona College of Medicine/Arizona Health Sciences Center in Tucson and author of *Natural Health, Natural Medicine.*

Athlete's Foot

Soothing Ways to Stop the Itching

You don't have to be an athlete to have athlete's foot. You don't even have to wear sneakers. Wearing shoes of any kind can be enough to cultivate this exasperating itch. That's because the fungal infection that causes athlete's foot loves warm, dark, damp places—like inside sweaty footwear.

Even deerskin moccasin wearers apparently are not immune, since we received a Native American remedy for this condition. "Before you get into bed for the night, spread raw honey on your freshly washed and dried feet and put your socks on over this," suggests Margaret, 74, of La Puente, California. "I haven't tried this myself," she admits. "I heard it from a friend of a friend, who said that it was an Indian remedy. Yes, it does sound messy."

Soaks, powders and creams topped the list of more orthodox remedies, along with tips about shoes and socks. A number of people minister to their feet with household cleaning products, such as chlorine bleach, cleansing powder or Lysol spray. Although they report no harm, doctors warn that use of these strong products on your feet could easily increase irritation and redness, especially if those products contain ammonia.

All told, the remedies reported to us address almost every conceivable aspect of athlete's foot prevention and treatment—from scrubbing shower stalls to wearing different shoes on alternate days.

Here are the details.

BLEACHING IS ONE SOLUTION

Footbaths top the list of cures. People use quite an array of ingredients in their soaking solutions. Chlorine bleach, vinegar and salt are most popular, but red clover tea, cayenne pepper, baking soda and Fels-Naptha soap all get votes of confidence.

Those who use a laundry bleach solution on their feet emphasize that it works when everything else failed, including over-the-counter remedies.

"After picking up a very bad case of athlete's foot in a public bathhouse in Florida, I tried everything," says Elizabeth, of Elmira, New York. "My medicine chest was full of powders and creams, and I even tried boiling my socks. Finally, someone suggested I soak my feet in Clorox bleach. It didn't cure my problem overnight, but I could quickly see an improvement. Within about a week to ten days, my athlete's foot was gone, and it never came back."

Elizabeth says she mixed about half a cup of bleach in a gallon of water and soaked for about 15 minutes, twice a day. "It did sting a little bit at first," she says.

"I use bleach, and it works better than anything else I've tried," adds Ben, 58, a small-engine repairman in Hill, New Hampshire. "I developed a terrible case of athlete's foot one day when I was flying to Florida. My feet were sweaty, and I didn't have a chance to remove my shoes for about 16 hours. That night, I soaked my feet in a bleach solution, and by the next morning the skin was clear. Now, the minute my feet begin to itch, I get out the Clorox," he says.

Ben uses a fairly strong solution. "I mix about a quart of bleach in a gallon of water," he says. "I soak for 15 or 20 minutes with the water completely covering my feet." When he's done, he pats his feet dry without rinsing. The next morning, while he's showering, he uses a washcloth to rub some of the dried skin off his feet.

Other people who use bleach stick with weaker solutions—anywhere from two tablespoons to half a cup per gallon of water. "Chlorine is certainly a strong antiseptic, and it will kill athlete's foot fungus along with other bacteria, both good and bad, on the skin," says Glenn Copeland, D.P.M., podiatrist for the Toronto Blue Jays and author of *The Foot Doctor*. "I can't tell you exactly what dilution of bleach would be best, but certainly, weaker is better."

EDITOR'S NOTE: Chlorine bleach used to come with guidelines for using it in the treatment of athlete's foot. The label of a bottle from the early 1950s gives these directions for athlete's foot: "Thoroughly mix a solution of two tablespoons of Clorox with each quart of warm water. Soak feet daily for five minutes, remove loose skin, continue soaking 15 minutes and dry."

However, modern-day foot doctors discourage its use, saying it may be too strong a remedy, especially for irritated, cracked skin. "I find nothing in the current medical literature that would give any indication of a safe dilution to use," says Glenn Gastwirth, D.P.M., deputy executive director of the American Podiatric Medical Association in Bethesda, Maryland. It's true that stubborn athlete's foot is sometimes

*accompanied by a secondary bacterial infection—not just a fungus—and may re-
spond to a chlorine soak when over-the-counter remedies have failed. "But I believe
you would be better off having the infection identified and using the appropriate antibiotic to kill the bacteria," Dr. Gastwirth says.*

A VINEGAR SOAK WORKS WONDERS

The people who use a vinegar soak say it works well, too. "All the kids in
my family used vinegar foot soaks when they had athlete's foot," says Viola,
of Detroit. "I only needed to use it once myself. I mixed about half a cup of
white vinegar in a gallon of water and soaked for five to ten minutes, twice a
day. After a few days, my athlete's foot was gone, and it never did return."

"Vinegar makes an excellent soaking solution," Dr. Copeland agrees.
"It's acidic enough to kill athlete's foot fungus, but even a concentrated solution is so mild it won't hurt your skin." For best results, he suggests soaking for 10 or 15 minutes, then letting your feet air-dry.

AN OCEAN NOTION

Several people suggested a saltwater soak, and one California man has
found a way to make this remedy truly invigorating. "I walk barefoot along
the beach, allowing the salt water to lap at my feet," says Peter, of La Jolla,
California.

For those who can't get to the ocean so easily, two teaspoons of table salt
per pint of warm water makes an excellent soaking solution for athlete's
foot, experts say. "The salt kills fungus and helps to dry up surface skin
cells," says Dr. Copeland. "Simply soak your feet for five to ten minutes at a
time, repeating often until the condition clears."

DRUGSTORE PRODUCTS DELIVER RELIEF

Many people have tried nonprescription athlete's foot medications with
good results.

"I use a medicated powder on my feet regularly. I sprinkle it on, just like
baby powder," says Cris, 54, of West Haven, Connecticut. "It keeps my feet
dry so I don't have any itching."

"My husband powders his feet and his shoes every morning with an athlete's foot powder, and it seems to work," says Edith, 47, of Schenectady,
New York. "If he stops doing it, he usually develops a problem."

Other antifungal powders, creams or sprays, such as Desenex and Tin-
actin, are also frequently mentioned. A common ingredient in these prod-

ucts is tolnafate, an antifungal agent. "I tell my patients to first try a product containing tolnafate, and if it doesn't work in a week or two, to switch to one containing clotrimazole, another antifungal agent," Dr. Copeland says. "I also think it helps a lot if you soak your feet in salt water for a few minutes prior to applying the medication," he adds.

CREAMS ARE SOOTHING

Some doctors think that powders work better than creams, because the creams can trap moisture between the toes. That seemed to be the consensus of survey participants, too: They preferred powders over creams three to one. "Creams do have their place, though," says Dr. Copeland. "They are very soothing if your skin is cracked and sore."

WORMWOOD TO THE RESCUE

Roy, 74, a retired cattle and sheep farmer living in Riverton, West Virginia, has used another over-the-counter product, Absorbine Jr., for his foot problems. "I just follow the directions on the bottle. It smarts a bit, but it works pretty well," he says. Absorbine Jr. contains a derivative of wormwood (*Artemisia absinthium*), an herb that may have analgesic and antifungal action.

THOROUGH DRYING IS THE KEY

People prone to inner toe itchiness know that keeping their feet bone-dry is essential. They've already found out the hard way that just a few hours of dampness can trigger an episode of athlete's foot. So they've come up with a number of ways to ensure dryness, even between the toes.

"After a shower or bath, I dry between my toes with a paper towel," reports Michael, 38, a Shreveport, Louisiana, interior designer. "I think it works better than a regular towel. It's certainly easier to slide between your toes."

"I turn on a blow-dryer and use it on my feet. Believe it or not, that's the only thing I have to do," says Phillip of Bensalem, Pennsylvania.

Other people dry their feet thoroughly, then powder them with cornstarch or baking soda to absorb perspiration moisture.

UNDERARM PROTECTION WORKS FOR FEET, TOO

The same wetness-stopping ingredients that make underarm antiperspirants so effective can help prevent or cure athlete's foot, several people tell us. In fact, this and many other brands of deodorant, including those marketed for feet, contain aluminum chlorohydrate or a related compound, which stops sweating and creates an inhospitable environment for the athlete's foot fungus, Dr. Gastwirth says.

A pharmacy-prepared solution of aluminum chloride, another strong antiperspirant ingredient, was very successful at clearing a stubborn case of athlete's foot, reports Max, 58, of Corvallis, Oregon. "My son Matthew had the problem for a while before he came to me about it," Max says. "He actually had tiny holes in his heels where the fungus had eaten away his skin."

Although Matthew had spent more than a year trying "anything and everything," even replacing all his shoes with new ones, his athlete's foot was actually growing worse. "I was absolutely and totally desperate and began to investigate further," Max says. "I started doing some reading and came across the aluminum chloride remedy. I asked the pharmacist to mix up a five percent solution. I swabbed it on my son's feet, then gave him the bottle and told him to keep using it. Three days later, his feet were starting to clear up, and within two weeks they were cleared up for good."

But you needn't go through the added expense and trouble of having a pharmacist specially prepare such a solution. Over-the-counter antiperspirants can have up to 15 percent aluminum chloride concentration. Besides, pharmacists may be unwilling to prepare the solution without a prescription.

Be aware, however, that aluminum chloride is stronger than aluminum chlorohydrate and may be more irritating to the skin.

A RUBDOWN FOR SORE FEET

Several people note that rubbing the dead skin off their feet seems to help clear up their problem. "I soak my feet in a baking soda solution, then rub them with a rough towel, especially between the toes," says Al, 52, of Ipswich, Massachusetts.

SOCK IT TO THE FUNGUS

Several people mention that they wear white socks to counter the athlete's foot fungus, and some also have a special cleaning ritual for those socks—hot water and bleach.

"My husband wears white socks to work every day," says Rose, of Jessup, Pennsylvania. "The socks, along with powders and careful foot drying, really do seem to keep his athlete's foot away."

White socks may be helpful because they contain no dye to irritate tender, sore skin, Dr. Copeland says. He recommends choosing socks made of cotton, wool or a synthetic material such as polypropylene, which wicks wetness away from the skin. "Nylon is absolutely the worst thing to wear," he contends, "because it traps moisture."

THEY BARE THEIR SOLES

A few people suggest the cheapest, simplest preventive of all—they just take off their shoes and air their tootsies.

"I slip my shoes off whenever I have the chance," says Suzanne, 40, of Seattle. "It airs out my feet and shoes and keeps my socks dry." She admits she does occasionally hear some comments around the office when she sheds her shoes. "But most people don't mind at all," she says.

Back Pain

Teaming Up against Nagging Aches

There's more than one way to skin a cat—more than one route to grandmother's house—and more than one fish in the sea. And for people who have back pain, there's more than one technique to fight the ache and agony of a belligerent back.

Consider Joyce, of Warren, Texas. A retired insurance salesperson, Joyce misses the challenge of the business world, but her treatment of low-back pain can only be described as businesslike.

When the pain really flares, Joyce tries a triple whammy—mineral ice, an ice pack and moist heat. Joyce has also been helped by daily walks around her farm or walks on a treadmill, and she works out using videos to help strengthen her back muscles. Joyce also listens to relaxation tapes. And she uses a bed with a firm mattress to insure that she gets the kind of rest that keeps the kinks out. "Through trial and error, I've been forced to learn how to manage my pain," she says. "It hasn't been easy, but I've come a long way since the pain started."

Diverse treatment techniques may very well be the key to back pain relief, says Fred L. Allman, Jr., M.D., an orthopedic surgeon and director of the Atlanta Sports Medicine Clinic. Activity, heat and ice and a firm mattress all have their benefits, he points out.

"There are many, many different things that can cause a back to hurt—but often it's a muscle or ligament strain or pull," says Dr. Allman. "Some people go to the doctor for their problem. Others want to do something on their own that helps, and many times they are able to avoid seeing a physician." In addition to Joyce's remedies, our survey takers have recommended many others.

RELIEF WITH ROCK 'N' ROLL

All kinds of exercise score high on our hit parade of back-pain relief methods.

Minnabel calls her treatment rock 'n' roll yoga—but that doesn't mean this 72-year-old Covington, Kentucky, woman pops in a Bruce Springsteen CD every time she assumes the lotus position. "I'm a little old for that—the music I mean," she laughs.

Minnabel's version of "rock 'n' roll" begins with her lying on the floor. She pulls her knees to her chest, wraps her arms around them and gently rocks back and forth. Within minutes, she says, her pain is gone. "I don't rock very vigorously—it doesn't take much to make me feel better," she says.

Minnabel is doing exactly the right thing with her mini yoga session, says Dr. Allman. "She's stretching the muscles in the lumbar—lower back—area that are probably tight," he says. "In fact, that particular movement is virtually identical to the best exercises doctors recommend for back trouble."

SHE'S FEELING THE CRUNCH

While strengthening the stomach muscles is a great way to help prevent lower-back pain, Cynthia from Tampa learned the hard way that there's a right and a wrong way to get the job done.

"I spent years trying to strengthen and treat my painful lower back, and sit-ups were always a part of my routine. I did the kind of bent-knee sit-ups that are widely recommended, but my back pain persisted and was often worse after exercise," she says.

"Then, on the advice of an aerobics instructor, I started doing crunches—modified sit-ups in which you raise your upper body only partly off the floor. I found them to be just as effective as regular sit-ups at keeping my belly tight. And guess what? My lower back pain has vanished."

Keeping your lower back firmly on the floor during a sit-up does help prevent strain to weak back muscles, confirms Charles Kuntzleman, Ed.D., Ph.D., adjunct associate professor of kinesiology at the University of Michigan in Ann Arbor and author of *Maximizing Your Personal Energy & Personal Productivity*. "It's also extremely important to fold your arms across your chest instead of behind the head," he says. "Hands can pull too hard and damage neck muscles."

Just don't get fixated on strengthening your stomach and forget about your back, says Dr. Allman. "Improving your abdominal strength is part of spine stabilization. But it stabilizes just one side of the spine and doesn't strengthen the extensors, which are probably more important than the stomach muscles," he says.

If you are going to do crunches, make sure you add movements that ease your back in the opposite direction. "One way to do this is to put your hands on the back part of your hips just below your belt and arch backwards slowly as far as you can," he says.

EDITOR'S NOTE: Crunches can pose potential problems. "If you do a sudden flexion movement like a crunch, and you already have a damaged disk in your back, this could cause the disk to become acutely painful or even herniated," warns Dr. Allman. Check with your doctor before beginning any new exercise program for back pain.

THEY TELL PAIN TO TAKE A HIKE

With two severe back injuries, Linda would probably be one of the last people you'd expect to briskly walk six or more miles every evening.

In fact, the 48-year-old Granite City, Illinois, housewife says that her back actually feels worse if she misses her nightly jaunts. "When I don't walk at all I can really tell," says Linda. "I'm in a lot of pain."

Linda says she has carefully developed her own special walking technique that minimizes the stress and strain on her back. "I have to be aware of every step—being careful to avoid uneven pavement, for example," she says.

An airline reservationist, Amelie spends her workday at a computer punching in travel arrangements. But if the 51-year-old Aurora, Colorado, resident didn't take walks during her break, her back would be ready to take a vacation without her, she says. "I always feel better when I return from my walk," she says.

Amelie's work schedule only allows her enough time to go around the block during a break. When she's not on the job, however, she tries to take at least a three-mile walk as often as possible.

There is evidence that when you walk, your abdominal and back muscles become stronger. "The stronger the muscles, the more support they'll provide for your back," says Dr. Allman. "Walking is a very good exercise and one that we recommend for all of our patients who can walk without too much pain," he says. "Motion is good because it lubricates the joints, and you have many joints in the spine."

EDITOR'S NOTE: If you have a bad back, don't start a walking program unless you have a doctor's okay. Rest for a couple of days is usually the prescription for acute back pain. And walking can worsen problems like degenerative disk disease, says Dr. Allman.

MASSAGE TO THE RESCUE

The soothing comfort of massage is also a favorite back pain treatment among the people we surveyed. For some, massage is essential in helping to recover from injuries.

Snorkeling in the bright blue waters off the Virgin Islands was the highlight of a dream vacation for Carol, 51, of Princeton, New Jersey—until it almost spelled doom for her lower back.

While Carol was snorkeling, the dive boat pulled up anchor and started to cruise away. Fearing she'd be left behind, Carol swam frantically for the boat. Spotting her just in time, the crew stopped the boat and pulled Carol aboard. She was safe. "But I really overdid it trying to get back to the boat," she says.

Days later, back at work, Carol was bending over a low table in the mail room when she suddenly felt a spasm of pain in her back. The pain was so severe that she was forced to visit an orthopedic surgeon.

After diagnosing disk degeneration, the surgeon steered her to a physical therapist. For a year, Carol followed the therapist's recommendations. She performed back and stomach exercises, applied her heating pad and stayed on a low-fat diet (she lost 48 pounds at her doctor's request). In addition, she got her husband to massage her back. And she says her husband's massages have provided the most soothing form of back pain relief.

Using his thumbs, Carol's husband gradually rubs the length of her spine, moving out from the center. He finishes by rubbing the muscles on either side of the spine. "It really does help me a lot," she says.

Charles's need for back massage came as a result of an uncooperative roof truss at work. The 73-year-old Eau Claire, Wisconsin, man was helping load a 1,000-pound truss on a cart when the equipment shifted, knocking him off the cart and onto the concrete floor.

For the next four years, Charles says he visited his chiropractor regularly and took Anacin when the pain was intense. But it was the massages lovingly provided by his wife that seemed to ease the pain the most, he says. "There was nothing really scientific about it," says Charles. "She would just rub my back until I felt better or until her hands got tired."

Because massage stimulates circulation of both blood and lymphatic fluid (which tends to pool around the site of an injury), it can help reduce swelling and even promote healing, says Dr. Allman. "Massage also helps by relaxing tense muscles. Aching back muscles are often tight and in spasm. Massage helps reduce the spasm," he says.

THESE TREATMENTS RUN HOT AND COLD

People in our survey aren't lukewarm about hot and cold treatments. Roughly 25 percent said they use one or both when they are in pain.

But it took an extraordinary week-long trip through the Copper Canyon in Mexico for Helen, 62, to try these backache beaters.

Owners of a motor home, Helen and her husband didn't just tour through the Mexican countryside looking for cacti. They joined 43 other owners who loaded their campers onto a flatbed train and rode through the canyon—which, in some spots, features sky-high trestles and mile-long tunnels.

The scenery, Helen says, was spectacular. But as you might imagine, lurching along on a train through treacherous terrain presented more than a few anxious moments. "It's really a worthwhile trip, but it was nerve-racking," says the 62-year-old Hendrum, Minnesota, resident.

Between the stress of the trip and the constant bouncing, by the time she and her husband arrived in Apache Junction, Arizona, to visit her aunt and uncle, Helen's back was literally in knots.

Her aunt recommended a chiropractor who advocated a two-step plan for dealing with her pain. On the chiropractor's orders, Helen placed an ice pack on the sore area for 20 minutes every hour. The next day, she stepped into the shower and turned up the heat, allowing the hot water to wash over the painful area for as long as she could stand. The combination worked.

Today, Helen's trip is only a memory, but she still turns to the cold-and-hot treatment routine whenever she feels twinges of back pain. "I use it all the time," she says, "and it really seems to help."

Warm Epsom salts soaks also got a thumbs-up from some. "Whenever I had muscular aches or pains, my grandmother would tell me to soak in hot water and Epsom salts," one woman told us. "And then when I went to a physical therapist, she said the same thing."

After filling up her bathtub with hot water, she pours in some Epsom salts and relaxes for 20 minutes—the same amount of time her physical therapist used to apply moist heat to her back.

Moist heat relieves a lot of stiffness and discomfort and may allow some people with back pain to get into an exercise program, says Dr. Allman. Ice, on the other hand, can help to relieve the effects of fatigue and get rid of pain at the end of the day.

EDITOR'S NOTE: Be careful not to overdo it. Leaving a heating pad on too long or applying a moist towel that's too hot can burn your back, cautions Dr. Allman. "You also need to be careful with ice. After more than 10 to 12 minutes of ice treatment, you can run the risk of frostbite," he says. Use ice the first 24 hours after an injury, ice and/or heat thereafter, he says.

SHE GETS TO THE ROOT OF THE PROBLEM

A victim of several back-jarring accidents, Claudia suffers pain in no fewer than three places: her lower back, her midback and her lower neck.

When stress or overuse cause a flare-up, the 46-year-old Hopewell, New

Jersey, resident heads straight to one of nature's strongest medicinal herbs—valerian root. "Taking valerian root is a lot like taking a sedative," she says. "It's very, very relaxing."

Claudia says she takes valerian root two ways: in capsules and brewed in hot water to make a tea, which she sweetens with honey. She purchases both forms of the root at a local health-food store.

Within 15 minutes of taking valerian root, she says her pain is gone. The pain stays away for at least two hours afterward, she says. And a cup of the tea before bedtime ensures a great night's sleep, she adds. "It's certainly not the best-tasting thing you can drink, but it does the job," says Claudia.

EDITOR'S NOTE: Don't get carried away with your home dose. A powerful sedative and sleeping aid, valerian depresses the central nervous system. Large amounts of valerian may cause headaches, blurred vision, nausea and morning grogginess. If you notice any of these symptoms, cut back your dosage.

HELPED BY AN ASPIRIN RUB

While tending to his cattle and corn, Roy had little time to worry about his sore back. But before the workday started—or after his chores were done—this 74-year-old Riverton, West Virginia, farmer often turned to an unusual remedy his wife learned from one of her friends.

Roy says he combines a pint of rubbing alcohol, about two ounces of wintergreen and a dozen aspirin in a half-gallon container. When the aspirin have dissolved, Roy has his wife rub the liquid on painful parts of his back.

"I'll try things out and sometimes they won't work real good, but this did. It burns a little bit, but it seems to give me relief," he says. "I expect I've been using it for eight to ten years."

Although Roy's remedy doesn't deal with the cause of back pain, it still sounds like a winner, says Dr. Allman. "It's like a massage, but in a different way—it's altering the threshold of the pain," he says. "And the aspirin in the mixture may also provide some pain relief."

EDITOR'S NOTE: If you are allergic or sensitive to aspirin, do not try this remedy. Rubbing aspirin into the skin could cause a reaction.

DRIVEN TO FIND A CURE

A few people report that minor changes in their driving habits delivered major back pain relief.

"For years I had an annoying lower-back problem," says Ken, of Dayton, Ohio. "About a year ago, I described it to a truck-driving friend. He said many drivers have similar problems from sitting long periods of time on their wallets. I moved my wallet and have had noticeable improvements in my back."

Experts agree with Ken. They point out that extended periods of sitting on a wallet—particularly a fat one—can aggravate nerves in the buttocks and cause pain.

A CUSHION GIVES RELIEF

Paul found out that a long commute can lead to lower-back pain. When he joined a growing publishing company and started doing an hour-long commute, his lower back began to complain.

"It didn't bother me much when I was out of the car, but when I was driving, it was really hard to get comfortable," he says.

A chiropractor suggested that Paul place a wedge-shaped cushion behind him on his car seat to help support his lower back. Since using the cushion, the symptoms have virtually vanished, Paul says.

Thrown from a horse when she was a child, Anne has been dodging bouts of back pain ever since. And strangely, sometimes just lying down was enough to bring on the ouch. But when the 74-year-old Oswego, Illinois, resident heard that a strategically placed pillow might soothe her pain, she was all ears.

"The pain used to bother me quite a bit," Anne says. "But now I just put a small pillow under my knees when I go to bed, and I don't have any problem. I use the pillow every night—and that seems to keep away the pain."

Back supports help to prevent slouching—another cause of back pain—while you're driving or resting, says Dr. Allman.

Bad Breath

How to Make Life a Little Sweeter

It seems terribly obvious. If you have bad breath, you brush and floss your teeth regularly, pass on the onions and see your dentist on a regular basis.

While these tried-and-true techniques are the norm, people who responded to our survey had a bit more to offer on this subject, including a popular skunk-spray cure that apparently also deodorizes the breath—tomato juice. One also had a suggestion that we weren't quite sure was meant for people—milk bones. Hmmmm . . .

Here's what the more than 100 survey takers who answered this question say works for them.

SHE BRUSHES HER TONGUE

Some of us—if we're really conscientious—will spend a good three to five minutes each day polishing our pearly whites. The rest of us barely bother—we spend less than two minutes with a brush in our mouths. Such neglect can lead to a buildup of bacteria that cause gum disease and tooth decay, not to mention breath that can peel off wallpaper.

More than half our survey takers say that good oral hygiene is their cure or preventive for bad breath. Their idea of good oral hygiene? What the dentist orders, and more.

Merry, 42, a college instructor in Pensacola, Florida, figures she brushes two to three minutes twice a day, cleaning not only her teeth but her tongue, and sometimes the roof and sides of her mouth as well. "No one told me to do it. I had to take medicine when I was a child, and I started brushing my tongue to get rid of the taste. I just kept at it." She also flosses her teeth once a day.

In fact, Merry's instinct is right on course. Dentists say that the velvety-textured tongue is loaded with food particles and bacteria that can cause bad breath, and that brushing your tongue, or even wiping it with a rough towel, is a good way to clear off the germs that cause bad breath.

BACK TO BAKING SODA BASICS

Long ago, in the days before sparkle toothpaste and pump bottles, there was baking soda. Baking soda was cheap and effective. It cleaned teeth so well, in fact, that some toothpaste manufacturers now include baking soda in their toothpaste. More than 10 percent say they also rely on baking soda to help freshen their breath.

"My dentist suggested I brush with baking soda and hydrogen peroxide to help control gum problems, and it seems to help sweeten my breath, too," says Doris, 73, of East Northport, New York. She's been using it, off and on, for a few years, as necessary.

"When I was a little kid, when we'd run out of toothpaste, our mother would have us use baking soda, and I've always preferred it," says Frank, 45, a mail handler living in Indianapolis. "I think my mouth feels cleaner and my breath feels fresher when I use it than it does with toothpaste." Frank says that only once has he been told that his breath offends. "I think that's pretty good, considering I'm a smoker," he says.

Baking soda actually changes the acidity in your mouth and makes it a less friendly environment for the bacteria that help cause bad breath, experts explain.

THEY GO FOR THE GREEN

Twenty percent of our survey takers say they chew parsley, and five percent say they chew mint leaves to sweeten their breath.

"When I'm out in my herb garden, I always break off a few stems of parsley to chew on. I can tell that it immediately freshens my breath," says Shirley, 57, of Ione, California. She's also the type to clean her plate, right down to the parsley garnish. "I figure it's there for that reason," she says. In fact, that's exactly why it's there. The parsley garnish originated with the Romans, who munched on sprigs at banquets to freshen their breath.

"Whenever I feel the need, I chew on peppermint," says Marcie, 43, of Allegan, Michigan. There's no shortage of this aggressive plant in her large formal herb garden. "It's practically a weed," she says. Besides freshening her breath, the mint seems to clear her sinuses, she says. "I chew it for a few minutes, then spit it out."

Both parsley and mint have long been used as breath fresheners with good results, experts say.

These plants contain strong-scented oils that mask mouth odors when they are chewed. Those who swallow the leaves get an additional breath-freshening benefit, says Ronald Bogdasarian, M.D., an otorhinolaryngologist and clinical assistant professor at the University of Michigan Medical School in Ann Arbor. "The same oils that freshen the breath when you chew are digested and exuded through the lungs some 24 hours later. So you get long-term breath freshening."

Both parsley and peppermint also have a history of use for digestive upsets and constipation, which many of the people in our survey believe also contributes to bad breath. Both these plants apparently help to reduce the formation of intestinal gas and aid digestion by stimulating the flow of bile.

GIVING UP BREATH BLASTERS

Those of us who cannot imagine life without garlic happily endure the odoriferous emanations that come from our bodies as a result of sucking down a plate of, say, Polish kielbasa. While garlic and onions are mentioned as obvious breath-altering foods, people who responded to our survey also have a few less common culprits in mind: meat and cheese. "I find that staying away from meat keeps my breath fresher," writes one survey taker. "No dairy products," says another.

It may be that the high-fat versions of these foods are causing bad breath in some people, says Robert Sataloff, M.D., professor of otolaryngology at Jefferson Medical College in Philadelphia. "Fatty foods take longer to move through your stomach and so can sour in your stomach, causing bad breath," he says. And certain fats contain aromatic substances that we metabolize and exhale, which changes the breath's smell, he adds.

SWEETENING WITH FRUITS AND VEGGIES

More than a dozen survey takers say they add foods to their diet specifically to counteract bad breath. Fruits (especially apples), vegetables (especially leafy greens), and psyllium (a popular natural bulk laxative), along with yogurt and wheat grass juice, topped the popularity poll.

How might these foods work? Well, our survey takers think that foods such as these help to keep things moving right along and generally "detoxify" the bowel, which in turn sweetens the breath. "It's true that bowel problems can cause bad breath," says Dr. Sataloff. "These foods may help prevent constipation, which can contribute to bad breath."

Some of these food also contain chlorophyll, which has its own deodorizing effect. A form of chorophyll called chlorophyllin copper complex is approved by the Food and Drug Administration as a safe and effective de-odorizing compound. This product, sold in tablet form, can be used by in-continent people to neutralize the odor of urine and feces.

CHLOROPHYLL TO THE RESCUE

Although chlorophyll product manufacturers do not make the claim that their products can improve bad breath, four people report that they work well in that regard. One survey taker, in fact, says that chlorophyll tablets worked when all else had failed.

"My son is healthy. He has wonderful teeth and gums, no cavities, and no apparent gastrointestinal problems," says Mary, of Furlong, Pennsylvania. One thing her son did have until recently, though, was bad breath. "Yes, he knew he had it, and so did everyone else," his mother says. "He tried breath mints and just about everything else, but nothing seemed to help."

Then, one day, Mary read about chlorophyll tablets in a magazine she'd picked up at a local health-food store. "It said they were supposed to help bad breath, and I figured, 'Why not buy some and let him try them?' " she says. "Well, they work better than anything he's ever tried. He takes one tablet a day, and if he skips a few days, we all know it, including his girlfriend."

Bed-Wetting

Drying Up an Aggravating Problem

Sometimes it's tough to tell who's hurt more by bed-wetting: the little boy who hides his sheets in shame or the concerned parents who can't believe their son hasn't yet mastered his bladder. (Although girls sometimes wet the bed, it's far more common in boys.)

Fortunately, the people who provided bed-wetting remedies for our survey recognize that exasperation is not among the best techniques for keeping junior dry. Rather, most know the key is simply helping their son or daughter learn how to control the bladder. "Kids who wet the bed often have more frequent and more intense bladder contractions, and if they can't respond to that by tightening their anal sphincter muscles, it's surf city time," says Martin Scharf, Ph.D., director of the Sleep Disorder Center of Mercy Hospital in Cincinnati and author of *Waking Up Dry: How to End Bed-Wetting Forever.*

SHE CHAMPIONS THE WAKE-UP CALL

Several readers favor waking the child up for one last trip to the bathroom a few hours after he goes to bed.

For Sandy, of Champaign, Illinois, the trick was to get her five-year-old to the bathroom before midnight. Once the habit was formed, her son began waking himself up when he needed to go.

Waking a child up before he wets the bed works, but you can speed his progress by helping strengthen his bladder muscles, says Dr. Scharf. "According to research, 30 percent of the kids get dry just from doing stream interruption and bladder-stretching exercises. That means having them stop and start in midstream at least ten times, every time they go to the bathroom. Kids can also hold back urination as long as they can during the day to help stretch their bladder," he says.

SHE ENFORCES LIQUID CURFEW

With 4 children, 10 grandchildren and 12 great-grandchildren, France-line knows a thing or two about keeping kids from springing a nighttime leak. The 76-year-old West Branch, Michigan, native says a liquid curfew is among the best ways to control bed-wetting.

"Over the years, I've just learned that the ones who go to bed at 8:00 P.M. shouldn't have anything to drink after 6:00 P.M.," she says.

While dealing with a grandchild who occasionally violates the no-drinking policy, Franceline says she has also learned that quietly repeating, "I will not wet the bed tonight," with the child just before bed can help.

"You don't want to embarrass the child—you just want him to start thinking about taking control of the situation," she says.

While Dr. Scharf doesn't support outright fluid restriction, he does see the need to control soda and milk. "What you need to do is eliminate anything that fizzes, whether it has caffeine or not, before bed," says Dr. Scharf. "When the kids drink soda, within a few minutes they have to go to the bathroom." Some children also stop wetting after their evening glass of milk has been removed from the menu, he says.

SHE SAYS THE BUZZER CAN'T BE BEAT

Judith, a 55-year-old child psychologist, wasn't too concerned about her son's bed-wetting when he was younger. But after his sixth birthday, she decided it was time to find a solution.

At her pediatrician's recommendation, she bought a device that sets off an alarm when the sheets get wet, prompting the child to get up and go to the bathroom.

Within a week, Judith says, her son's bed-wetting stopped. "It really was a quick and easy solution," she says.

Using a bell-and-pad alarm works best with an assist from parents, explains Dr. Scharf. "The bell and pad works wonderfully in three-quarters of the kids. But the rest of the kids don't hear it," he says. "The problem is that they are wetting early in the night when their sleep is the deepest. So if the parents will wake the kid up an hour or two after bedtime, with the intention of delaying wetting until later in the night when their sleep is lighter, the child will have a better chance of responding to the alarm. You can tell when the child starts responding to the alarm because the wet spots get smaller. At that point, the parents can stop waking the child up. Then it's just a matter of time before the child stops wetting the bed."

ENDING STRESS STOPS THE STREAM

Alice, a 72-year-old South Bedford, Iowa, resident, knows stress is harmful—even for kids. But it wasn't until she was taking care of her 2½-

year-old granddaughter that she discovered a possible link to bed-wetting.

A few months after the child was successfully potty-trained, a relative offered to take her roller skating during an upcoming visit. For whatever reason, the child became fixated on the thought of the trip, constantly bringing it up—and to Alice's surprise—began wetting the bed again.

When the day of the trip finally arrived, they visited the relative but were unable to go roller skating. Alice thought this might upset the child. But in fact, the next day, she discovered that the child had not wet the bed—and never did again.

"The more nervous and stressed out they are, the more likely they're going to have an accident," says Alice.

Stress can indeed cause bed-wetting, says Dr. Scharf. Stress does not play a role in all cases, but if stress is the cause, the bed-wetting will stop when the stress is removed, he explains.

SHE FOUND TOYS REWARDING

Back when her daughter was three, Joy used a multifaceted approach to get her daughter to stop wetting the bed.

Just before she went to sleep, Joy would wake the child and take her to the bathroom, running the water in the sink to encourage her to go.

"I think the sound of water really helped, but don't ask me where I heard about that," says the 71-year-old Smokerise, Alabama, resident.

The real breakthrough, however, came when Joy linked the child's potty performance to a new toy she wanted. Joy informed her daughter that only big girls who didn't wet the bed were allowed to have this particular toy. When the child insisted she would stop, Joy bought the toy and she did stop—for a few days. When she asked for another toy for her birthday, Joy repeated her assertion, and once again the child insisted that she would stop. But this time, all the mornings after were different: no wet sheets.

Rewards work, says Dr. Scharf, but they must be used carefully. "You can't beat a reward system to get the child to try, to focus. In fact, we use a gold and silver star chart in our office," he says. "But if you say to a child, 'Good boy, you're dry,' then there's a converse that's implied and that's 'Bad boy, you're wet.' And bed-wetting has nothing to do with being good or bad. The message I try to give the kids is that you can wet the bed and still be president someday. We keep track of so many different things—their bladder capacity, the number of dry nights, even the size of the wet spots— we make sure the kid has some success every visit. That's what keeps them motivated."

Bee Stings

Soothing Away the Ouch

Maybe you're minding your own business, maybe you're not. Maybe you're roofing a house or mowing a lawn. Maybe you're robbing a beehive of its golden stash of honey or walking barefoot through the grass for the pure pleasure of it. Whatever the case, you wind up on the receiving end of a buzzing varmint—or two or three.

Most people, our survey revealed, take it for granted that insects and people will occasionally collide. Many have gardens and so have come to a kind of truce, figuring the bugs have as much right to be there as the people do.

"We just seem to have a lot of yellow jackets around our house, so I get stung every once in a while when I'm mowing the lawn," explains John, 75, a retired Department of Commerce statistician living in Forestville, Maryland. The insects seem to prefer hairy, sweaty, knobby-kneed legs, he's convinced.

But some have been taken very much by surprise, whether by inadvertently settling their derriere down in hornet territory or imbibing a bee along with their Dr. Pepper.

Luckily, no matter where or how they were stung, our survey takers were able to find something that soothed the pain. "When we'd get stung, we'd go racing across the field to Pa, and he'd put a bit of chewing tobacco on it for us," says Patti, of Slidell, Louisiana.

One man recalls learning about his remedy—rhubarb juice—from an old-timer who came to his rescue when a bee nailed him in his backyard. "You break off a stalk, bust it open and rub the juicy end on the sting," says Allen, a heavy equipment operator from Minong, Wisconsin. Yes, but does it work? "You betcha. It gets the hurt and swelling out fast. You don't believe me, try it next time you get stung."

Our survey participants say that not all the remedies they use get the seal of approval from their doctors. But that certainly hasn't stopped them from using them—or finding relief. Here's what they say works.

GETTING OUT THE STINGER

Removing an embedded stinger is a priority when you've been stung. If it's left in, the tiny venom sac attached to the stinger continues to contract, pumping venom under your skin. The trick is to remove the stinger without squeezing the venom sac, and our survey takers suggest a number of ways to do just that.

"Draw a moist bar of soap across the sting. It will pull the stinger right out," suggests one person. "Scrape out the stinger with the edge of a credit card or the dull side of a knife," offers another. "Use your fingernail to scrape the stinger out," advises a third. "Scrape out the stinger with a popsicle stick," recommends one mom.

"We used to live in Hawaii, where a flowering vine on our apartment terrace attracted a lot of bees," says Rebecca, of Corpus Christi, Texas. "Some of the bees would find their way into the apartment, and sometimes they'd end up stinging someone. We'd always get an ice cube and hold it on the sting for a few minutes. When you remove the ice cube, the stinger sticks to it, and the cold helps to keep down the swelling."

BAKING SODA SOOTHES

What can you do once the stinger is removed, and you're left with an angry welt? Our survey takers had a veritable picnic basket full of suggestions for things to apply: onions, mustard, honey, oatmeal, cucumber, lemon juice. Tops on the list, however, is a paste of baking soda.

"I've used baking soda paste dozens of times, and it's always worked for me," says Amy, 43, of Mount Clemens, Michigan. "It's all I ever used when my kids were growing up, and I've used it on my grandson, too. It says right on the box that it's good for minor skin irritations."

"The soothing qualities of baking soda have been known for centuries," says Ara DerMarderosian, Ph.D., professor of pharmacognosy and medicinal chemistry at Philadelphia College of Pharmacy and Science. "It works because a paste made with water retains moisture and produces an alkaline medium. That means it can neutralize things that are acidic, such as the irritating venom of an insect sting."

"I'm convinced baking soda saved my life when I was stung by a bee as a youngster," says Linda, 48, of Nyssa, Oregon. "We lived quite a way from the doctor and, by the time my mother found me, I was swollen all over. When my mother called the doctor, he told her to bathe me down with a paste of baking soda. She did. I've used baking soda paste ever since, making sure I get it on as fast as possible."

THEY SWEAR BY MEAT TENDERIZER

Thirty-three of the 212 people who offered remedies for stings suggest applying a paste of meat tenderizer. "I'd use it any time one of my children got stung, and it did seem to reduce the pain and swelling," says Rosetta, of Seattle. Her husband was a rose enthusiast, so their yard was loaded with bug-enticing blooms. Their children shared their play space with plenty of busy bees.

"Look for a meat tenderizer that contains papain," suggests Philip Koehler, Ph.D., entomologist at the U.S. Department of Agriculture Laboratory at the University of Florida in Gainesville. This is an enzyme, derived from papaya fruit, that breaks down protein. Since the inflammation-producing toxins in insect venom are made of protein, applying a paste of meat tenderizer as soon as possible neutralizes the venom and helps you avoid pain and swelling, Dr. Koehler says.

One woman uses papain straight from the papaya. "I tried this for the first time when I was in Hawaii, and it worked so well, I figured out how to have it available to me year-round," says Arlene, of Columbia Station, Ohio. "I freeze squares of papaya skin. When I get stung, I take a square out of the freezer, run it under water to thaw it out a bit and put it on the sting. It works very quickly to relieve the pain, and I think it works better than meat tenderizer."

MUD PLASTERS PAIN

Mud is usually handy if you're stung outdoors, and 15 percent of the people who responded to this question said plastering a bit of mud on a sting worked for them.

"If you don't have mud, make it, even if you have to use saliva to do so," urges Alice, 83, of North Hollywood, California. "You can just mix it up in your hand, put it on the sting, and let it dry. I think it draws out the toxin, and sometimes it draws out the stinger, too."

Icy cold mud from a tiny creek flowing nearby was the antidote for bee stings at Greta's childhood home in Easton, Pennsylvania. "We'd get stung playing in the fields, and our mother always said to put mud on the sting," recalls Greta, a landscaper still living in Easton. "It did seem to help, although I think it was the cold as much as anything that eased the pain."

Experts contend that mud has no ability to draw toxins out of a bee sting. "Mud may offer some pain relief by cooling the skin as the water in it evaporates," Dr. Valentine says. Others say that applying mud may also keep you from scratching the sting for a while, which will also reduce the pain.

ICE AND COLD FREEZES THEIR PAIN

Ice is as popular as mud with our survey participants. Some 15 percent say applying cold to a sting stops pain and swelling. "I've tried a few things for stings, but as long as it's handy, I think ice works the best," says Henry, 76, of Pensacola, Florida. "The trick is to get it on fast and to continue to use it, off and on, until the pain is gone for good."

In fact, experts say this straight-from-the-freezer remedy is one of your best choices for insect stings. The cold constricts blood vessels, which delays the absorption of venom and puts a clamp on swelling and inflammation. That means less pain. If you don't have an ice cube handy, a cold can of soda, an icy brook or even a liquid that evaporates rapidly, causing the skin to cool, such as alcohol or vinegar, may do the trick.

THEY'D GO FOR A WAD OF CHAW

South of the Mason-Dixon line, tobacco has traditionally been a popular remedy for bee stings. Twenty-one of those surveyed recommend chewing tobacco for stings; two more suggest snuff, which is powdered tobacco.

"It sure did come in handy if you were out in the yard or field," says Daphne, an oil company secretary living in Garland, Texas, who says this remedy was popular when she was a kid. It didn't matter if the tobacco was from a cigarette, chew or snuff, and it didn't matter if you wet it with spit or water, it worked to draw out the pain and swelling, she says. And others agree. "Of course, it's a lot harder these days to find a cigarette, much less chew," says Daphne.

We asked a number of experts about the possible medicinal properties of tobacco, and all seemed to think that tobacco would be no better—or worse—for a sting than any other wet, pasty material. "As far as I know, it would simply provide a cooling effect," says Varro E. Tyler, Ph.D., professor of pharmacognosy at the School of Pharmacy and Pharmacal Sciences at Purdue University in West Lafayette, Indiana, and author of *The Honest Herbal.*

AMMONIA NEUTRALIZES THEIR PAIN

Twelve survey participants suggest applying ammonia to a bee sting to ease the pain.

"I've stepped on bees several times," admits Connie, 76, a gardener in Voluntown, Connecticut, with a penchant for going barefoot. "I limp right into the house, soak a piece of cotton with ammonia and dab it on the sting for a few minutes, until the pain goes away. I'm not sure exactly why I tried it in the first place—I guess I just figured it might help, and I think it does."

In fact, ammonia "pens," or dabbers, used to be sold for just for this purpose. Like baking soda paste, ammonia is alkaline, so it apparently helps to neutralize the acid toxins in bee venom, says Dr. Tyler. If you do use ammonia on a sting, make sure you keep it away from your eyes, he adds.

AN ASPIRIN PASTE EASED HER PAIN

Only two people suggest making a paste of aspirin to apply to a sting, and one of those women is convinced the aspirin saved her day.

"We were on our way to a family reunion and stopped at the old homestead, which had been empty for about six months," explains Patti of Slidell, Louisiana. "I sat down on a swing on the porch—the same swing I used when I lived there as child. Well, I didn't see the wasp's nest under it, and before I knew it, a couple of wasps had flown up my skirt and stung me. The only thing we had with us that we thought might possibly help was aspirin. We put the aspirin on our tongues to wet them, then put them on my stings, and they relieved the pain in a matter of minutes. I had no swelling, either."

Experts say that rubbing a wet aspirin on the area where you were stung can provide pain relief and help neutralize some of the inflammatory agents in the venom.

EDITOR'S NOTE: People who are allergic to aspirin should not rub aspirin on their skin. You don't have to ingest aspirin to have an allergic reaction. Even rubbing an aspirin on the skin can cause a serious reaction in people who are allergic to it.

Bladder Infections

Techniques for Flushing Out Bacteria

G uys get them, of course. But bothersome bladder infections are anything but an equal opportunity annoyer. In fact, women are 25 times more likely than men to come down with a case.

Why the gender bias? No quotas here—just a pesky bacterium named *Escherichia coli*. While both men and women have *E. coli* living in their intestines and rectum, it's a shorter trip from a woman's rectum to her urethra—the urinary tube that leads to the bladder. And when *E. coli* overruns the bladder, it causes all kinds of unpleasantness—a constant urgent need to go to the bathroom, a burning sensation upon urination and sometimes blood in the urine. Left untreated, a bladder infection can even travel to the kidneys, where it can cause serious complications.

Judging from our survey, most women are willing to do just about anything to avoid going through this painful scenario. "After you've had one of these, nothing you've heard to prevent them is out of the question," says Linda, of East Canton, Ohio, who swears by kidney bean juice as her bladder cure.

While doctors continue to debate the reputed curative powers of assorted juices—cranberry tops the list—there's no question that simply boosting the amount of liquid you're drinking can be of some benefit.

"Most women drink one or two glasses of water a day, and that's just not enough," says Yvonne S. Thornton, M.D., professor of obstetrics and gynecology at Columbia University College of Physicians and Surgeons in New York City. "We should be drinking six to eight glasss of water during the fall and winter and eight to ten glasses in the spring and summer," she says.

Why pour in the liquid? "It flushes the bladder out, preventing residual urine from becoming a breeding ground for the bacteria that cause infection," she says.

KUDOS FOR CRANBERRY JUICE

The tart liquid of choice for over 80 percent of the women who responded to our survey: cranberry juice. Clara, of Jacksonville, Florida, says she relies on cranberry juice because it works for her, and because she's tried just about everything else.

With just one functioning kidney, Clara has been in and out of the hospital for decades—at last count 30 visits. But now when an infection strikes, instead of getting ready for an emergency room visit, the 53-year-old Mohawk Indian says she looks to the ever-present bottle of cranberry juice in her refrigerator.

Clara says she begins self-treatment when she gets a distinct tingling sensation in her hands and a slight burning on urination that almost always precedes her infections. During each day of treatment, she drinks a 64-ounce bottle of cranberry juice, filling a typical 8-ounce glass three-quarters of the way with juice and a fourth with water.

Also plagued with chronic bladder problems, Verna has used more than her share of doctor-prescribed antibiotics to beat bladder infections. But if she starts gulping cranberry juice and water at the first sign of a bladder infection, the 63-year-old Nicholasville, Kentucky, resident says she can fend one off. "If I catch it early, I'm usually okay," she says. "It seems to do the trick."

Verna doesn't fuss with exact amounts, however. She simply stocks her refrigerator with an ample supply of cranberry juice and has a glass every few hours until the threat is gone. The only problem: draining the glass. She doesn't like the taste. "It's much too sweet," she says.

While cranberry juice advocates are legion, not all researchers are convinced. Some tests, however, have intimated that drinking cranberry juice might increase the acidity in the bladder, thereby killing the bacteria that cause infections. Other researchers say that cranberry and blueberry juice contain ingredients that seem to prevent bacteria from sticking to the bladder walls, making it easier to flush them out.

A six-month study of 153 older Boston-area women makes a strong case for this folk cure. Half the women drank ten ounces of cranberry juice a day for six months, while the rest drank a look-alike beverage fortified with vitamin C but devoid of cranberry. By the end of the study, those who drank cranberry juice were half as likely to suffer from a bladder infection as their cranberry-less sisters, says Mark Monane, M.D., project director of the study and an instructor at Harvard Medical School.

Varro E. Tyler, Ph.D., professor of pharmacognosy at the School of Pharmacy and Pharmacal Sciences at Purdue University in West Lafayette, Indiana, and author of *The Honest Herbal*, recommends drinking 3 ounces of cranberry juice daily as a preventive and upping that amount to between 12 and 32 ounces if infection occurs.

SHE BRAGS ABOUT BAKING SODA

Rusha says her home town of Sitka, Kentucky, an old coal mining burg, is little more than "a wide spot in the road." And when she was growing up, they hadn't even built the road yet—let alone the wide spot.

"If you had to see a doctor, you'd have to ride for a few miles by horseback just to get to a place where the ambulance could come and pick you up," she jokes.

As a result, Rusha's mother had home remedies "down to a science"—including her baking soda and water cure for bladder infection. "Mother would mix a teaspoonful of baking soda in a glass of water and drink the contents once a day for three days," says the 65-year-old grandmother. "It had a peculiar taste, but that would take care of it."

Rusha may have armed herself with a bacterial hammer, according to Kristene E. Whitmore, M.D., chief of urology at Graduate Hospital in Philadelphia and coauthor of *Overcoming Bladder Disorders*. "I've had lots of patients tell me it relieves the burning quickly," she says. At the first sign of symptoms, Dr. Whitmore recommends drinking 16 ounces of water and then 4 ounces of water with a tablespoon of baking soda mixed in. Then she recommends drinking 8 ounces of plain water every hour for the next eight hours.

EDITOR'S NOTE: It's best to avoid taking baking soda after a large meal. In a few rare cases, people have suffered stomach rupture by taking baking soda when their stomachs were overfull.

SHE GETS RELIEF FROM HERBS

When Carolyn discovered her remedy, a bladder infection was the least of her problems.

Dying from kidney failure, the 50-year-old Medford, Oregon, resident faced an operation to make it possible for her to receive dialysis—daily blood-cleansing treatments. But when she arrived at the doctor's office, she learned her operation had been canceled: Her doctor had suffered a stroke.

On the way home, Carolyn's car had a flat tire. By a strange and miraculous twist of fate, an herbalist and a doctor stopped to help her with her tire. During the repairs, she told them about her kidney problem, and they recommended that she drink tea brewed from the dark green leaves of the prince's pine plant.

The story gets better. Because her own doctor was sick, she had to go to a different doctor about her kidneys. And when the new doctor did his own tests, he discovered that her kidneys had started to function again. Carolyn is convinced that the tea cured her. "It was unbelievable," she says.

The herbalist also introduced her to uva ursi to prevent bladder infections, and she continues to rely on it.

"Because I'm prone to bladder infections, I don't know how many times this tea has prevented me from getting one," she says. "But since then, I've only had one that was severe enough to send me to the doctor's office."

For just such occasions, Carolyn says she keeps a few quarts of brewed prince's pine and uva ursi tea in her refrigerator and drinks four cups a day when she feels the symptoms of a bladder infection coming on.

While Carolyn's case seems extraordinary, both prince's pine and uva ursi do have a long history of use for treating urinary tract problems.

Uva ursi leaves are taken from a short evergreen plant that grows in northern Europe and North America. To promote healing of the bladder, use two capsules of dried uva ursi extract three times a day or one dropperful of tincture in a cup of warm water three times a day and continue this treatment until the symptoms disappear, suggests Andrew Weil, M.D., associate director of the Division of Social Perspectives in Medicine at the University of Arizona College of Medicine/Arizona Health Sciences Center in Tucson, in his book *Natural Health, Natural Medicine*. Uva ursi products are sold in many health-food stores.

Also called pipsissewa, prince's pine grows wild in hardwood forests. It was used during the Civil War to relieve rheumatism and kidney disorders and was at one time listed as an ingredient in Hire's root beer. And, according to herbalist Michael Moore, it can be taken several times a week for extended periods to remedy weak kidneys. It, too, is available in health-food stores that sell herbs.

GIVE THEM A C

After liquids of all varieties, vitamin C is the second most popular choice among those surveyed for beating bladder infections.

But if the mighty vitamin needs a spokesperson, Amelie is it. On the last leg of a trip to Europe, the Aurora, Colorado, resident felt a bladder infection coming on. She hadn't been drinking enough water, and transatlantic flights can dehydrate anyone. Amelie didn't want to take antibiotics for the infection, because, she says, they always seem to lead to a yeast infection.

So when her airplane finally touched down at Denver's Stapleton Airport, one of her first stops was her neighborhood health-food store. The store's owner suggested 1,000 milligrams of buffered vitamin C a day and Cranactin, a cranberry-based capsule, to help prevent a full-blown infection. Amelie says she starting taking her new supplements that day.

"The first thing I noticed was that the pain was gone within 24 hours," says Amelie. "And before long, there was no sign that I had any problem at all."

Nearly a year after she started taking 1,000 milligrams of vitamin C a day, plus the vitamin C contained in her multivitamin, Amelie says she still hasn't had a bladder infection. "I just don't do drugs well, but I prefer this anyway."

Amelie apparently got good advice at that health-food store. Experts say about 1,000 milligrams of vitamin C taken throughout the day will acidify the urine enough to interfere with bacterial growth, particularly in those who have recurrent bladder infections.

Amelie's flight-flogged immune system also probably got a much-needed boost from the vitamin C, says Dr. Whitmore, while her Cranactin provided all the bacteria-fighting benefits of cranberry juice—with less acid.

It's important, however, to check with your doctor if you're taking antibiotics prescribed for bladder infections; some of them don't work well when urine is highly acidic, says Dr. Whitmore.

EDITOR'S NOTE: The recommended Daily Value for vitamin C is 60 milligrams—less than what you'd get if you ate a single orange. Too much vitamin C is known to cause diarrhea in some, but researchers say you can safely take up to 1,000 milligrams a day long term and up to 1,500 milligrams a day for up to two months. But it's best to take it over the course of a day. If larger doses cause cramping or diarrhea, cut back the amount you're taking.

SHE GRABS FOR THE GARLIC

Glenna says she uses garlic for everything: spider bites, athlete's foot, even shingles. So it's no surprise that when any member of her vast family (including 25 great-grandchildren) has a bladder infection, she reaches for a clove or two.

"I fell in love with the heavenly stuff when I was teenager in Reno, Nevada—a real strong Italian town," says the 74-year-old Spokane, Washington, resident. "I don't get bladder infections because I peel and eat garlic like some people eat apples."

When preparing garlic for others, Glenna says she mixes a pressed clove into a serving of yogurt or sour cream that's destined for a baked potato. Two servings a day for three straight days is usually enough to banish their bladder infection, she says.

"Usually by the third day, they've gotten over their temperature, and that cranky feeling and their urine has cleared up," she says.

And while she's tried garlic pills, Glenna doesn't think they work nearly as well. "There's no comparison—for me, anyway," she says.

Glenna's zeal for garlic is certainly real. But can the stuff subdue a bladder infection? Experts say garlic's antibiotic properties have been confirmed in dozens of studies. Among its proven uses: killing the bacteria of women's bladder infections.

GETTING A LITTLE CULTURE

Merry eats nonfat yogurt like some people drink coffee—at least a cup every day. But when a bladder problem threatens, she's discovered that boosting her yogurt intake—as well as drinking cranberry juice and eating garlic—seems to ward off an infection.

"I wouldn't hesitate to go to the doctor if I had a serious bladder infection," says the 42-year-old adjunct junior college professor. "But since I've been trying this, I haven't needed to."

Once she feels an infection coming on, Merry alters her diet just a little: Instead of her usual cup, Merry says she downs three to four cups of yogurt and three to four cups of cranberry juice a day, while an extra garlic clove makes its way into her evening meal.

Eating massive amounts of yogurt won't cure a bladder infection, but it could prevent one, says Dr. Whitmore. In a study of women with a history of recurrent vaginal infections, a daily cup of yogurt reduced the incidence of vaginitis threefold. And women who have fewer vaginal infections seem to have fewer bladder infections, she says. Doctors theorize that acidophilus, the friendly bacteria found in yogurt, somehow prevent unfriendly bacteria from establishing themselves, she explains. Look for yogurts that have active cultures, or consider acidophilus supplements that also contain them, says Dr. Whitmore.

THE CLEANER, THE BETTER

She knows she's a clean freak. "They're going to put 'She Tried to Be Hygienic' on my tombstone," says Doris, a 72-year-old former school teacher and Long Island, New York, resident. But she firmly believes that careful attention to hygiene can aid in reducing the frequency of bladder infections.

"It seems so obvious, but it's very, very, important," she says.

Part of Doris's regimen includes using only unscented white toilet paper or wipes and keeping washcloths and towels separate—even from her husband.

"Community involvement is great when you're living in a youth hostel, but when you get older and become more susceptible to opportunistic infections, then you have to be more concerned," she says. "That's why we have hot water and soap."

Doris may sound a bit extreme, but she's likely to stay free of bladder infections as long as she keeps hygiene a top priority, says Dr. Thornton. "If you're allergic to the inks and dyes in toilet paper, that can cause inflammation in your bladder," she says. "If you have inflammation, then you're going to have bacteria. And if you have bacteria multiplying like crazy, you're going to have an infection."

Using inappropriate cleaning techniques after going to the bathroom can also cause bladder infections. Women should wipe themselves from the front to the back, says Dr. Thornton. "You want to take the tissue from a sterile area, which is the bladder, to the least sterile area, which is the rectum," she explains.

If you're overweight and have trouble wiping this way, you should try taking a bath in a tub once a week or using a hand-held shower to help clean the area more thoroughly, she says. And because sharing soap, towels and other bath items with your husband or guests has been linked to bladder infections, she says it's a good idea to keep them to yourself. Other techniques: urinating before and immediately after sex, leaning slightly forward when urinating, and changing immediately out of a wet swimsuit.

Body Odor

Clearing the Air

Most people think sweat causes body odor. In fact, real sweat— the kind that pours off you when you're cranking up a bicycle or pounding the pavement—is clear, clean and odorless, unless it's scented by foods such as onion, garlic, coffee or booze. Although copious sweat may contribute to odor by helping to disperse body secretions, it's usually not the main cause.

So what causes the smell? A milky substance, secreted in very small amounts from special glands called apocrine glands, found under the arms and in the groin. Once it hits the skin, this secretion quickly undergoes bacterial decomposition. That's what causes the bad smell.

Unlike sweat glands, which up production when the heat's on, apocrine glands respond mostly to emotional stress. The substances these glands produce are thought to have once served as sexual turn-ons. Nowadays, however, most people are more likely to find the smell they produce more of a turnoff.

Nearly 100 people in our survey offer suggestions for dealing with body odor. Whether it's caused by a healthy workout, brow-beating stress or nothing in particular, here's what they say leaves them smelling good enough for polite company.

BAKING SODA SNUFFS THEIR SCENT

Chances are you could take away their deodorant, toothpaste, soap, baby powder—just about anything that lets them smell good and feel clean. But the one thing our survey participants simply won't do without is baking soda. "Of course it works," says one ardent user. "It says right here on the box that it helps to control odors."

Some 26 people recommend baking soda for body odor, and more than a few say it outshines much more expensive products. People use it in the bath, as an abrasive paste on their skin and as a powder.

"Years ago, when I was a teenager, I was having real problems. I sweated a lot, and I would break out under my arms when I used deodorants," says

Shirley, of Virginia Beach, Virginia. "I tried quite a few things, and finally, my mother said, 'Let's try baking soda. That's what my mother used.' So I did. I put about four tablespoons in the bath water, and I also used it under my arms, and it worked beautifully. I continued to use it for a few years, and eventually my sweating problems resolved."

"We were camping this summer in Canada, and it snowed, so we were a little reluctant to jump in the lake to clean off," says Jerry, of Rock Hill, South Carolina. Being inventive and not wanting to offend, he and his buddies neutralized their "eau de P.U." with baking soda. "You just pour some of it in your hands and rub it on. You don't have to worry about it; it just falls off. Even though we were making do with what we had, we found it to be very effective. At least, nobody complained about the close quarters."

Baking soda works because it kills odor-causing bacteria and absorbs moisture, says Arthur Jacknowitz, Pharm.D., professor and chairman of the Department of Clinical Pharmacy at West Virginia University School of Pharmacy in Morgantown. "Many people find it's just as effective as deodorant."

ANTIESTABLISHMENT ANTIPERSPIRANTS

Speaking of deodorant, some 17 people recommend using it for body odor. Makes sense, since that's what these products are designed to do.

A typical deodorant contains an ingredient that inhibits odor-causing bacteria on the skin, such as triclosan chloride. Most also contain some sort of fragrance to help mask odors. And some contain moisture-absorbing powders such as cornstarch or talc.

Antiperspirants, however, contain an additional ingredient that inhibits sweat secretion. "A common sweat-stopping ingredient is aluminum chlorohydrate, which seems to work simply because the pasty material plugs up sweat glands," says Donald R. Miller, Pharm.D., an associate professor of pharmacy at North Dakota State University in Fargo. "Many of the products on the market are both deodorant and antiperspirant."

Not all our survey takers use a typical over-the-counter deodorant, however. Several people suggested using chunks of mineral compounds. And one woman said she gets good results using a long-acting deodorant that contains zinc oxide, a thick white paste that is better known as a nose-protecting sunblock than a deodorant.

"I started using a crystal rock because I simply didn't like the way most deodorants smelled or how they clogged up the glands under my arms," says Regina, of St. Augustine, Florida. "The rock is very easy to use. After you shower, you simply dry your armpits, then dampen the rock and rub it under your arms or anywhere else you want. It works well on feet, too." The rock doesn't keep you dry, she says, but it does prevent odors from developing. It has no smell of its own. One rock lasts about a year for her. She buys them at a health-food store.

These rocks are sold under a variety of trade names. They are made from potassium alum, a mineral salt obtained from bauxite that is said to be less irritating than the usual deodorant ingredients.

THEY'D RATHER LATHER

"Use a good, strong deodorant soap like Lifebuoy," suggests a Connecticut man. "Try Dial soap," recommends a woman from Florida. These and other deodorant soaps contain an antibacterial ingredient such as triclosan or triclocarban.

"These soaps work by depositing the antibacterial ingredient on the skin, where it remains active for a time," Dr. Miller says. "How long it really lasts depends on how active and sweaty you are. The more you sweat, the shorter amount of time it works."

ZINC ZAPS THEIR STINK

About 10 percent of the people who responded to our question about body odor recommend zinc supplements.

This is a remedy that has been around for quite some time but has yet to be proven or disproven in any sort of scientific way. It's true that zinc is contained in some antiperspirants, where it helps prevent perspiration by acting directly on the sweat glands, perhaps both as an antibacterial and by plugging sweat gland pores. But experts say that, taken in oral form, it probably doesn't work the same way.

"It's possible that some of the people who say zinc supplements help their body odor do have a zinc deficiency," says Robert I. Henkin, M.D., Ph.D., director of the Center for Molecular Nutrition and Sensory Disorders at the Taste and Smell Clinic in Washington, D.C. "If so, they may develop changes in their perception of taste and smell, so that they think they smell bad and have bad breath, even if others cannot detect an odor." That's because zinc plays a major role in the proper function of the body's taste- and smell-perceiving cells. Suppplemental zinc can correct this problem, Dr. Henkin says.

Several of those we contacted say they simply take zinc supplements as a health measure, not to combat a case of B.O. Nevertheless, they feel their body odor is slight, compared with those around them.

"I take several kinds of supplements, including zinc, just to make sure I get enough, and my body odor has practically vanished as a result," says Norma, of Ottumwa, Iowa. "Even when I sweat a lot during the summertime, I don't tend to smell." She takes 50 milligrams a day.

And at least one survey taker takes zinc specifically for body odor and feels it has provided significant benefit.

"Taking zinc supplements hasn't completely cured my problem, but it has helped a lot," says Linda, 47, of Worcester, Massachusetts. "I had had a problem with body odor for years. I'd tried just about every deodorant out there and sometimes was using two different deodorants at the same time. I was desperate."

She decided to try taking zinc after she read in a magazine how it had helped someone with body odor. "I noticed a big improvement within a few days," she says. "It didn't seem to affect how much I sweat, but the odor was reduced considerably."

She's continued to take zinc supplements every day. "I still use deodorant, and I avoid most synthetic fiber clothing, which seems to retain odors," she says.

EDITOR'S NOTE: If you decide to try this remedy, it's best to take no more than 15 milligrams a day without medical supervision. That's because high levels of zinc can interfere with absorption of copper, another essential trace mineral. If you have a true zinc deficiency, your doctor may initially prescribe amounts as high as 150 milligrams, then cut back as your zinc status returns to normal.

PARSLEY AND ALFALFA: SPECIAL EFFECTS

A small but vocal contingent of participants suggests nibbling on plants believed to have deodorizing effects—parsley, alfalfa and other green leafy vegetables—to neutralize strong body odor. Hey, bet you've never seen a rabbit with B.O.!

"Parsley did the trick for me," says Mary Ann, a retired nurse living in Glenshaw, Pennsylvania. "I was going through a period of extreme stress— my daughter was getting divorced—and I just started to perspire a lot. I was talking to a friend about herbs one day, and she suggested I try eating parsley. I did—just a few sprigs a day—and it did check my perspiration odor. It took maybe a week for me to notice a difference. I ate it as long as I needed it, probably for about four or five months."

Parsley also came through when deodorants failed for a busy Texas woman. "Years ago, I was going to school and working nights in a fast food place, and it was a hectic pace," says Johnnie, of Dallas. "I'd sweat a lot, and nothing I did seemed to help." One night, a fellow employee suggested she munch on the parsley that was used to garnish plates. "I started to eat some every night, and from then on I never had a problem with body odor," she says. "My daughter uses it, too, and it works for her."

"Since I've been taking alfalfa tablets, my body odor is very slight," says Pauline, a retired hospital accounts auditor from Boyertown, Pennsylvania. "I didn't start taking the alfalfa because of body odor. I did it just because I thought it would be a healthy thing to do. Not having to use deodorant or worry about body odor is a pleasant side effect."

Both parsley and alfalfa contain good amounts of chlorophyll, which apparently has some sort of deodorizing effect. A form of chlorophyll called chlorophyllin copper complex is approved by the Food and Drug Administration as a safe and effective deodorizing compound. This product, sold in tablet form, can be used by incontinent people to neutralize the odor of urine and feces.

"I haven't used chlorophyll tablets myself, but I do give them to my female dogs when they are in heat, and especially if I have to take them to shows," says Lee, a breeder of Siberian huskies living in Eagle Creek, Oregon. "It keeps the odor down, which makes it more pleasant to be around the dogs and helps keep the male dogs from becoming too interested." She says many professional breeders use chlorophyll tablets for this purpose.

MINTY SOAK DISSOLVES HIS ODOR

Need we be reminded that bathing regularly might just be our best bet against body odor?

There's an art to fine bathing, and Ben, a small-engine repairman living in Hill, New Hampshire, seems to have mastered it—with no need for embellishment.

"Sometimes during the summertime, I'll be out in the woods all day, getting wood ready for the next winter," he says. "I'll be sweating up a storm. So when I come home, I'll draw a hot bath and drop in it a nylon stocking containing fresh mint leaves from our garden. It makes the water smell great, it's very relaxing, and when I get out . . . well, I don't smell like a rose, which I'd just as soon not, because it attracts bugs. I do smell like mint."

Boils

From the looks of your shopping list—eggs, oatmeal, onions, potatoes, bread, bacon, milk and tea—you could be planning a breakfast buffet. But did you know you've also selected some of America's favorite treatments for boils?

That's right, boils. When bacteria invade a microscopic break in your skin and infect a blocked oil gland or hair follicle, your white blood cells fight back. This intra-skin skirmish produces pus and pain as the boil swells (it seems) to biblical proportions.

The best way to beat the annoying and often painful skin eruptions: Most doctors say apply a warm, wet compress. "When you are using a warm compress, you're attempting to increase the blood flow, to get more of your body's immune response to accumulate in that area to fight the infection and bring the boil to a head," explains William Dvorine, M.D., chief of dermatology at St. Agnes Hospital in Baltimore and author of *Dermatologist's Guide to Home Skin Treatment.*

Here's where that shopping list comes in. Rather than settling for a warm washcloth, those who suggested remedies for boils for our survey opened their kitchen pantries and revealed a plethora of homemade poultices that they say work for them.

Is there any reason why this wide assortment of pantry items might work? "Anything and everything you can imagine has been applied as a poultice. Why, I've even had patients tell me they use warm cow manure to treat boils," says Dr. Dvorine. "The important thing is that anything that is going to be of help provides warmth and moist heat and anything else is probably superfluous." If you want to try a poultice from the pantry, fine. "But also use common sense," urges Dr. Dvorine.

MAKING THINGS WET AND WARM

Of course, just over 25 percent of the people who suggested remedies for boils did take the warm water route.

Repeated hot compresses at morning and night work best for Stephanie, of Llano, Texas. "I get the water as hot as I can stand it, dunk a washcloth in there, squeeze the cloth out and then put it on the boil," she says.

After the washcloth cools, the 71-year-old grandmother says she repeats the treatment for 15 or 20 minutes.

When the boil breaks, she covers it with an over-the-counter antibiotic cream like Neosporin and a bandage. And if the water from the tap isn't hot enough, Stephanie says she heats some up on the stove.

When he's treating boils, Dr. Dvorine also turns up the heat. "The best possible thing is a hot, moist compress made with a clean washcloth and water, as hot as you can stand, applied several times a day for 10 or 15 minutes. If the boil is in an inaccessible area, you could soak in a tub of hot water, again being very careful not to scald the skin; and if the boil appears to be developing a white head, it should be opened up, preferably by a medical professional, because it should be done under sterile conditions if at all possible."

SOME LIKE EGGED BOILS

Several people say they get cracking when they get a boil—not because they're in a big hurry but because they need the lining of a boiled egg to treat their boils.

Ed, a semiretired artist from Orlando, Florida, explains: "Just inside the shell, there's a lining that I peel out of there," he says. "It doesn't seem like much, but one time I wrapped it around my finger and as it dried out, the piece started constricting, cutting off the circulation. That convinced me these things have some squeezing power.

"I lay that piece of egg right over the boil and put a Band-Aid over it," he says. "Overnight it squeezes, bringing the boil right to the surface— sometimes it will even pop. My mother used it on me when I was a child, and we used it on our children. It works."

In fact, the remedy works so well for Ed that peeling the lining out of the egg may be the most difficult part. "It's sort of like peeling a decal," he says.

EDITOR'S NOTE: Although Ed and other egg users crow about their remedy, there is cause for concern. Salmonella bacteria are common in raw eggs and can cause digestive illness if applied to an open wound, experts say. The egg should be boiled for a full 15 minutes to sterilize it before applying any part of it to an open wound.

SHE PACKS IT WITH A TEA BAG

The way Cherie, of Napa, California, tells it, by the time her parents reluctantly took her to the doctor, her left eye was swollen shut—the victim of an infected boil in her eyebrow.

But even the doc was stumped, Cherie recalls. "There's not much we can do," the doc said. "If I try to lance it, she could lose her sight in that eye."

Arriving home, Cherie's mother went to the bookshelf and pulled out a slim volume—a handwritten compilation of home remedies passed on by her mother, a French Quaker immigrant. Quickly paging through it, she spotted an entry: Carbuncles. "It was quite a book," says Cherie, now 68. "There were all kinds of old-fashioned remedies in there."

After brewing a cup of tea that night, Cherie's mother called her into the kitchen and asked her to apply the still-warm tea bag to the swollen mass. Meanwhile, her mother cracked an egg, carefully peeling away a piece of the lining. After ten minutes of heat treatment with the tea bag, Cherie's mother placed the egg lining over the boil, covered it with a bandage and sent her to bed.

When the bandage came off the next morning, the tea and egg lining had apparently done their job. Cherie's face was still swollen, but the infection had come to a head. Within a day of lancing the boil with a sterilized needle and wiping the wound with alcohol, her eyebrow was fine, says Cherie.

A properly placed tea bag might just do the trick, says Dr. Dvorine.

"Tea has no medicinal effect in this case, but a warm, moist tea bag is just the right size for a warm compress—and that's what you need," he says. In addition, tea contains tannins—astringents that are effective against some forms of bacteria.

HOW ABOUT BREAD AND MILK?

Violetta, 70, can't remember exactly how old she was when she had her first boil. But she'll never forget where they were—or how her grandmother treated them. "Let's just say I couldn't sit down for a few days," says the Topeka, Kansas, resident.

A registered nurse, Violetta's grandmother would mix up a poultice that combines Fels-Naptha soap, milk and bread.

"She'd take about a tablespoon of chopped-up soap, a tablespoon of milk and half a piece of bread and mix it up into a paste," says Violetta.

"Then she'd put it over the boil and keep it on with a cut-out bandage and some tape." After two days of application, the contents of the boil would pop right out, she says. "I'm not sure why it worked, but it really did," she says.

John, of Midland, Michigan, also creates a paste out of bread and milk for his home boil remedy, but he insists on bread baked at home. "I wouldn't use any of that bread that you get in the store," he says. "It's got to have plenty of yeast and none of those artificial ingredients."

THEY TAP SAP

Some families keep a bottle of alcohol handy for treating skin infections. But for Patricia and Robert, of Fargo, Georgia ("as the crow flies, 20 miles from the Okefenokee Swamp"), there's no better way to beat boils and other infections than a mixture of pine sap and beef tallow.

"We keep a couple of ounces around at all times," she says. "The sap just pulls the impurities out of a boil or any other infection."

To make the remedy, which has been passed down in Robert's family for generations, Patricia says she scratches the bark off of a pine tree until the sap begins to run and then collects it in a small jar. Next, she trims the fat from a piece of beef and sears it in a skillet. When the fat melts, she pours it into the jar containing the pine sap.

"I blend it together until it becomes creamy and spreadable and then cover the boil or whatever with it," she says. After applying the gooey mixture, Patricia says she covers the sore with gauze. She repeats the application twice a day and waits for the boil to pop on its own.

Could this treatment help bust a boil? "Actually, the pine sap may work as a mild irritant, stimulating blood flow to the boil and helping bring it to a head," says Dr. Dvorine. "But as far as the beef fat goes, it's purely a vehicle for this remedy; it has no medicinal value."

THEY PREFER PORK

Not since the ribeye was touted as a cure for a black eye has a slab of meat received so much medicinal acclaim. Several of our survey takers who suggest a remedy for boils recommend bacon.

Between her mother's and grandmother's applications, Hazel, of Franklin, North Carolina, says she's seen literally hundreds of boils treated with bacon fat.

"We'd take a tiny piece of the fat and put it over the boil with a Band-Aid," she says. "By the next morning, the boil would be ruptured. I don't quite remember how we used to clean it up afterward, but hydrogen peroxide would probably work just fine."

Linda, of Canton, Ohio, says her mother used bacon fat to cover her boils. But she also wrapped the fat in a piece of gauze that had been soaked in warm water and Epsom salts. "You keep changing the bacon fat until it stops turning green," says Linda.

Also a common folk remedy for splinters, bacon fat may act as an irritant to increase the flow of moisture to a boil, bringing it to a head, experts say.

OATMEAL WORKS FOR HER

Oatmeal gets high marks from Wilma, of Lebanon, Missouri, for beating boils. For years her grandmother applied warm oatmeal like a poultice over boils and left it overnight, only to discover that the boil had popped the next morning—without squeezing or pricking. "It works for me every time," says Wilma.

Her approach: Just before she goes to bed for the night, Wilma covers the boil with a gob of warm oatmeal, then wraps the wound with a bandage and a piece of tape or an Ace bandage. The next morning, Wilma removes the bandage and the oatmeal, usually discovering the boil is broken, she says.

The use of this popular grain for boils may stem from its success as a facial mask, says Liza Ovington, Ph.D., director of the University of Miami Wound Care Information Institute. "In addition to the heat, the oatmeal may be doing some constricting there," she says. "When you squeeze a boil, you're distributing the pressure unequally, often forcing as much pus in as out. The whole concept here, I believe, is that there's a constriction over a broad area, so nothing is forced back in." The warmth of the oatmeal may also help bring the boil to a head, she says.

TRYING THE BOTTLE TRICK

Paul was plagued by boils on his neck as a child, but his mother's treatment came to the rescue. Instead of poking him with needles or prodding him with tweezers, she used an innovative extraction technique that called for a small glass bottle the size of a liquor sample, says Paul.

"She would fill the bottle halfway with warm water—not too warm that I couldn't stand it," says the Little Rock, Arkansas, resident. "Then she would carefully tilt the bottle so the mouth of the bottle was placed firmly over the boil. The cooling bottle creates a suction, and you can feel the pus being pulled out."

After the boil had been extracted, Paul's mother would wipe the area with rubbing alcohol, he says. "It may not work for everyone, but it sure worked on us eight kids."

Instead of putting water in the bottle, another reader suggests heating it and then placing the mouth of the bottle over the boil. "I get it as hot as I can stand it," he says. "It works every time."

While uncommon today, the bottle remedy has a solid basis in physics, says Dr. Ovington. "In physics, we learn that hot air expands and cool air contracts. This creates a vacuum that should pull the head out or at least to the surface of your skin."

EDITOR'S NOTE: If you decide to try the heated bottle method, make sure you don't get the bottle too hot. A good rule of thumb: If the bottle is too hot to handle with your bare hands, it's too hot to place on the boil.

BRINGING ONIONS AND POTATOES TO A BOIL

Mashed. French fried. Stuffed. Baked. Even boiled. But as a remedy for boils? Several of our survey takers with suggestions for beating boils recommend potatoes.

Jean says she and her twin sister learned about potatoes' curative properties after a day splashing in the local swimming hole yielded them each a legful of boils.

"My mother cut off some potato slices, placed them directly on the boils and then wrapped them good with a cloth to keep them on there," says Jean, now a 58-year-old Lakeland, Florida, homemaker. "It's hard to remember, but it seems like it brought them to a head overnight."

A thick, sauteed onion sounds more like a hamburger condiment than a boil remedy. But Arlene says she's flipped for it.

"Once, when my husband was away on vacation, a boil on my leg became infected. By the evening I could barely walk," she says. "So I sauteed some onion, put it on the boil, put a piece of wet gauze over it, and then put Saran Wrap around it to keep it moist. By the next morning, the redness was gone and my leg started feeling better. By the time I got to the doctor, you couldn't tell I had an infection. It worked that well and that fast."

To treat the boil, Arlene says she cooked a ¼-inch onion slice for about five minutes in a pan with water, just until the onion started to become transparent.

A retired bookkeeper, Genevieve also remembers her mother reaching for the onions when seven boils sprouted on her elbows. Her mother used several lightly sauteed slices of onion and changed them every few hours to keep them fresh, says the 72-year-old Monroe, Wisconsin, resident.

"She didn't fuss with the boils at all, they just broke open on their own," she says.

Breast Problems

Ways to Take Out the Ache

Swollen, lumpy, painful breasts. Breasts that pull at your back and neck. That make it difficult for you to sleep at night. That ache at the slightest bounce or bump. That's what some women suffer from, especially prior to their periods, when hormones stimulate fluid retention.

Many of the 20 women who answered our survey question about breast problems had seriously painful breasts. "I had considerable discomfort from engorgement," says Roberta, 49, of Midland, Michigan. "I had been taking diuretics for about ten years for this, but my doctor wanted me to stop taking the drugs because he was afraid I'd develop other health problems." (Diuretics help the body eliminate excess fluids.)

Like many of the women who responded to this question, Roberta found that a combination of things eased her breast pain. "I needed something that didn't involve drugs, and luckily, my doctor was able to suggest some things that worked for me," she says. Dietary changes and vitamin supplements top her list of remedies. And they are also what others with this same problem recommend.

THEY CUT CAFFEINE

Almost half of our survey participants say that cutting out beverages, foods and drugs that contain caffeine helps ease their breast pain. They've eliminated coffee, tea, cola drinks and chocolate, along with pain relievers that contain caffeine.

"I wasn't drinking a lot of coffee, maybe two cups a day, so it wasn't a big deal to cut it out completely," says Roberta.

"I did drink a lot of coffee," says Norma, a schoolteacher from Battle Creek, Michigan. "If I was home, the coffee pot was on all day long." Worried because she had developed a cyst in one of her breasts, she asked her doctor what might help. He suggested eliminating caffeine. "I went straight to decaf, and yes, I did have a bad headache for a while, but I noticed within a month that my breasts weren't swelling up like they used to, and my cyst disappeared within a few months."

Her daughter, who's had similar problems with swelling, didn't drink coffee. But she found that cutting back on her chocolate habit improved her monthly breast tenderness.

Not all researchers agree that caffeine can cause breast swelling. But some research suggests that eliminating methylxanthines—caffeine and other compounds found mostly in coffee, tea and chocolate—can reduce breast swelling for some women. The studies indicate that total abstention might be necessary to obtain noticeable benefits. In one study, women with a lumpy breast condition stopped consuming anything that contained methylxanthines. In more than three-quarters of the women, the condition went away completely.

Try eliminating caffeine for two or three months as a trial run, suggests David Rose, M.D., Ph.D., D.Sc., chief of the Division of Nutrition and Endocrinology and associate director of the Naylor Dana Institute for Disease Prevention at the American Health Foundation in Valhalla, New York. "If it works for you, then stay away from these things," he says. "If there is no improvement, obviously it is not going to help you—so you may as well go back to your coffee."

THE VITAMIN E EASE

Vitamin E supplements are the answer for 25 percent of the women with breast problems.

"I'd had a cyst in my breast off and on for over 20 years," says Arlene, 62, of Columbia Station, Ohio. "I was watching a TV talk show one day, and they mentioned taking vitamin E for breast cysts. I tried it, and in less than three months the cyst was totally gone. It never returned, and that was more than 10 years ago. I am a firm believer in vitamin E. I still take 400 IU (international units) every day."

Studies haven't proven that vitamin E makes cysts go away. But in one study, nearly half the women who took 600 IU of vitamin E daily for eight weeks said they felt less pain.

Most of the women in this survey who took vitamin E also did other things for their breast pain, and doctors say that multifaceted approach may be the best. Many of the women who cut back on caffeine also take vitamin E. And perhaps not so incidentally, they also frequently take other vitamins and minerals, including calcium, magnesium, vitamin B$_6$ and others. "These vitamins help to regulate the production of prostaglandin E, which in turn has a prohibitory effect on prolactin, a hormone that activates breast tissue," says Christiane Northrup, M.D., assistant clinical professor of obstetrics and gynecology at the University of Vermont College of Medicine.

EDITOR'S NOTE: Vitamin E is generally considered safe in doses up to 600 IU per day, but most experts recommend taking no more than 400 IU daily. If you want to take it for any therapeutic reason, do so only under supervision of your doctor.

THE LOW-SALT SOLUTION

Salty foods are bothersome to about 20 percent of the women who responded to this question.

"I noticed that whenever I ate a lot of snack foods, my breasts would get very tender, and I would have a lot of bloating," says Marie, 55, of Paradise, California, who with her husband owns a janitorial and housecleaning service. "This would happen just about any time of month, but it was particularly painful just before my period. I decided to try cutting out some of the foods that seemed to cause problems—pickles, potato chips, pretzels, which I love, lunch meats and popcorn—and had a noticeable improvement in symptoms. As long as I stay away from those foods, I have very little breast pain."

"If I'd eat even a few potato chips or a handful of popcorn, I'd quickly know I'd overdone the salt," says Roberta. "I would have considerable water retention and breast pain. So I cut out the salt and started using herbs and spices instead. I found thyme to be a good substitute for salt in some recipes. Now, I rarely have such pain, unless I eat out somewhere and indulge in something salty, like barbecued chicken."

Experts agree: Highly salted foods make you retain water, not just in your breasts but all over. They make it harder for your body to counteract the hormone-induced fluid retention that occurs during the two weeks leading up to your period.

"Try to keep your sodium intake to under 1,500 milligrams a day," advises Robert L. Shirley, M.D., gynecologist and clinical professor of medicine at Harvard Medical School. For most people, that means cutting way back on the use of table salt. Also, read the labels of processed foods and avoid the ones that have more than 300 milligrams of sodium per serving. There is this much sodium in just under a teaspoon of salt.

SLIMMING DOWN REDUCES THEIR PAIN

Several women mention that their breast pain seems to ease up if they are able to lose some weight. "It definitely improves when I weigh less," says a Trenton, New Jersey, woman who's been up and down on the scale. Another woman notes that losing just 8 of about 20 extra pounds reduced her breast pain considerably.

In fact, experts say it's not just the extra weight on the breasts themselves that can be contributing to pain. In women, fat acts like an extra gland, producing and storing estrogen, a female hormone that stimulates breast tissue. If you've got too much body fat, you may have more estrogen circulating in your system than is good for you.

Low-Fat, High-Fiber Works for Her

"The things that I've done to improve my health in general have also reduced my premenstrual symptoms, including painful, swollen breasts," says Linda, 44, of Ann Arbor, Michigan. Like many people, she's cut back on fat, eating less red meat and butter and switching to reduced-fat mayonnaise and cheeses and frozen yogurt instead of ice cream. She's also increased her intake of fruits, vegetables and grains.

Several studies suggest that cutting back on fat and increasing your intake of fiber, especially wheat bran, can reduce your blood levels of breast-stimulating estrogen. That's why these dietary changes are also recommended as a possible breast cancer preventive, Dr. Rose says.

The Right Bra Helps

"I'm convinced underwire bras contribute to breast pain," says Ruth, a diagnostic radiology technologist from San Antonio, Texas. Ruth has been having mammograms since 1976, and since she has solved her own problems with lumpy, swollen breasts, she offers advice to the women she sees with the same problems. (She also avoids coffee and takes vitamin E, along with other vitamins.)

Most experts recommend a sturdy sports bra. This sort of bra usually has a wide band of elastic—not wire—under the breasts. When you try on a bra for fit, jump in place, and buy the bra that most minimizes bounce, advises Kerry McGinn, R.N., author of *The Informed Woman's Guide to Breast Health*. "You want a bra that holds you firmly and comfortably, without biting and binding," she says.

They Go Hot or Cold

Both warm and cool compresses seem to relieve breast pain, our survey participants say. Four suggest applying a hot compress to an engorged, tender breast. Two suggest something cool—a compress or, in one case, cold cabbage leaves. (*Ah. A perfect fit.*)

"I nursed both of my children for quite a while, and when I had problems with breast engorgement or a plugged duct, I would use hot compresses," says Merry, of Pensacola, Florida. "I'd take a wet washcloth, wring it out, put it in a ziploc bag, and microwave it for a minute or so with the bag open. I'd close the bag and put it on my breast for a few minutes before I nursed. It did help resolve the problem."

In fact, experts suggest you try either heat or cold and see which works best for you. "And some women find alternating between heat and ice works best for them," McGinn says.

EDITOR'S NOTE: If you microwave a washcloth, be careful not to burn yourself. If you can't pick it up with your hand, you certainly can't put it on your breast.

Bruises

Draining Away the Black and Blue

They knock their shins against coffee tables, bump their elbows against door jambs, even get in the way of incoming baseballs. The result: an assortment of bruises—discoloration that results from bleeding from tiny blood vessels just under the skin.

It's impossible to avoid all of life's bumps, thumps, thwacks and swipes. So here's what people say they do when their soft places connect with the receiving end of something hard.

ICE ENDS THEIR PAIN

"I tried using a bucket of ice water to relieve a sprained ankle, and I was so impressed by how little bruising and swelling I had that I started to use ice on other bruises," says Sarah, 34, of Burlington, Vermont. One incident in particular she recalls—pinching her finger in a piece of tough firewood she was splitting. "As soon as I wiggled it out, I went into the house and stuck it in a bowl of cold water to relieve the pain as much as anything," she says. "I expected it to be bruised, but it hardly bruised at all."

"An ice pack, or better still, immersion in cold water, works because it constricts blood vessels, which leads to less blood spilling into the tissues around the injury," explains Hugh Macaulay, M.D., occupational and environmental physician at Holly Clinic in Denver. "That reduces inflammation and pain and makes it less likely that you will develop a blackish blotch."

EDITOR'S NOTE: To avoid frostbite, use an ice pack wrapped in a towel or cold (but not painfully cold) water. Chill your bruised area for no more than 15 minutes, then allow the skin to warm up for about 10 minutes before you ice it again. Apply the cold as soon as possible after the injury.

WITCH HAZEL WORKS WONDERS FOR THEM

"It's an old wives' tale, true, but it works," insists Pat, 42, a medical laboratory services salesperson from Cincinnati. She's referring to the use of witch hazel for bruises, and she says it even worked on the kind of bump that's sure to result in a show of colors—an encounter with a baseball. "Hardball, not softball," she adds.

She learned about this remedy one day while watching her son, an outfielder, get bopped in the arm by a bouncing ball that changed course at the last second. A woman sitting next to her suggested she try applying witch hazel to the bruise. "I did, liberally but lightly, in the evening after the game and again the next morning. Within 48 hours, the bruise was faded out, a lot faster than I would have expected," she says. This remedy was popular with other survey takers as well.

Studies show that witch hazel contains tannins, compounds that constrict blood vessels, which is why it is an effective home remedy for cuts, bruises, hemorrhoids and sore muscles. Commercial witch hazel products—made by steam distillation of the tree's twigs—do not contain much in the way of tannins. However, these products, largely because they contain alcohol, do have reported antiseptic, anesthetic, astringent and anti-inflammatory action.

If you have a witch hazel shrub on your property, you can make your own tannin-rich solution by boiling one teaspoon of dried, powdered witch hazel leaves or twigs per cup of water for ten minutes. Strain and cool. Apply directly or mix with an ointment, such as petroleum jelly.

COMFREY GIVES THEM COMFORT

A few people told us that they use the herb comfrey to stop bruising. "Take a handful of comfrey leaves, boil them for 10 minutes, let the mixture cool, pour it in a foot tub and soak your bruised or swollen ankle or other body part for 15 to 20 minutes," advises one survey participant.

In fact, comfrey has long been used for bruises and wounds, mostly as a poultice, and it has two ingredients that may make it useful in this regard, according to Varro E. Tyler, Ph.D., professor of pharmacognosy at the School of Pharmacy and Pharmacal Sciences at Purdue University, West Lafayette, Indiana, and author of *The Honest Herbal.* It contains allantoin, a compound that promotes cell growth and is found in some over-the-counter skin creams. It also contains blood vessel–constricting tannins.

VITAMIN C STOPS HER BRUISES

"Vitamin C is the best preventive measure I know of for bruises," says Janice, 38, a computer operator from Virginia Beach, Virginia. She normally takes about 1,000 milligrams of vitamin C a day. (She smokes, she says, and there is evidence that cigarette smoke depletes the body of vitamin C.)

When Janice gets a cut or bruise, she immediately takes an additional dose of vitamin C, about 500 milligrams. "It does seem to work," she says. "I used to have bleeding gums, gingivitis, and bruise easily. I've been using vitamin C for about 17 years, and I don't have any of those symptoms."

Vitamin C is essential for the body to make collagen, a tough connective tissue that, among other things, helps to form the outer cover of blood vessels. Vitamin C deficiency can lead to capillary fragility, making these tiny blood vessels under the skin leaky and prone to injury from even slight bumps. In fact, a major symptom of scurvy—the classic vitamin C deficiency disease—is widespread capillary hemorrhaging.

EDITOR'S NOTE: While the recommmended Daily Value for vitamin C is only 60 milligrams, medical experts say that taking several times that much a day is safe for most people. But taking large dosages of any vitamin should be done only under the supervision of a physician.

Burns

Putting Out the Flames

Grok: "Gosh, darn, burned myself again on this freakin' fire. Now what do I do?"

Gloid: "Quick, Grok, stick your hand in the creek. I'll go get the mastodon grease to put on after it's cooled down."

Ever since hominids learned how to tame a flame, they've been singeing their digits on everything from hot rocks to barbecue grills. And no doubt, they've been looking for ways to douse the pain quickly and effectively and to help the burn heal faster.

Minor burns—those confined to a small area that simply leave behind painful, red skin and perhaps an occasional blister—respond well to home remedies. Deeper burns, with extensive blistering and oozing or whitish, charred skin—whether painful or not—require prompt medical attention.

We found that our survey participants have survived their share of minor, moderate and occasionally severe burns. Some 248 people offered remedies, many variations on the same basic treatment—cool it down fast, then smear on something that soothes and protects the damaged skin. Here's what they say works.

THEY REACH FOR SOMETHING COOL

It makes sense to chase heat with cold, and that's what the majority say they do.

"That's a standard first aid recommendation, and it seems to be what most people do instinctively if they have the chance," points out Robert, 60, of Indiantown, Florida, an auxiliary coast guard volunteer. "We're told to put the burn in cool water as soon as possible, even sticking a hand or foot over the side of the boat if necessary to cool it down." At home, he treats a minor burn by putting it under the cold water faucet.

The key here is cool, not icy water, experts say. As anyone who's ever plunged into a mountain stream will tell you, extreme cold can be as much of a painful shock to your body parts as heat.

In addition to water, people suggested a number of cooling liquids, including milk and plain iced tea.

"Whole milk is an effective compress for minor burns because its fat content is soothing and promotes healing," says Stephen M. Purcell, D.O., chairman of the Division of Dermatology at Philadelphia College of Osteopathic Medicine and assistant clinical professor at Hahnemann University School of Medicine, also in Philadelphia.

And tea, rich in compounds called tannins, may help to form a mildly antiseptic protective coating over the burn, says Varro E. Tyler, Ph.D., professor of pharmacognosy at the School of Pharmacy and Pharmacal Sciences at Purdue University in West Lafayette, Indiana, and author of *The Honest Herbal.*

THEY PICK ALOE

Topping our participants' list of preferred burn remedies is aloe vera gel, harvested from the spiky leaves of this fleshy succulent. Aloe vera is mostly grown indoors as an ornamental, and it seems to soothe so well that it's also known as "the burn plant." Many of the people who use it keep it close to their stove—on a windowsill in the kitchen. More than 100 people said they smear their damaged skin with the slippery sap from this plant.

"I begged, borrowed and bought aloe vera plants from a local greenhouse and friends when my husband was undergoing radiation therapy for cancer," says Josephine of Spokane, Washington. "He was experiencing horrendous radiation burns, and the aloe vera gel really did some fantastic things for him."

She simply sliced the leaves and rubbed the gel on his face. "I don't know if the burns would have gotten worse if I hadn't used the aloe, but I do know it relieved the pain he was experiencing, and it took the redness away, while the cortisone cream the doctor gave us simply made the pain worse."

Josephine says she told the people who were giving her husband the radiation treatments what she was doing. "They simply said I should continue doing it, as it appeared to be working," she says.

"I've found that applying aloe vera takes the pain right away and keeps the burn from turning white and from blistering," says Fern, 63, a retired nurse from Berrien Springs, Michigan. "We used aloe vera when my sister-in-law poured boiling water on her hand. We covered her whole hand with it and wrapped it lightly in gauze. The accident happened at noon, and by nightfall her hand looked normal."

There are good reasons aloe vera gel is helpful for burns. "Evidence indicates that aloe contains a substance that reduces inflammation and swelling," Dr. Tyler says. "The gel inhibits the action of bradykinin, a peptide that produces pain in injuries like burns. It also inhibits the formation of thromboxane, a chemical detrimental to wound healing." Aloe also contains allantoin, a substance thought to stimulate skin cell growth.

Our survey takers use both fresh aloe gel and liquid aloe juice available from health-food stores. If you're planning to use an aloe vera cream, stick with one that contains at least 70 percent aloe, recommends John Heggers, Ph.D., director of clinical microbiology at the Shriners Burn Institute in Galveston, Texas, professor of surgery in the Division of Plastic Surgery, and a professor of microbiology and immunology at the University of Texas Medical Center, also in Galveston. One cream that fits the formula is Dermaide, which is used by some radiation therapists to treat radiation burns. Another is a product called After Burn Plus.

VITAMIN E OIL EASES

After aloe vera, people are most likely to apply vitamin E to burns. Some 31 people said they use vitamin E oil, and a few felt they got dramatic relief and prevented the formation of blisters and peeling skin with this remedy.

"My nephew was playing around with gasoline and got his arm pretty badly burned," says John, 75, of Forest Hills, Maryland. "The doctor said he might need a skin graft, but we started using vitamin E on the burn. We'd completely cover the arm with it a couple of times a day, then lightly wrap the arm in gauze. When my nephew went back to the doctor in a couple of weeks, the doctor said his arm had healed so well he didn't need the skin graft after all."

"I burned my upper arm pretty badly cooking," says Margaret, 64, a part-time sewing machine operator from Fall River, Massachusetts. "I had lifted the lid on a hot pan, and steam just poured out of it. I had read about using vitamin E for burns, but I'd never tried it before. I decided to try it this time, and I was very impressed with how well it worked. I'm sure my burn would have blistered if I didn't use the vitamin E. But it didn't. I was amazed at how quickly the pain went away, too."

There is little in the way of scientific proof on the use of vitamin E for burns, Dr. Heggers says. "But there is good reason to believe it could be helpful," he says. Vitamin E is well known for its role as an antioxidant. "It helps to limit biochemical reactions that involve oxygen. So it may help to neutralize some of the nasty biochemicals that produce an inflammatory reaction after a burn," Dr. Heggers explains.

OVER-THE-COUNTER OINTMENTS HELP SOME

About 15 people turn to over-the-counter products to relieve burn pain and speed healing.

"I use A and D Ointment," says one woman. "It's great for healing minor burns."

Many products marketed as burn ointments contain a topical anesthetic such as benzocaine or lidocaine. Some also contain an antimicrobial such as benzethonium chloride to help fight infection. Some contain aloe vera. And a few have vitamins A and D or zinc oxide, all substances said to promote healthy skin.

EDITOR'S NOTE: One product not principally marketed as a burn ointment nevertheless makes a wonderfully effective covering for minor burns. That product is good old petroleum jelly, says Albert Kligman, M.D., Ph.D., professor of dermatology at the University of Pennsylvania School of Medicine. In fact, Dr. Kligman says that petroleum jelly may be the most effective of all. Burn ointments containing anesthetics may cause adverse reactions (such as swelling) in some people.

IS BUTTER BETTER?

Although a few people said they use butter on a burn, doctors advise against it. Although butter may be temporarily soothing, most butter contains salt that can cause additional tissue damage, Dr. Heggers says. Applying salt to the skin draws water out of skin cells, which could be fatal to cells that are burn-damaged.

SHE USES RAW POTATOES

A woman from Dawson Creek, British Columbia, describes using layers of sliced raw potatoes on a burn. "Work as quickly as possible to get them on, and then change them every two to three minutes," she says. This is a remedy that provides cooling first and then a protective layer of starch on the skin. One reason people say things like potatoes, laundry starch, baking soda, eggs and flour help burns is that all of these form protective layers on the skin, which makes them soothing for a burn, Dr. Tyler says.

EDITOR'S NOTE: You might be better served by cooling the burn with water, then applying a protective coat of aloe vera gel or a simple gauze cover, Dr. Heggers says.

Bursitis

Quick Relief for Little Troublemakers

Unbeknownst to you (probably), your body is literally bursting with bursas—small, but strategically located sacs of sticky fluid. Like the tin man's oil can, your bursas silently help lubricate those places where friction can develop between your bones, muscles and tendons—shoulders, elbows and knees, for example. Bursas are silent, that is, until problem areas get overworked during activities that call for repetitive movements—like painting ceilings, gardening, playing tennis or tossing a baseball. Then they scream with pain.

Painful inflammation sets in, and in some cases, calcium deposits begin to form, causing even more pain. Chances are, however, you'll need a doctor to tell whether you have bursitis or that other "itis"—arthritis.

A hefty contingent of survey takers with bursitis told us that they rely on an over-the-counter anti-inflammatories like aspirin or ibuprofen to knock out pain. Others have developed a grab bag of tactics to ease the ache.

Treatment Leaves Them Cold ... and Hot

Nearly 25 percent of the people who provided remedies for bursitis recommend either one or both of that soothing tandem: heat and ice.

Take Art, for instance. A news photographer and videographer for the past 43 years (he's still freelancing), the 77-year-old Bradenton, Florida, resident often suffers from bursitis while carrying his heavy camera bag on assignment.

No matter. First, he stretches out his tight shoulder joint by grabbing a wall, shelf or rail above his head and gently pulling down. Then he opts for a heat or an ice treatment—either by soaking a towel in hot water and placing it on his shoulder for relief or by slapping on an ice pack for 20 minutes. "Dry heat never did a thing," Art says. "But alternating hot and cold like that seems to force more blood through the area."

Other methods mentioned in our survey include using heating pads and hot water bottles and heating up a damp towel briefly in a microwave.

Either heat or ice is a nice way to beat the pain, but ice may be the best, confirms Robert Sallis, M.D., assistant program director of the family medicine residency program at Kaiser Permanente Medical Center in Fontana, California, and the author of several studies on chronic shoulder pain.

"I think the main thing to remember is that you reduce swelling by constricting blood vessels with ice. You want to get rid of swelling because it slows healing," he says. "If the injury is more than 24 hours old, you can use moist heat, like a hot shower. But don't use either heat or ice for more than 20 minutes at a time." Only ice should be used within the first 24 hours after an injury.

EXERCISE GETS THEIR NOD

Exercise is another bursitis beater favored by some of our survey takers—but none more so than Barbara.

When her shoulder started aching, the 58-year-old Gulfport, Mississippi, housewife initially thought muscular soreness caused by her new workout program was to blame. Later, she learned she had bursitis.

Did she bench her barbells? Do you spell Mississippi with an *E*?

"I toned things down a little bit, but I didn't stop working out. I stayed with the routine and now my shoulders are much more durable than ever. My arms used to go numb when I carried anything heavy. Now I can handle shopping bags and things like that with no problem."

Barbara's weight-lifting regimen includes several sets of shoulder presses with light dumbbells, bent-knee push-ups and tricep extensions, among other things, she says.

Working in the coal mines of Virginia for over 30 years, Walter was what you call a wire man—he strung the wires overhead that brought electricity into the shaft.

And with that job came at least two health problems for Walter: bursitis and black lung.

"The doctor said he had the worst case of bursitis he had ever seen," says his wife, Helen. "It got so bad he couldn't even lift his arm over his head."

First came a cortisone shot, a common drug treatment for bursitis. Then, armed with an inexpensive pulley weight system in his home and a routine provided by his doctor, Walter went to work on his bursitis, sometimes exercising his shoulders as many as three times a day. With the help of the pulley, he'd carefully raise his arms as high as he could until the pain stopped him—at first that was no more than shoulder height. In a little over six weeks, Walter's painful bursitis was just a bad memory, says Helen.

In fact, doctors have developed several exercises specifically for bursitis. "The most important initial treatment for bursitis is to reestablish full range of motion," says Dr. Sallis. One helpful technique to improve range of motion with severe bursitis involves leaning your chest on a stool with your arms dangling free. Swing your arms in large circles in both directions. Dr. Sallis recommends doing this exercise several times a day. You can also do this one by letting one arm at a time dangle over the edge of the bed.

"Another technique is to stand with your shoulder facing the wall. Use your fingers to walk your arm up the wall like someone in a commerical might use his fingers to walk through a telephone book," says Dr. Sallis. "When your shoulder muscles are inflamed and sore, using your fingers and wrist will allow you to lift your arm higher than you probably could otherwise."

While workout programs can do wonders for stabilizing the shoulder joint—perfect for defeating bursitis—you should probably take some time off following the initial injury to recuperate before forging ahead, says Dr. Sallis.

"People tend to push themselves. Most shoulder pain is caused by overuse, folks trying to push through the pain," he explains. "The only other species that do that are racehorses and greyhounds. Weekend athletes who are having problems need to back off, rest until the pain is gone and then gradually regain range of motion and then gradually resume activity."

SHE LETS HER FINGERS DO THE HEALING

It was a rare day on the softball diamond when a runner successfully stole a base with Pat playing catcher. And, thanks to a chiropractor who taught her how to use acupressure, Pat is even less likely to succumb to bursitis when it flares in her throwing shoulder.

"Whenever the pain is getting to me, I use my index finger to press where it hurts for as long as I can five or six times," says the 45-year-old Tempe, Arizona, resident. "It feels better almost immediately. In an hour, you might have to try it again, but it's better than taking some kind of pill for it."

A 73-year-old Pennsylvania woman said she also champions acupressure—even though she prefers to press the problem area with her knuckles rather than her fingers.

While results often range from person to person, there's no harm in trying acupressure, says Dr. Sallis.

"I've seen some people get relief from it for everything from bursitis and headaches to back pain and others who have had little or no benefit," he says. "Acupressure has been around for thousands of years—it seems like there has to be some validity to it."

Activating the acupressure points that control bursitis pain in your shoulder may be even more effective, says Michael Reed Gach, Ph.D., founder and director of the Acupressure Institute in Berkeley, California, and author of *Acupressure's Potent Points*. These pressure points, he says, are located on your shoulder muscle (which runs from your neck to your arm on both sides), a half-inch above the upper tip of your shoulder blade. Feel for a tense muscle that will be sore upon pressure. Hold at a depth that "hurts good" for at least three minutes. Although only one side may ache, have a friend find the points on both sides. "You want to press on that gradually but increase pressure until it hurts just a little. It will be a good kind of pain. You'll feel some relief if you hold this point steady for three to five minutes," he says. Properly done two to three times a day for a month, this can give relief to your shoulder bursitis, says Dr. Gach.

SHE GIVES ARNICA AN A+

Most of the time, playing classical music on her cello doesn't bother Ruth's bursitis. But when she plays too much or she's forced to tighten the strings repeatedly, it's enough to make her change her tune—to the blues.

"It's the worst when I haven't played for a long time and then overdo it," says the 61-year-old Urbana, Illinois, native.

That's when she pulls out a homeopathic ointment containing arnica she purchased at a local health-food store on her sister's recommendation. A resident of Switzerland, Ruth's sister gave the herb rave reviews after she used it successfully for injuries she suffered in a bicycling accident.

"I just rub it in two or three times a day, and in a matter of just a few moments it feels better—a very natural, cool feeling," says Ruth. "I can't say that it's magic, but it's sure not a drug or a muscle relaxant or something like that."

Both Europeans and Americans—or at least the native ones—have been familiar with arnica's soothing qualities for some time. American Indians used the herb to prepare healing ointments and tinctures. Natural healing experts say massaging with arnica reduces pain and swelling of bruises, sore muscles and sprains. It is not recommended for broken skin.

While he's never treated anyone with arnica, Dr. Sallis says it may be of some benefit. "If it has anti-inflammatory properties, that would work well because bursitis is characterized by inflammation," he says.

EDITOR'S NOTE: Never take tincture of arnica internally. The plant is toxic when ingested. (Homeopathic arnica tablets are dilute enough to be safe.)

SHE KEEPS HER ARM OUT OF THE WAY

Janet wasn't really sure what caused the persistent bursitis-like pain in her shoulder and arm—maybe a bump or a fall—until she mentioned it to a friend.

"Don't sleep on your arm," the man said.

By following that simple recommendation, in a few days her pain went away, she says. And she hasn't had any problem with either since. "It worked for me," says the 66-year-old Rochester, New York, resident. "It gave great relief."

Ordinarily, just sleeping on your arm shouldn't cause bursitis, says Dr. Sallis. But if you persistently sleep on your arm with it over your head, you might have problems, he says.

Calluses and Corns

Smoothing Away the Rough Stuff

Do your feet take you where you want to go, without complaining every step of the way? If so, you're among a lucky minority—as people in our survey can attest. Most people have some problems with their feet—often pain caused by a callus or corn.

A callus is your body's way of protecting itself from pressure. Prolonged pressure or rubbing causes skin to build up more layers than normal. The thick, insensitive, yellowish layer that forms a callus is dead skin, designed to protect more sensitive layers below from breaking down or being worn away, explains James McGuire, D.P.M., director of physical therapy at the Pennsylvania College of Podiatric Medicine in Philadelphia.

If you often grip things in your hands, for instance, you may get calluses across the palm of your hand, just below your fingers. And if you're on your feet a lot, you may get sheets of calluses on the ball and heel of your feet.

Calluses usually don't hurt unless they become so thick that they press on underlying bones or nerves in the feet. So you need not disturb a callus unless it's causing you pain, or unless you know from previous experience that it will cause pain later if not reduced in size, Dr. McGuire says.

Corns are a different, meaner story. They, too, are layers of skin built up as a result of pressure. Unlike calluses, which are flat, corns are cone-shaped, and involve an additional, deeper layer of skin, called the corium, which is well supplied with nerves. "That's one reason corns are so painful," Dr. McGuire says. The tissues between the bone and the area immediately under a corn may become tender and irritated," he says. "This is a condition that for many people becomes chronic and painful."

Corns are almost always caused by friction or pressure from bony prominences or poorly fitting shoes rubbing against a toe or bunion. Sometimes two toes on a foot rub together, causing "soft" but nevertheless painful corns, usually between the fourth and fifth toes.

Of the people who answered our survey, 76 have suggestions for dealing with corns or calluses. Most involve routines of soaking the feet, rubbing away the corn or callus, and then using a soothing, softening lotion or oil.

And several point out that nothing you can do will permanently banish a corn or callus unless you also eliminate the cause—usually shoes designed with fashion, not comfort, in mind.

Here's what those "who've been there" say works for them.

SOOTHING SOAKING SOLUTIONS

A third of our sore feet sufferers rely on foot soaks to soften up their corns and calluses. They use a variety of fluids, including plain warm water or water containing vinegar, iodine, Epsom salts or baking soda.

"I soak my feet in plain water that's just hot enough to notice it's very warm," says Francine, 43, of Denver. She'll soak for about five minutes, then rub her calluses with a pumice stone.

"I find that adding about a quarter cup of vinegar to the hot water helps my corns soften faster," says Dolores, 34, of New York City, a busy waitress who's on her feet all day. "I don't have much time to baby my feet, and what helps me the most is wearing comfortable shoes."

EDITOR'S NOTE: Soaking in water is temporarily soothing, and will soften a corn or callus, making it easier to remove. But repeated soaking removes natural oils from the foot's skin, making calluses more likely to become hard and dry and to crack, Dr. McGuire says. "For this reason, we tell people with diabetes or poor circulation not to soak their feet in water," he says.

But healthy people whose sweaty feet are prone to friction-generated corns may find soaking in a solution of table salt, Epsom salts or vinegar helps their problem. "These soaks temporarily reduce sweating and help to control sweating and therefore relieve corn and callus problems," Dr. McGuire says.

PLASTERS, POULTICES AND OTHER OFF-BEAT SOLUTIONS

As a variation on the soak, some people like to soften their calluses and corns with oils, plasters or poultices, applying the remedy, then wrapping the area in plastic, bandaging it or simply wearing socks to bed.

One self-proclaimed tenderfoot, Viola, of Detroit, uses a family remedy passed down to her by her mother. "When a callus is really bothering me, I put a thin slice of lemon on it, secure it with a Band-Aid, and leave it on overnight. It softens the corn or callus so well that I don't have to do anything else."

Other people use lemon juice, vinegar or salicylic acid, an ingredient found in aspirin and also found in some wart-removing patches and some acne treatment pads. You can make a solution of salicylic acid by dissolving six crushed aspirin in one tablespoon of water.

Lemon juice tea and vinegar work to soften corns because they are weak acids that help break down dead skin, Dr. McGuire says. "They're fine for most people and are about the mildest acid you can use."

EDITOR'S NOTE: If you use this treatment, make sure you put the solution only on the callus itself, not the surrounding skin. If you are allergic to aspirin, do not put salicylic acid on your skin. People who are sensitive to aspirin can have an allergic reaction just from coming in contact with this substance.

OILS AND CREAMS THAT WORK

Castor oil tops the list of foot softeners, with five people saying it works for them.

"I rub my feet with castor oil before going to bed, then sleep in socks to keep the linens from getting stained," says June, 67, of Dover, Delaware. That's a remedy she has relied on since she was a teenager, when she worked as a waitress and a clerk in a five-and-dime store. She stills uses it when her feet start to bother her. "I soak them in water, rub them with a rough towel and then apply the oil." A week or two of treatments generally does the job for her.

In fact, a nighttime oil treatment is also what many experts recommend to soften corns and calluses, Dr. McGuire says. "You can soak a cotton ball with mineral oil, put it over the corn, tape it in place and leave it on overnight. In the morning, the corn will be all soft and gooey and you can remove it easily," he says. Any kind of oil will work, he says—mineral, vegetable, even shortening.

Some experts, however, prefer a water-based cream. "These are the typical moisturizing creams you'd use on your hands or face, and I think they penetrate and soften better than oil-based creams," says Suzanne M. Levine, D.P.M., a clinical assistant podiatrist at Mount Sinai Hospital in New York City.

Dr. McGuire also recommends a product called Carmol 20. "It's a cream containing urea." Urea, as those with a bit of chemistry background will know, is a chemical found in urine. "Years ago, in Russia, they noticed that people who handled horses and accidently got horse urine on their hands had their calluses peel off," he explains. "Today, we have been able to synthesize the ingredient in the urine that worked and produce a pleasant-smelling cream that removes calluses gently without using an acid."

THEY GO FOR THE GRIT

Corn-softening soaks or poultices are only the first step, say our survey participants. Next, they work at removing the corn or callus using a variety of techniques.

Rubbing a corn or callus with a gritty, glassy volcanic rock known as pumice stone came out on top as a safe and effective way to remove the dead skin that's creating the toughened spot.

"After I'm done soaking, or in the bath or shower, I use a white porous foot stone, which is coarser than the gray pumice rock," Francine says. "This keeps my calluses from returning."

Dr. McGuire suggests a kind of laboratory-concocted pumice stone, a Personal Pumi Bar distributed by Teregen Labs. "It's a little square bar that looks like a pumice stone but is much more effective," he says. "It's gentle enough that you can't really do yourself any harm with it, but it does remove a lot of callus."

Want to smooth out your feet and get a workout at the same time? Lorraine, a retired physical education instructor from Savannah, Georgia, goes for a barefoot stroll on Tybee Beach. "I walk a mile each way, and it was quite by accident that I discovered the abrasiveness of the sand had whittled my corns down to zero," she says. In fact, experts say that gritty sand acts just like a pumice stone.

THEY THROW IN THE TOWEL

Some people say they use emery boards on hard-to-reach between-the-toes corns and calluses. "That's probably the best implement you can use in these spots," Dr. McGuire agrees. Just be careful not to damage the skin. "There are more bacteria between the toes than anywhere else on the foot, and cuts and cracks in these areas can easily become infected."

And some people—apparently those who don't use clothes softener—find that simply rubbing their feet with a towel sloughs off enough dead skin to keep their feet comfy.

THEY MAKE SURE THE SHOE FITS

More than one survey participant can trace foot problems back to a pair of shoes designed by the Marquis de Sade.

"I bought a pair of sandals last year, and I regretted that I wore them as long as I did before I got rid of them, because they really aggravated a corn on my little toe," says Violetta, 43, a Spanish language professor living in

Yamhill, Oregon. Since she's on her feet teaching and runs or walks for exercise, she's learned the hard way to always buy shoes that are comfortable. "At home, I wear Birkenstock sandals. When I need to dress up a bit more for work, I wear Rockport dress shoes. When I'm not wearing either of them, I wear running shoes."

Says beachcomber Lorraine: "Like most people, my feet are longer at the big toe than the middle toe, so I never buy shoes that come to a point at the middle of the shoe. I also stick with heels that are no more than about one-half inch high. I search forever for shoes, and when I find a pair that fits well, I'll buy them in two or three colors. When I'm not dressed to go out, I wear a good all-purpose tennis-type shoe."

Buy shoes that allow plenty of room for your toes and that fully cushion the bottom of your feet, Dr. McGuire recommends. "I tell people to look for a shoe with a high toe box, and with Vibram soles, which do a good job of absorbing shock." He also suggests shoes with replaceable insoles. Shoes that flex easily at the ball of the foot also help reduce pressure on feet, he adds.

Canker Sores

Taming the Meanest Mouth Sores

I
f you think about it, canker sores are, at worst, a parking ticket in the Supreme Court of life—unimportant, really, yet undeniably annoying. So just who wrote you this citation, anyway?

One theory suggests that stress and certain foods like chocolate, strawberries, even cinnamon provoke bacteria living in your mouth's salivary glands to kill a small amount of surrounding tissue. The result is an irritating sore inside your mouth that can make eating miserable for the next two weeks. Our survey takers insist that by using the right home remedies, they can—and do—cut healing time and pain.

ALUM ADVOCATES ABOUND

Who would have thought you could find a remedy for canker sores in the bottom of a pickle barrel? Not us, at least until some of our survey participants said they use alum—the same ingredient that keeps pickles crisp—to crack down on their canker sores.

As a matter of fact, unleashing alum on canker sores—and, of course, pickles—was common at Helen's childhood home. "I remember watching my mother add about a fourth of a teaspoon of alum to each jar," says the 62-year-old Hendrum, Minnesota, resident. "And when I had a canker sore on my tongue, she'd dry it off with a cloth and then put a drop right on the sore. It took the soreness away and a few days later, the sore would be healed."

Barbara, of Homewood, Illinois, also fondly remembers watching her mother pack a peck of pickles—and fight canker sores—with alum. "My mother would use the little lumps that formed near the top of the box of alum to put on our canker sores," says the 54-year-old seamstress. "It burns like crazy for a minute and makes your mouth pucker up, but it seems like it cauterizes the sore and within a day, you can eat salty things, even lemons, no problem."

While her children object to having a dash or lump of alum—available in the spice aisle of grocery stores—placed on the sore, "the pain of having a canker sore for a couple weeks is worse than 15 minutes of puckering up," she says. "I figure if I can eat it, then it should be safe to use," she says.

Is using alum against a canker sore kosher? In fact, the preservative may indeed help draw fluid from the wound, easing pain, says Dan L. Watt, D.D.S., a dentist in Reston, Virginia, and chairman of the International Dental Health Foundation, also in Reston. "If you dry up the area, you might remove some of the fluid that's causing the soreness," he says.

THEY SWISH WITH SALT WATER

A human wave of folks who responded to our survey said they are sweet on salt water for fighting canker sores.

John, a retired statistician for the U.S. Census, even scores salt water higher than hydrogen peroxide, another commonly named cure. "Either salt water or peroxide works for me—but to tell you the truth, salt water is my choice because it doesn't taste as bad," he says.

After dissolving a tablespoon of salt in an eight-ounce glass of warm water, the Forestville, Maryland, resident swishes the mixture around in his mouth for a few minutes twice a day and then spits it out. "It will sting, now. It will hurt a little bit, but it heals it. Salt water dries it right up in a few days," he says.

Minnabel, of Covington, Kentucky, also swears by a mixture of salt and water to heal her canker sores—but she prefers more frequent treatment.

"Growing up in the country, we used salt water for a lot of things, like gargling, for example," she says. "When I have a canker sore, if I just swish some salt water around in my mouth three or four times a day, that's usually enough to heal it."

Salty water works because it helps draw fluid through tissues, which speeds healing, says Dr. Watt. His recommendation: two tablespoons of salt per six-ounce glass of warm water. "It needs to be nice and briny," he says.

SHE BREWS HER RELIEF

Growing up on her grandparents' farm in De Ridder, Louisiana, Vera became well acquainted with her granny's home remedies at an early age. "Whenever you had an ailment, she had something for it. The benefits might have just been psychological, but she had one," says the 60-year-old Denver resident. Among her granny's repertoire: tea bags for canker sores.

"I'd enjoy the tea first and then take the bag and tuck it in my mouth on the sore there like you would some chewing tobacco," she says. "As I understand it, the tannic acid in the tea is supposed to help heal the sore faster."

Can the tannic acid in tea tame a canker sore? "It's not that far-fetched," says Dr. Watt. "In fact, tannic acid is the active ingredient in an over-the-counter canker sore treatment called Zilactin."

THEY SUPPORT SUPPLEMENTS

Nutritional supplements—like vitamins B and C—also get hearty recommendations for their so-called healing properties.

Like the stock market, the reputation of vitamin C has waxed and waned over the years. But Lucille still stands by oranges, lemon juice or vitamin C supplements for canker sores.

"They seem to all have the same positive effect," says the 86-year-old Lawrence, Kansas, resident, who faithfully takes at least two 500-milligram vitamin C tablets a day. She hasn't had a canker sore in decades, she says.

Kathie, a vitamin supplement distributor in McKinleyville, California, says many of her customers ask for B-complex vitamins when they are suffering from canker sores. "The people who have more than one canker sore a year seem to have the most success treating them with B-complex," she says.

Vitamin C supplements and juices containing citric acid both get Dr. Watt's vote for prevention as well as treatment. On the treatment side, "a canker sore is an open wound, and the acid in the juice will kill any bacteria living there," he says. "And it's well documented that vitamin C will help healing."

In this case, Andrew Weil, M.D., associate director of the Division of Social Perspectives in Medicine at the University of Arizona College of Medicine/Arizona Health Sciences Center in Tucson and author of *Natural Health, Natural Medicine*, is partial to B vitamins. B-complex and a mouth rinse made with ¼ teaspoon salt, ½ teaspoon goldenseal powder to 1 cup warm water are his preferred canker sore treatments. You can find goldenseal powder in health-food stores, loose or in capsules.

THEY REACH FOR BAKING SODA

What's good for the inside of your refrigerator—baking soda—is also good for the inside of your mouth, according to some of our survey takers.

Even though she doesn't like the taste, Marian's been using baking soda ever since her mother treated family ills with the powdery, all-purpose stuff. "Mother did a lot of doctoring at home," says the 78-year-old Selinsgrove, Pennsylvania, grandmother. "I guess because we didn't have a whole lot of money."

Marian says her mother taught her to place a pinch of baking soda directly on the sore. "It stings a little, but it doesn't take long for it to heal after that," she says.

Alice of Sherwood, Oregon, says she prefers to make a paste out of baking soda before applying it to her canker sores. "Baking soda is a really good healer. I put about a teaspoon in a bowl, add just a tiny bit of water to it, and mix it up to form a paste," she says. "Then I scoop a little out and put it right on the sore."

When the paste dissolves, Alice applies another scoop of baking soda, repeating the procedure several times throughout the day. After two days of treatment, the canker sore is usually on the mend, she says.

Not only is baking soda great at preventing all kinds of periodontal disease, but it's also shown promise fighting future canker sores, says Dr. Watt. "If used on a regular basis, baking soda reduces the amount of bacteria in the mouth, and we think it probably lessens the ability of bacteria to get into the salivary glands in the first place," he says.

EDITOR'S NOTE: Because baking soda contains high levels of sodium, people who have to limit their sodium intake must rinse their mouths thoroughly after using it.

MILK MEETS THEIR NEEDS

Born in England, Margaret naturally feels that the British are more sympathetic to home remedies than Americans. "They're more old-fashioned, you know," says the 67-year-old Aurora, Colorado, grandmother, "less willing to use all kinds of drugs and things."

So it makes sense that she's partial to something as simple as a cold glass of milk for canker sores. "The best way I've found is to keep the milk in your mouth and swish it around a few times before you swallow. You only have to do that a couple of times before it will clear up." Avoiding chocolate also seems to prevent them, she says.

A 61-year-old woman who answered our survey says she swishes buttermilk around in her mouth three or four times a day, also to defeat canker sores.

Although milk or buttermilk may make your canker sores feel better, there's no evidence that either promotes healing, says Dr. Watt.

THEY HYPE HYDROGEN PEROXIDE

After years of watching her mother rinse her mouth with hydrogen peroxide to treat canker sores, it's no surprise that Rose encouraged her daughter to give it a try when one appeared in her mouth.

"Of course, it tastes terrible," says the 49-year-old Jessup, Pennsylvania, middle school secretary. "But after swishing a capful around her mouth twice a day for a couple of days, the sore was gone."

Quinton and Marie of Potlatch, Idaho, have not only found hydrogen peroxide effective as a rinse for canker sores, but virtually any kind of mouth sore. "You just slosh it around through your teeth and squish it back and forth," says Quinton. "It has kind of a weird taste and it will foam up on you, but it doesn't hurt at all and definitely seems to make any mouth sore heal faster."

Hydrogen peroxide is so good at killing bacteria in the mouth that you have to be careful how much you use, says Dr. Watt. "If we kill off too much bacteria, then we can have yeasts and other things growing—and the only times I've run up against people with yeast infections in the mouth is when people are rinsing with hydrogen peroxide," he says. "I would say if you are going to use it, only use it sparingly and occasionally." And, of course, never swallow hydrogen peroxide, he says.

SHE SEES GREEN

Fern, a registered nurse and our survey's resident aloe vera fan, says she's even used gel from this succulent plant on her canker sores.

"By the time I got home from the dentist the other day, I had a canker sore, a sore throat and swollen glands," says the 63-year-old Berrien Springs, Michigan, resident. "But after swishing around some aloe vera gel in my mouth like mouthwash two or three times a day, it was gone in two days."

Fern buys aloe vera gel by the gallon jug at a local health-food store. "We just have to get back to more natural remedies," she says. "Lots of people just can't handle all these medicines."

Aloe apparently contains salicylates, the same painkilling and anti-inflammatory compounds found in aspirin, says Dr. Watt. "It's well documented that aloe eases pain in burns," he says. "It's also antibacterial—even if it's not the strongest antibacterial around."

THE SOUR SOOTHER

Yogurt and acidophilus, the Bobbsey Twins of friendly bacteria, are cited by several survey takers for helping stop canker sores.

Meet Chris, a vociferous acidophilus advocate. Whenever the 52-year-old Pekin, Illinois, resident gets a canker sore, she mixes the contents of an acidophilus capsule into a glass of milk. Two glasses a day do the trick. "It definitely soothes the sore and speeds up healing," she says.

Yogurt gets a creamy okay from at least one farmer's wife, who appreciates the soothing qualities of the dairy dish in more ways than one. "Canker sores can make your mouth pretty sore—it's literally uncomfortable to eat, but yogurt is just right," she says. "It also seems like yogurt adds friendly bacteria to your mouth, which has got to help your immune system fight canker sores."

Cleveland dermatologist Jerome Z. Litt, M.D., author of *Your Skin: From Acne to Zits*, recommends four tablespoons of plain yogurt a day for chronic canker sore sufferers. The bacteria in yogurt actually help healing by competing with the bad bacteria in your mouth, he explains.

MAKE HERS MYLANTA

Plagued with canker sores and an upset stomach for most of her life, Ann has downed her share of Mylanta, an over-the-counter antacid. But it wasn't until the 62-year-old Baltimore bartender discovered both can be caused by excess acid that she started using Mylanta for her canker sores, too.

"I took a big drink and just left it in my mouth for a little while and did that a few times a day for a couple days," she says. "Within three days, it was healed."

Ann shared the remedy with her two daughters, who also seem to be prone to canker sores, and several friends at work. Sure enough, all have reported good results, she says. "One of my daughters had one that felt like it was the size of a nickel in her mouth, and the doctor prescribed her an antibiotic," she says. "The antibiotic didn't do a thing, but within a few days of taking Mylanta, it healed up."

EDITOR'S NOTE: A spokesperson for the manufacturers of Mylanta said his company does not endorse the use of its product for anything other than its intended purpose. Robert Goepp, D.D.S., Ph.D., professor of oral pathology at the University of Chicago Medical Center, says it's okay to try swishing a little Mylanta or milk of magnesia around in your mouth.

MERLA'S MAGIC ACT

Merla, of San Francisco, says she made her canker sores disappear simply by changing her diet.

"After years of suffering from these painful little monsters, I found to my delight and amazement that when I stopped eating sugar they disappeared," she says. "I've been sugar-free for six months now, and for the first time in years, I'm free from this problem."

EDITOR'S NOTE: Experts have noted that in addition to sweets, nuts (including coconut and peanut butter) can trigger canker sores. Try cutting out suspected items for a few weeks and then reintroduce them to your diet one at a time to see if the breakouts recur. Then simply avoid whatever's causing them.

Carpal Tunnel Syndrome

Turning Off Hand and Wrist Pain

Carpal tunnel syndrome has been dubbed the disease of the computer age. It's common among people who spend their days pecking away at a word processing keyboard.

"I bet people had it years ago, too, but just didn't know what it was," says Susan, a bank teller from Harrisburg, Pennsylvania, who is all too familiar with the pain, numbness and tingling in the hands that is typical of this problem. In fact, just about anyone who uses his hands repetitively with the wrists bent can develop carpal tunnel syndrome. It hits carpenters, musicians, painters, typists, butchers and meat packers, auto workers, gardeners, construction workers and supermarket checkers.

"Just about everything I do makes me a candidate for this condition," says Jeremiah, 53, of Redwood, Washington. When he's not busy hammering nails or driving screws, he's riding his bicycle. All these activities have the potential to put a painful twist in your wrist.

Carpal tunnel results from too much crowding in too little space. It occurs when tendons in the wrist become inflamed and swell up, compressing the median nerve, a major nerve that leads from the arm into the fingers. This is the nerve that signals some of the small muscles in the hand and also provides sensation to the thumb and first three fingers. Squeezing the median nerve leads to pain and numbness, morning stiffness and impaired movement in the fingers, and sometimes even temporary paralysis.

Survey participants who offer remedies for carpal tunnel syndrome say they've been able to keep a mild case from getting worse. And a few believe they've been able to avert surgery by employing one or more methods to relieve the pressure on this nerve.

Here, then, is what they do.

B_6 ENDS THEIR SYMPTOMS

Vitamin B_6 tops our participants' list of suggestions—it is recommended by about one-third.

"I'd had carpal tunnel syndrome in both wrists for about two years, and it was really quite severe," says Susan, 55, a teacher and writer living in Oregon. "I was wearing wrist braces most of the time, and always at night, and sometimes it was difficult for me to even use my hands."

She happened to discuss her problem with her brother, a vocational rehabilitation counselor. "He told me that vitamin B_6 was very effective for this problem. I asked my doctor about it, and he said it was okay to try, but not to take more than 250 milligrams a day. I started taking 50 milligrams once a day, but soon increased it to twice a day. After only two or three days on that dose, the pain and other symptoms started to ease off." She noticed, though, that if she doesn't take the vitamin every day, her symptoms are more likely to flare up.

Richard, 66, a retired utility company cable splicer living in Scotia, New York, recalls that his symptoms of carpal tunnel didn't appear until after he retired. "I don't know exactly what caused it, but I am very active—digging stumps, cutting wood, doing carpentry work—so it could have been lots of things," he says.

"I didn't do anything about my symptoms for a long time," he says. But then he read about vitamin B_6, and started taking 100 milligrams a day. About that same time, he saw his doctor about the problem. "The doctor just shrugged when I told him about the B_6," he says. The doctor wanted him to wear immobilizing splints on both wrists all the time. "That wasn't something I was prepared to do," he says. "You can hardly even drive a car wearing those things." Instead, he started to wear the splints only at night.

But after a few weeks, he found he no longer needed the splints— only the vitamin B_6. "As long as I continue to take it, I do pretty well," he says.

Several studies do indicate that, at least for some people, vitamin B_6 can improve symptoms of carpal tunnel syndrome. In a study by Allan L. Bernstein, M.D., chief neurologist at Kaiser Permanente Medical Center in Hayward, California, pain and numbness were significantly reduced in people with carpal tunnel who took 200 milligrams of vitamin B_6 a day. Improvement took about three months to become apparent. However, Dr. Bernstein adds, 50 to 100 milligrams may be a more appropriate dose for long-term usage.

Some researchers speculate that carpal tunnel syndrome is actually B_6

deficiency–related nerve damage, and that taking higher-than-normal doses of the vitamin corrects the deficiency.

ACTIVE EXERCISES HELP THEM

Exercises that flex or strengthen the wrist or that stimulate circulation to the hands also win a few votes. About one-fifth of our survey participants say that exercise improves their symptoms of pain and numbness.

Jeremiah, 53, the West Coast carpenter-bicyclist, relieves his pain with a few simple wrist exercises he perfected during the nights when the aching in his wrists and hands would keep him awake. He developed them with the help of some reading and talking with physical therapists.

For one exercise, he gently circles his hands at his wrists, first in one direction, then the other. For another, he bends his arms at the elbows, points his fingers upward, and presses the palms of his hands together. Then, with his hands clasped and fingertips pointed downward, he presses the backs of his hands together. He does both, several times, each for a count of five.

"I'll do these exercises when my wrists start aching, or when my fingers or hands start to go numb," he says. "It does seem to help."

Susan, 44, who spends her days counting money, also hit on an exercise that works for her during a painful, sleepless night. "I hold my arms straight up in the air and rotate my arms and wrists at the same time," she says.

Elva, 57, a secretary from Brooklyn, New York, developed her symptoms of pain and numbness soon after she took a job that required constant typing and offered only the minimum number of breaks required by law. Other women in her office, one as young as her early twenties, had the same symptoms.

"I'd deliberately drop things just so I could stop typing for a few seconds and stretch my arms out," she says. At home at night, she would do wrist rotations and bends. It wasn't until she lost her job, though, that her symptoms slowly cleared up over the course of a year. "I felt bad at first when I lost that job. Now I realize how awful it really was." She's since gotten a new job that requires less typing.

Exercises such as these are exactly what physical therapists recommend for relieving the symptoms of carpal tunnel syndrome, says Susan Isernhagen, P.T., a Duluth, Minnesota, rehabilitation specialist. "It's important to do them at least four times a day, not just during your painful sleepless nights," she adds.

THE SPORTS CONNECTION—AND CORRECTIVE

Karen, 43, a psychotherapist from Napa, California, first noticed a problem with her hands soon after she'd graduated from a light to a moderate weight-lifting program. "I noticed that it would feel like I'd hit my funny bone when I did certain exercises," she says. "I figured out what was happening, and I also discussed it with my chiropractor, who is also a sports trainer."

Karen found she didn't need to stop lifting weights. But she started using a curved rather than a straight bar for certain lifts to keep her wrists straight. She also started doing wrist rotations using three-pound weights to strengthen her forearm muscles and so help to stabilize her wrists.

There's no doubt that carpal tunnel syndrome can be aggravated by some sports, says David Troppy, D.C., of Napa, California. Dr. Troppy is a certified chiropractic sports physician who teaches for the American Athletic Trainer's Association. "I have many patients who develop this condition as a result of weight lifting," he says. "It is pretty common if the hands tend to be cocked back while someone is lifting weights." Using a curved bar changes the angle of the wrist slightly and so makes it less likely to bend back as a weight is lifted, he says.

Leaning heavily on bicycle handlebars or the rails of a stair climber or incorrectly gripping a racket can also put the squeeze on this wrist nerve. "With biking, it is extremely helpful to change hand position often or to use a training bar that allows you to put some weight on your elbows," Dr. Troppy says.

In some cases, getting guidance from a sports medicine specialist may be in order.

REST PLAYS A ROLE

Some people find resting the wrists just as important as exercise. In fact, several of the people who do exercises for their carpal tunnel symptoms also use rest when appropriate.

"I'd lay my arms on pillows to rest and relax them," says Elva.

"I back off now whenever I need to," says Richard, of Scotia, New York.

"I take frequent breaks at the first twinge of pain," says an artist. "Instead of painting or drawing, I simply do something that doesn't involve wrist motion for a while."

Several people rest their wrists by wearing an immobilizing splint designed by a physical therapist. "You should try splints at night first, and you may find that's all you need," advises Isernhagen.

But nobody should wear immobilizing splints unless medically applied by a physical or occupational therapist, stresses Isernhagen. These professionals are qualified not only to fit you with a splint, but they can also analyze your work and help you make adjustments in your daily activities. In fact, redesigning your activity should be your first course of action, while wearing an immobilizing splint should be your last resort, because you may place stress on other parts of the body, such as your elbow or shoulders, when you compensate for the loss of wrist motion, explains Isenhagen.

EDITOR'S NOTE: Although several people also mentioned the use of an elastic bandage, experts point out that these may not help carpal tunnel syndrome. Pressure from such a bandage can restrict circulation, and since it restricts motion, you may fight against it, creating additional stress, says Isernhagen. And these soft bandages don't provide the stiff support you need to help keep your wrist straight, she explains.

Cataracts

Antifog Devices

Like a descending fog, untreated cataracts gradually reduce the eyesight to an incomprehensible blur. But cataracts steal more than a person's vision, according to a study of 1,021 ophthalmology patients conducted by Johns Hopkins School of Hygiene and Public Health in Baltimore. Researchers there discovered that the quality of people's lives actually mirrors the quality of their eyesight.

When their vision declines, people's view of life grows dim, the study shows. When their vision improves—in this case, through cataract surgery—their outlook brightens. After surgery, nearly all of the study participants started taking better care of themselves.

"It's clear that improving vision increases quality of life. The greater the improvement, the greater the gain," says Alfred Sommer, M.D., dean of the Johns Hopkins School of Hygiene and Public Health and an author of the study.

Of course, home cataract surgery isn't an option. But several of the people who took our survey have focused their efforts on preventing cataracts. And a few who've developed the condition have found ways to cope with discomfort following surgery. With remedies ranging from vitamin supplements and sunglasses to celery juice, here's what they say keeps the fog from rolling in.

SHE LIKES C

Don't tell Pauline, 84, that failing eyesight is one of the costs of aging. This Boyertown, Pennsylvania, resident attributes her good vision to vitamin C. "I feel like I have created a barrier of vitamin C around my body, I take so much," she says.

Pauline upped her vitamin C dose about a year ago after her doctor discovered two telltale spots in her eye. Averaging about 2,250 milligrams of vitamin C a day, Pauline says she takes 500 milligrams at breakfast, lunch and dinner and 750 before bed. Since she began taking megadoses of C, she says, her doctor reports that the spots haven't grown at all.

Pauline is smart to take vitamin C for cataracts, but she might want to reconsider the amount, says Ben Lane, O.D., nutritionist, optometrist and director of the Nutritional Optometry Institute in Lake Hiawatha, New Jersey. Dr. Lane is one of the country's leading experts in the field of nutrition and the eye.

"It's well established in the literature that vitamin C deficiency is linked to cataracts," says Dr. Lane. "But for the most part, between 500 and 1,000 milligrams seems to be ideal for most people. The dose she's taking may be perfect for her, but I've found the risk for floaters and retinal detachment statistically increases when taking more than 1,500 milligrams of vitamin C a day." (Floaters most usually are harmless bits of cellular debris in the eyeball that cause spots.)

EDITOR'S NOTE: The recommended Daily Value for vitamin C is 60 milligrams—less than you'd get by eating a single orange. Many researchers recommend taking no more than 1,000 milligrams per day long-term. Too much vitamin C can interfere with how the body uses calcium and, especially, chromium and copper. It can also cause diarrhea and cramping. If you find that larger doses of this vitamin cause digestive discomfort, cut back your dose. You can also try taking the vitamin with plenty of liquid and a bit of wheat bran, suggests John Weisburger, M.D., Ph.D., senior member of the American Health Foundation in Valhalla, New York.

BONNIE'S APPROACH IS BROAD-BASED

With several family members suffering from cataracts, Bonnie decided about a decade ago that she wasn't going to take any chances. As a result, the retired Boulder, Colorado, resident implemented her own cataract prevention program that features vitamins E and C and wearing sunglasses.

"I'm still cataract-free," says Bonnie. "I really feel like the preventive measures that I've taken have helped."

Bonnie says that in addition to a multivitamin, she takes 200 international units of vitamin E. She also makes sure to eat plenty of foods packed with vitamin E, such as sunflower and sesame seeds, pine nuts, walnuts, almonds and cashews. To increase her vitamin C, Bonnie takes 600 milligrams and does her best to eat fruits such as oranges, kiwi and strawberries as often as possible.

"Bonnie's aggressive dietary (food) and vitamin strategy can pay dividends," says Dr. Lane. Vitamin E has a major antioxidant function. Antioxidants are substances that help the body eliminate naturally occuring toxic substances known as free radicals. "Light coming through the eye creates free radicals," Dr. Lane explains. "But when our diet is excellent, we can get appropriate concentrations of antioxidant vitamins like vitamins E and C and selenium, and our bodies can synthesize the natural enzymes that protect us from the free radicals, which can cause cataracts."

"Beta-carotene is another good antioxidant choice in the battle against cataracts," says Dr. Lane. "The best advice is to eat lots of fresh, ripe fruits and green leafy and yellow vegetables; wash them quite well and peel them when you can."

SHE PREFERS TO WEAR SHADES

Before she learned about the hazards of ultraviolet rays, Alice worked on her father's farm for decades, all the time squinting into the bright Iowa sun. Alice's extended time in the sun could have been a factor in the cataract that developed in her left eye ten years ago. And since the surgery to remove the cataract, she won't go anywhere without her sunglasses on, she says. So far, Alice hasn't had any more eye problems.

"A short time after the surgery, it snowed and the sun came out and it was so bright and pretty I just had to take a look without the glasses on," says the 72-year-old grandmother. "But after I stopped looking, everything had a reddish tint to it—it literally looked rosy. The doctor told me later I had burned my eyes and that it would take a few days to get my full sight back. Now I don't go out without my dark glasses on."

"Most people would be best served to have protective lenses when they are out in the sun for long periods," says Dr. Lane. "They should wear blue blockers that block not only ultraviolet, but also a portion of the blue spectrum light that can damage eye tissues without our realizing it. This potentially higher-energy part of the spectrum penetrates into the eye deeper than ultraviolet. Sunglasses that block the blue spectrum will have a yellow or orangish or reddish tinge to them in addition to a basic brown, green, grey or other color."

CELERY JUICE TO THE RESCUE

Joy will never forget her 92-year-old mother-in-law's nighttime reading sessions in their Smokerise, Alabama, home: curled up in bed in the dark reading without glasses. Or banging out gospel tunes on the piano—also without glasses.

Her remedy for cataracts also got Joy's attention: For at least two decades, Elizabeth swore by a mixture of celery juice and water. "She told just about anyone who listened that it had given her sight back," says Joy.

Although no one is sure where she got the idea, Elizabeth apparently mashed the celery into a pulp with a fork, removed the juice, added some water, and then put it in her eyes with a dropper. How precise was the procedure? Even the fork and water were sterilized by boiling before each treatment, Joy says.

And not just any piece of celery would do. A strict vegetarian, Elizabeth insisted that the celery had to be fresh and green, says Joy. When she was younger, Elizabeth apparently used the mixture a few times a week but only applied it a few times a month later in life.

"I saw her brewing it up from time to time, too," confirms George, Joy's brother and an M.D.

Elizabeth died from pneumonia while in the hospital for hip replacement surgery. "She was an amazing woman," says Joy.

But would her remedy work? "It is theoretically possible that celery juice, extracted from very fresh celery, picked from her garden and that hadn't been sprayed with pesticides, could have remarkable healing properties for the eye," says Dr. Lane. "We know of people using vitamin C drops in their eyes and claiming good results. There is a chemical in celery called psoralen—an active ingredient that reacts strongly with light—that may provide benefit in some tissues. But it could also possibly contribute to cataracts. It would require much more study. And for this reason, it's not something I would recommend that other people start doing."

Chafing

Putting an End to the Irritation

Purse straps, bicycle seats, poorly fitted shoes, scratchy waistbands, heavy thighs, even the up-and-down motion of bouncing breasts can rub you the wrong way, making your skin red and sore. That's uncomfortable enough in itself. But it's also a signal that, if you don't do something to protect your skin, you may end up with blisters, an oozing rash or worse.

Those painful consequences aren't likely to happen to the 94 survey participants who offered home-care tips to prevent chafing. They have it under control. Their suggestions include a number of skin-protecting creams, ointments, and powders—some of which you probably have right in your kitchen pantry. Here's what works for them.

CORNSTARCH IS NUMBER ONE

Tops on the list of no-chafe solutions? Cornstarch, the silky-smooth moisture-absorbing white stuff you use to make no-lump gravy and lemon meringue pie. More than 40 percent said cornstarch was their first choice when it comes to adding some slide to the old hide.

"I use it just as I would use powder," says Althea, 66, of Richmond, Virginia. "After I bathe and dry off, I sprinkle a little cornstarch in my hands and rub it wherever I need it—under my breasts and arms, between my legs and on my feet. It feels great and it helps to keep me dry and comfortable. Plus, I like that it has no odor, since I tend to be sensitive to perfumes."

Another woman says her twist on the cornstarch method has withstood the test of time for at least three generations.

"I bathe the chafed area with baking soda water, dry it well, and then dust it with cornstarch," says Patricia, of Fargo, Georgia. "Almost everyone has those two items in the cupboard, so they're always handy."

She's used the baking soda–cornstarch combination on her babies in the past to relieve painful diaper rash, and now she finds that the same method relieves the chafing she sometimes gets in the folds of her skin. "I'm diabetic and stout, and I chafe pretty badly when my sugar is up," she explains.

"I have used this many times, and I believe it helps keep my skin healthy."

Cornstarch relieves chafing by forming a protective, absorbent layer on the skin, explains Stephen Purcell, D.O., chairman of the Division of Dermatology at Philadelphia College of Osteopathic Medicine and assistant clinical professor at Hahnemann University School of Medicine, also in Philadelphia. "It makes skin less tacky, so surfaces that come in contact aren't tugging at one another," he explains.

POWDERS PAMPER THEIR HIDES

Trailing cornstarch, with about half as many recommendations, are powders of all sorts—baby powder, bath powder, medicated powder, talcum powder. Only one brand name was mentioned more than once, Gold Bond, a mentholated talcum recommended for life's little itches.

"I use it all over my body," says Gilbert, a retired printer from Taunton, Massachusetts. "It's especially soothing for hot, tired feet if you've been standing all day long, and I think it helps to reduce itching and rashes."

Several people mention a few other powdery substances. Some dust baking soda on their skin. And two say they use white wheat flour.

These also work by absorbing moisture on the skin, Dr. Purcell says. "If someone has mild chafing primarily from sweating, any one of these powders will work just fine."

SHRINKING THIGHS END HER PAIN

Trying to walk on a hot summer day when every step is chafing the skin between the thighs is a problem Violetta, 70, a retired day care mother from Topeka, Kansas, would rather not have. "I've used cornstarch to help relieve the problem, but I've found if I can lose 10 or 15 pounds, my chafing stops," she says.

Losing weight may help resolve chafing thighs, breasts and arms, even chafing that occurs under that pouch of fat some people develop on their bellies, Dr. Purcell says.

SOME LUBE UP WITH OIL

As any mechanic can tell you, oil or grease reduces friction on moving parts simply by coating the surfaces of contact points. So if it can extend the life of your crankshaft, think what it can do for constantly rubbing thighs or anywhere else you get the grind.

Eight of our survey takers rely on petroleum jelly to reduce wear and tear on body parts. "I'm a long-distance runner, and I've learned the hard way that a little rubbing can become a major problem when you have to put up with it for 15 or 20 miles," says Marjorie, 41, a San Francisco landscaper and occasional marathon runner.

Before she hits the road, she applies a thin coat of petroleum jelly to the spots that usually bother her—the backs of her heels and between her thighs. And sometimes, she'll stash a small tube of the stuff in a tiny pocket in her running shorts in case she needs to apply more while she's out. "It helps, especially when I'm sweating a lot," she adds.

An equal number of our survey takers use vitamin E oil, an expensive alternative to petroleum jelly that can soothe irritated skin. "I use a cream that contains some vitamin E oil. I just rub it on wherever my skin feels raw, usually my upper thighs," says Lucille, 83, of St. Louis, Missouri.

Others found soothing relief from aloe vera lotion, A and D Ointment (a diaper rash and minor burn cream), cocoa butter and Bag Balm—thick, petroleum-based goop in an attractive tin you're more likely to find at a feed store than a drug store. It's a remedy for cows with sore udders, but farmers with sore hands say it works for them, too.

One person suggests calendula lotion, a product you're likely to find in a health-food store. Calendula, commonly known as pot marigold, is a bright orange flower used in creams to treat minor burns and skin irritations. It may have some anti-inflammatory properties.

SOME SWEAR BY ZINC OXIDE

Most people chafe "where the sun don't shine," but it turns out that the thick white paste lifeguards dab on their noses to prevent sunburn—zinc oxide—works well for chafing. Several people mentioned it specifically as an ingredient to look for in a skin-protecting product. Zinc oxide is found as an ointment in Desitin, a diaper rash and prickly heat remedy, and as a powder in Gold Bond and Balmex baby powder. "Both paste and powder are very effective for chafed skin," Dr. Purcell says. Zinc oxide absorbs moisture and deters bacterial growth on the skin.

THEY FIGHT FRICTION

Bicyclists know all about chafing—and how to avoid it. The shorts they wear are designed to cushion their bottoms and reduce chafing as they pedal.

"I was about ready to give up on bicycling because I'd gained some weight that really made my legs raw when I biked," says Susan, 37, of Providence, Rhode Island. "I'd refused to buy biking shorts because I thought they looked so strange. But I finally did purchase a pair, and I was very pleased to discover how well they worked to alleviate this problem."

People who find that regular biking shorts reveal a bit more than discretion allows can purchase double-layered shorts that hide the padding and skin-tight Lycra under a pair of baggy shorts.

Super-large sizes (up to 72-inch hips or bust) of Lycra leotards and tights are available by mail order from: Women at Large Fitness Clubs, 1020 South 48th Avenue, Yakima, WA 98908. "All of our exercise wear is designed to support the body tissue during exercise. They glove the body without restricting movement," says Sharlyne Powell, founder of the company. "The slippery surfaced nylon-Lycra tights work especially well to prevent chafing inner thighs during aerobic exercise, biking or walking, and some women wear them daily instead of pantyhose."

Hikers know about chafing, too. For them, the cause is likely to be stiff boots rubbing tender tootsies. "I use two pairs of socks—friction-reducing, moisture-wicking liner socks under a pair of thick wool socks," says Vivian, 64, a long-time hiker and outdoors enthusiast from Tallahassee, Florida. These liner socks are typically made with soft synthetic wicking materials such as polypropylene or treated polyester fiber. Capilene by Patagonia and Coolmax by DuPont are good examples.

"Wear cotton," one survey taker wrote. Dr. Purcell agrees: "An excellent choice for people with sensitive skin."

You may want to cultivate the disheveled look, too, if your clothes give you the rub. A study showed that the chemicals used to make some fabrics wrinkle-resistant are a more common cause of skin irritation than previously realized. In the study, 12 of 17 people with skin irritation in areas where clothes came in close contact with skin, such as around the waist, were found to be sensitive to the formaldehyde resins used to make permanent-press clothes.

THEY LAUNDER WITH CARE

Chafing around the waist, crotch and upper thighs or anywhere else where clothes come into tight contact with the body can also be a reaction to skin-irritating chemicals or soap residues in fabrics.

"I use Shaklee's laundry soap, called Basic L," says Kathie, of McKinleyville, California. "It contains no phosphates, perfumes, fillers or softeners, so it's great for people with sensitive skin." Other environmentally friendly laundry soaps will tend to be friendlier to your skin as well, she contends.

If you don't use such a soap, simply double-rinse your clothes, Dr. Purcell says. And avoid using fabric softener in the dryer. "It leaves a residue on clothes, and when you sweat, the residue can leach out and irritate your skin."

Cold Hands and Feet

Relief That Goes Out on a Limb

Keeping your tootsies toasty probably doesn't rate on your to-do list today—unless you're already shivering. If that's the case, then your cold hands and feet are probably all you can think about.

Actually, having hands and feet that simply won't warm up—or that tend to chill out at inappropriate times—is a fairly common complaint. Some of our survey participants are all too familiar with this icy predicament. And they say they've come up with remedies that will kill the chill—whether you're suffering from poor circulation or the effects of Old Man Winter. Beyond the basics—like wearing warm gloves, dry socks and waterproof boots—here's what they had to say.

SHE APPRECIATES VITAMIN E

No fewer than four of our survey participants are excited about the results they get from using vitamin E.

After years of suffering from cold hands and feet, Connie surprised even herself last winter by walking around the house barefooted.

This Romulus, Michigan, resident claims to have improved circulation in her extremities by taking two 400 IU (international units) vitamin E capsules a day. "All I know is that it works for me," she says. "I used to have to wear socks, slippers, everything just to stay warm."

And if she's accidently skipped her dose for a few days and feels a little chilly, Connie says she takes her vitamin E and then enjoys a hot shower or foot soak until the supplement takes effect.

EDITOR'S NOTE: While its effect on cold hands and feet has not been studied, a daily dose of 300 to 800 IU of vitamin E has been found to gradually improve intermittent claudition—a painful condition caused by the narrowing of leg arteries. Narrowed arteries in the legs may be a factor in cold feet, experts say. Vitamin E is found in vegetable oils, leafy green vegetables, nuts, and whole-grain cereals.

The recommended Daily Value (DV) of vitamin E is 30 IU. Although taking up to 600 IU is considered safe, most experts recommend taking no more than 400 IU daily without a doctor's supervision.

NIACIN HELPED HER SHED HER SOCKS

Alice, of North Hollywood, California, boasts of being able to go bare-footed around the house once again—and she credits niacin supplements for her newfound warmth.

"For the past 15 years, I'd been having trouble with cold hands and feet," says the 81-year-old great-great-grandmother. "It got so bad that I had to wear socks to bed! Well, I'm going around the house barefooted now, and it suits me just fine."

Alice say she began taking 100 milligrams of niacin three times a day after she read that the supplement might help her problem. Within a month, she noticed an improvement. She also discovered that taking niacin with a meal helped her prevent the sometimes unsettling facial flushing that's commonly associated with the vitamin.

EDITOR'S NOTE: Niacin has been shown to lower cholesterol, protect against cardiovascular disease and increase blood flow into certain parts of the body. These effects, however, are gained only through taking very large doses of the vitamin— several times more than the DV of 20 milligrams. Large amounts of niacin can produce unpleasant side effects, such as flushing, nausea and itching. While doses up to 100 milligrams have been shown to be safe, you should ask your doctor whether taking this supplement is appropriate for you. Food sources of niacin include lean meat, fish and poultry.

SHE LIKES IT HOT

Nicole, a resident of Fountain, Colorado, finds that the African cayenne pepper she buys at her neighborhood herb store is great for keeping feet warm. She doesn't eat it, however. She sprinkles it in her shoes.

In fact, she says it works so well that her son rarely leaves for work during winter without some of his mother's magic dust sprinkled in his shoes. "I don't remember how I found out about cayenne pepper, but it's really marvelous, absolutely great stuff," says the 55-year-old mother of two. "And African cayenne pepper is hotter than regular pepper."

Her son's interest in cayenne pepper began after he suffered from frost-bite on two of his toes, she says. So far, putting the pepper in a salt shaker seems to be the best way of sprinkling it on, says Nicole. To make sure she doesn't get any in her eyes, she says she uses gloves when filling the bottle.

Another survey participant reported that sprinkling dry mustard in socks and shoes can help keep hands and feet warm.

EDITOR'S NOTE: Applied externally, cayenne pepper has been found to be effective at bringing blood to the surface of the skin, and as a result, experts say it can help relieve cold feet if in the socks.

Special care must be taken not to get the pepper in your eyes—it will cause extreme discomfort. Also, you should not use cayenne pepper on broken skin or wounds or if you have athlete's foot.

THEY BOAST ABOUT BIOFEEDBACK

Two of our survey takers said they use biofeedback—a body-control technique that must be learned through special training—to turn up the heat in their hands and feet.

Pat, a customer service rep in Cincinnati, says she uses biofeedback while watching her son play junior varsity football.

"It gets pretty cold sometimes sitting in those bleachers," she says. "But all you have to do is put your mind toward getting your hands warm, and it works."

Pat says she visualizes her hands slowly glowing white-hot and within just a few minutes they're warm. She originally took courses in biofeedback to help get over painful migraine headaches, but has since adapted what she learned to help her with other physical problems.

Julia, of Huntsville, Alabama, is another ex–migraine sufferer who uses biofeedback to deal with both headaches and cold extremities. After counting backward from five, Julia visualizes a fiery ball moving from her head or chest to her hands or feet. In no time, Julia says she feels as warm as she would if she were basking in the sun. "It may just be in my mind, but I feel like it does help," says the 57-year-old.

During a typical training session to learn how to use biofeedback to control sensations of heat and cold, temperature sensors are connected to the skin—usually the fingers. The goal is to teach you how to actually raise and lower your skin temperature. The temperature sensors are hooked up to a machine that beeps. The sound quickens when your skin temperature goes up and slows when it goes down.

With the sound to help you, you begin to get the feel of what you need to do with your body and mind to make the temperature change. The biofeedback trainer gives helpful suggestions, which will probably include telling you about the kind of mental imagery that works for most people. Once you've mastered the technique—and some people find it easier than others—there's no more need for the equipment. And, medical experts say, you should be able to raise your body's temperature just by thinking about it.

Colds

Roughing Up Some Common Germs

The best way to treat a cold? "With contempt," according to Sir William Osler, one of modern medicine's founding fathers. That statement reflects the belief, still prevalent among doctors today, that there just isn't much you can do for a cold except ignore it.

Well, the people who responded to our home remedies survey aren't buying into that notion. They prefer to fight back with everything they have to ward off or weaken a cold. And they claim to have a lot of ammunition on hand, both to knock out the various viruses that cause colds and to relieve the runny nose, aches and pains, congestion and cough that accompany this common ailment.

To fight cold viruses, for instance, they add onions, garlic and lots of black pepper to their chicken soup and a shot of lemon juice to their hot tea. They take vitamin C and zinc, along with herbs that have an immunity-enhancing reputation, such as echinacea and goldenseal. They use salt water to gargle and to rinse out their noses. They smear their chests with mustard, guzzle orange juice, and inhale horseradish vapors. They even turn to hard spirits—for medicinal purposes only, mind you—to help "sweat it out."

Does any of this stuff really work? Here's what our participants have to say.

VITAMIN C STOPS THEIR COLDS

Among all these concoctions and cures, vitamin C clearly stands out as the most highly recommended defense against the common cold. Nearly 80 percent of our survey takers report that this essential nutrient relieves their symptoms, and several add that regular use has cut the number of colds they have.

"Because of illness, I have a weakened immune system," says Linda Mae, of Waco, Ohio. "I would normally have at least two colds a year, and twice I developed pneumonia that kept me in bed for months." About a year ago, however, she started taking 2,000 milligrams of vitamin C a day. "And last winter, for the first time in three years, I was not sick at all." No colds, no pneumonia, no nothing. Her self-care includes copious amounts of garlic, too, which we'll get to in a bit.

"I've been using vitamin C for colds ever since I read Linus Pauling's book, *Vitamin C, the Common Cold, and the Flu* back in the 1970s," says Orphy, 69, a self-professed "health nut" from Yucca Valley, California. "It's always worked for me."

She normally takes 300 to 500 milligrams of vitamin C a day. When she feels a cold coming on, however, she increases the dosage to 1,500 milligrams, three times a day, for a total of 4,500 milligrams a day. "I continue that dosage for several days, until my symptoms are gone," she says. "I also make sure I drink plenty of water. I haven't had a real cold for many years."

Mary, a jill-of-all-trades living in Bark River, Michigan, follows a similar regimen with slightly different amounts. "I normally take 500 milligrams of vitamin C plus bioflavonoids every day, but, if I feel like I am getting a cold, I double the amount I usually take—to one gram a day," she says. "I've found that doing this definitely relieves my symptoms and keeps the cold from progressing from sniffles to a full-blown head cold with lots of congestion. It's also reduced the number of colds I have, because I simply can't recall the last time I had one."

Bioflavonoids, sometimes part of a supplement marketed as C-complex, are compounds found in the same citrus fruits that contain vitamin C. Some studies suggest that they, too, can knock out cold and flu viruses.

Quite a few studies have now been done on vitamin C's effect on combating colds. An analysis of a dozen of these studies showed a 37 percent average reduction in the duration of colds treated with vitamin C. Most of the studies have found that vitamin C (often in 1,000-milligram daily doses) can reduce the severity and length of colds—but not the number of colds a person gets.

One thing most vitamin C enthusiasts agree on: Start taking the vitamin in larger amounts as soon as you begin to have cold symptoms. "If you wait until the cold's gotten a hold, the vitamin C won't help much," says Ophry.

EDITOR'S NOTE: Some researchers suggest you take no more than 1,000 milligrams a day as a long-term maintenance dose. One reason is the concern that continual high amounts of vitamin C may interfere with copper absorption in the body. High doses can also cause diarrhea and cramping in some people. If you do get cramping or diarrhea, try taking your vitamin C with plenty of liquid and some wheat bran, suggests John Weisburger, M.D., Ph.D., senior member of the American Health Foundation in Valhalla, New York.

Also, chewable vitamin C can erode tooth enamel, so stick with the stuff you swallow.

THEY'RE SOLD ON CHICKEN SOUP

Jewish mothers aren't the only people who rely on chicken soup for what ails them. Sixty percent of the people who answered our survey say this golden broth is a staple during the cold and flu season. "It's no cure, but it does make you feel better," explains one participant.

The benefits of this long-time folk remedy have been elucidated, thanks to the efforts of a few curious scientists. Researchers at Mount Sinai Medical Center in Miami Beach found that hot chicken soup got nasal mucus flowing significantly better than a cup of cold water. Hot water also outperformed cold, but didn't do quite as well as chicken soup. Because drinking either water or soup through a straw was not as effective as sipping it from a cup, the researchers believe the effect may be due, at least in part, to nasal inhalation of water vapor.

And in another study, researchers at the University of Nebraska in Omaha found that, in a test tube, chicken soup slowed the movement of neutrophils—immune cells activated by cold viruses. "When you have a cold, neutrophils normally migrate from the blood to the mucous membranes, stimulating such symptoms as inflammation and mucus secretion and perhaps fever and cough," says Stephen Rennard, M.D., chief of pulmonary and critical care medicine at the university's Medical Center. "Although we didn't test this in people, it's possible that eating chicken soup may provide some immune system benefits."

Vegetarians take note: While plain chicken soup provides immune benefits, Dr. Rennard also discovered that the vegetables added to the broth provided additional anti-inflammatory action. "We used onions, sweet potatoes, carrots, turnips and parsnips and found that each of these vegetables alone affected immune cells' activity," he says.

People who make their own chicken soup confirm that it's the extra added ingredients that put real cold-fighting power into this tasty broth.

"I'll make a bland chicken soup for an upset stomach, but when it's congestion and head cold I'm fighting, I throw in lots of onions and garlic and plenty of fresh-ground black pepper," says Ruth, a grandmother of six from Piscataway, New Jersey.

The best way to consume this head-clearing concoction? Slowly, hunched over a big steaming bowl, with someone, preferably a grandma, coaxing you on.

THEY GRAB THE GARLIC

Garlic, onions and hot spices are all hot weapons in the cold war, our survey participants report. And science backs them up.

Garlic, for instance, has been found to contain compounds with chemical actions similar to antibiotics. While it's considered to work best against fungal infections, garlic has antibacterial and antiviral effects as well.

"I add fresh garlic to just about everything I eat," says Linda Mae, who also used vitamin C to ward off her once-annual bouts with pneumonia.

Some say the best way to use this pungent bulb is to eat several cloves of raw garlic at the first sign of symptoms. You may want to chop it fine and add it to salads. Or try a cocktail suggested by a Patterson, New York, registered nurse: "To hot tomato juice, add the juice of one or two cloves of garlic, the juice of half a lemon, and about $\frac{1}{16}$ teaspoon of cayenne pepper. The results are amazing and sure to fight off any cold with force and speed." To neutralize the garlic smell, chew a few sprigs of parsley after you've downed your drink.

EDITOR'S NOTE: A clove of garlic, by the way, is one of the segments that make up a head or bulb. While capsules or pills made of dried garlic can offer some benefit, researchers say these products do not preserve the full activity of the fresh herb.

ONIONS GET KUDOS, TOO

People mention eating onions just as often as they do garlic. In fact, we got the recipe for an old-fashioned cough syrup made with onions from a Utah woman, who remembers her father making up a pot of the stuff when she was sick as a child.

"The nearest doctor was 10 or 15 miles away, so we did a lot of nursing ourselves," says Norma, 66, of Spanish Fork, Utah. "My father would slice a couple of big onions, sprinkle them with sugar and set them in a warm place on the stove. When the juice would start to come off the onions, he'd spoon it up and give it to me." The stuff didn't taste bad, she recalls. "It had so much sugar in it, that's all I could taste." And it did ease her cough and congestion.

Homeopathic doctors consider onions akin to "hair of the dog." This branch of medicine acts on the belief that like cures like. Since raw onion juice can make your nose run and eyes water, homeopathic doctors sometimes prescribe homeopathically prepared onion to treat colds and allergies with these same particular symptoms. Onions contain many of the same compounds found in garlic and may also stimulate the immune system.

HOT PEPPER GETS A VOTE

Speaking of hair of the dog, one woman suggests a remedy that might just singe your nose hairs if you're not accustomed to eating hot foods. "I make a tea using red pepper powder," says Viola, of Detroit. "It's excellent for relieving congestion and clearing out a stuffy nose. In fact, it works so well for me that often just one cup of tea is all I need to avert a cold."

How much you'll want to use in a cup depends on your taste, she says. Add just a pinch for starters, then increase the amount as your taste buds acclimate, she suggests. "I also use the tea as a gargle and find it very effective at loosening phlegm," she adds.

A substance in red pepper powder, capsaicin, causes you to perspire and can make your nose and eyes run, enabling you to cough up mucus or clear your nose when you blow.

MUSHROOMS WORK MAGIC FOR HIM

Living north of Chicago, where the winter winds stream down from the north, means hunkering down for the duration. "Oh yes, people do get lots of colds around here, but usually during times when the temperature is varying widely between warm and cold, not when it's bitterly cold," says Lothar, 57, a retired body-shop owner living in Deerfield, Illinois.

Guess who hardly gets colds at all, however? Lothar's cold-coming-on regimen contains several natural ingredients, including vitamin C and several herbs. One item he's added that he says does a good job on colds is shiitake mushroom capsules. "I take about six capsules a day when I notice symptoms, and this along with vitamin C knocks the cold out flat," he says. "I used to have a lot of problems with colds, but not anymore."

Certain mushrooms hold an important place in the treatment of illness in both China and Japan, and people in America have taken an interest in the potential healing properties of these fungi, especially their ability to stimulate immune function. "Mushrooms contain an array of novel compounds not found elsewhere in nature," according to Andrew Weil, M.D., associate director of the Division of Social Perspectives in Medicine at the University of Arizona College of Medicine/Arizona Health Sciences Center in Tucson and author of *Natural Health, Natural Medicine.* "And let's not forget that antibiotics are derived from closely related organisms—molds."

Of the food mushrooms with medicinal value, the shiitake is the best known. This large, meaty mushroom is most likely to be available dry. Soaked, then cooked, it makes a tasty addition to stir-fries or stews and holds its own in a soup.

HOT TEA'S THEIR COMFORT

You don't have to be a Brit to take comfort in a steaming hot cup of tea, our survey participants indicate. More than 50 people endorse a brew of one sort or another as a means of symptom relief. "You can sniff the steam, then drink the tea," explains a Boston resident, whose beverage of choice is black tea with honey and lemon.

Indeed, some research indicates that hot fluids help to loosen congestion, promote mucus flow and so unclog stuffy noses. Result: You feel better. But several people suggest herb or spice teas that apparently have additional benefits.

"I make mullein tea the way my grandmother taught me back in the 1930s," says Jean, a transplanted Midwesterner living in Vacaville, California. "I put about two teaspoons of dried leaves in a cup of hot water and steep it for about ten minutes, then drink it. This tea really does work for me. It helps to relieve the congestion in my chest and eases the coughing." If your throat is very sore, add a spoonful of honey for extra relief, as did her grandmother.

Mullein is available at some health-food stores. It's also a common roadside weed. However, Jean relies on her daughter, living in Oklahoma, to send her mullein leaves, since this plant does not grow in California.

In fact, the velvety leaves from this tall-stalked weed have long been used to treat coughs, colds and sore throats. Mullein contains a substance called mucilage, which swells and becomes slippery as it absorbs water, providing a soothing coating on the throat. It apparently also thins mucus, making it easier to cough up.

GINGER SPIKES THEIR BREW

A pungent spice, ginger is a favorite when it comes to head-clearing brews. "Cut thin slices of gingerroot into hot water and steep for about ten minutes," suggests one survey participant.

You can also use ginger powder to make a tea. Simply pour boiling water over a teaspoon or so in a cup. Or add a pinch of ginger to a cup of black tea.

The pungent oil found in ginger is similar to that found in capsaicin, or red pepper. Its slightly irritating effect on the nose and throat helps to thin mucus, making it easier to blow your nose or cough up mucus when you have a cold. Ingredients in ginger have also recently been found to reduce fever and relieve coughs.

And if that's not enough to send you scurrying to the spice rack, Chinese studies show ginger helps kill flu viruses, and an Indian report shows it increases the immune system's ability to fight infection.

TAKE TWO TENNIS BALLS . . .

Rest seems like an obvious antidote to a cold, and several busy people say that getting more rest was tops on their list of things to do for a cold. But two women say that they rev up to run off a cold.

"I developed pneumonia a few years ago, and as soon as I had enough energy, I started to walk for exercise, as I had before I got sick," says Corrinne, a retired executive secretary living in Fort Myers, Florida. "I might go five or six miles, and I'd be sure to take along a pocketful of tissues, because I'd cough up plenty of mucus." As far as she's concerned, exercise beats staying in bed any day.

Another Floridian couldn't agree more.

"I know that when they feel rotten, most people stay indoors and nurse themselves," says Jean, of Lakeland, Florida. "I do just the opposite. I usually go outside and play tennis, and I feel much better as a result." Indoors, she says, she'll be constantly reminded of her symptoms, with sneezing and coughing. "But once I'm outdoors, moving, my head clears and I have no symptoms."

In fact, exercise may be just what the doctor orders, a study from Loma Linda University in California suggests. The study found that a daily 45-minute walk or other exercise can help speed recovery from colds, because it mobilizes your body's first-line defense against infection—natural killer cells—sending them coursing through your bloodstream.

Don't overdo it, however, researchers warn. Exercising to the point of exhaustion depletes your immune system.

THEY SWEAR BY ZINC

Anyone who's ever sucked on a zinc tablet can tell you—it tastes yucky, and it suppresses your ability to taste for an hour or so after you take it.

This hasn't stopped a fair number of our survey participants from using zinc to knock out a cold or sore throat—or from raving about this trace mineral's impressive talents.

"I started using zinc for colds back in 1985, when I first heard about it on a radio talk show," says Irwin, a software engineer from Norristown, Pennsylvania, who admits he likes to try all sorts of different home remedies. "I've used it at least a dozen times since then, and it has always worked for me. It knocks the cold right out." He uses zinc gluconate tablets, letting them slowly dissolve in his mouth.

"I've used zinc for several years, and it has never failed me," says Bernice, 79, of Milwaukee. "At the very first sneeze, I put a tablet in my mouth and let it dissolve there. One tablet is all it takes to keep the cold away. Oh yes, it works, and not only for me. I have a couple of friends who can vouch for this, too."

A study by researchers at Dartmouth College has found that zinc gluconate does a respectable job at fast-forwarding a cold. The study found that students who took zinc after one day of symptoms had colds that lasted less than five days, compared with the usual nine. They also had less severe symptoms of nasal congestion, runny nose, sneezing, coughing and sore throat.

The researchers point out that zinc lozenges that contain flavor-improving substances such as sorbitol, mannitol or citric acid bind with zinc, making it inactive until it passes through the stomach—too late to act as a cold fighter. It seems zinc is only potent against colds when it dissolves in the mouth.

So use plain zinc gluconate tablets, or look for a new, tastier zinc product made with glycine, an amino acid that adds a sweet taste without interfering with zinc's healing power.

ECHINACEA ENDS THEIR MISERY

Pretty purple coneflower—the herb known as echinacea—wins votes among several of our survey participants as just the thing to knock out a stubborn respiratory infection.

Among herbalists, this plant has an impressive reputation as a natural antibiotic. It's often their first choice to treat colds and flu. The root of the plant is dried and used in capsules or as a tea. It is also available as a tincture.

"On the recommendation of a friend, I used echinacea for the first time last winter to treat a dry cough that had lingered for weeks after I'd had a cold," says June, 48, an Indiana social worker. "I took about eight capsules a day for a week. By the middle of the week, my cough started to ease off. By the end of the week, it was gone. It might have simply been ready to go; I can't say. But I'd certainly be willing to try echinacea again for this problem."

Studies show that a compound found in echinacea helps kill a broad range of disease-causing viruses and bacteria.

German researchers report success using echinacea to treat colds, flu, tonsillitis, bronchitis, whooping cough and ear infections.

EDITOR'S NOTE: Although evidence suggests that echinacea is safe, it's best to use it only in consultation with your doctor. Pregnant or nursing women should use it only with their doctor's approval.

GOLDENSEAL WINS THEIR SEAL OF APPROVAL

A flower that's a member of the buttercup family, goldenseal is recommended by a few people. "I drink a tea that contains goldenseal several times a day when I begin to develop cold symptoms," says Helen, 40, an assistant bank officer from Chattanooga, Tennessee. "It seems to help keep the cold from getting so bad that I can't go to work."

Like enchinacea, goldenseal apparently acts as an immune system stimulant, studies show.

To make a tea, use ½ to 1 teaspoon of dried, powdered root per cup of boiling water. Steep ten minutes. Goldenseal tastes bitter, so you'll want to add honey, sugar or lemon or mix it with a beverage tea to improve its flavor.

EDITOR'S NOTE: Women who are pregnant or nursing and people with high blood pressure, heart disease, diabetes, glaucoma or a history of stroke should not use this herb. High doses of goldenseal can irritate the skin, mouth and throat and cause nausea and vomiting. So stick with no more than two cups a day.

ASPIRIN, MENTHOL RUBS ARE TOP CHOICES

You'd think that with this cornucopia of natural pharmaceuticals, people would have no need to turn to over-the-counter remedies for relief of cold symptoms.

And indeed, many people prefer to avoid such drugs. "I started using herbs because cold medicines made me nauseated and tired," one woman explains.

Those who did mention cold medicines tended to stick with the basics. Aspirin is mentioned most often, followed by Vicks VapoRub, a mentholated petroleum that can be rubbed on the chest or throat to warm the skin, while the vapors provide some relief from congestion.

"I take aspirin for a lot of little aches and pains, including those that accompany a cold," says Jean, the Lakeland, Florida, woman who walked off pneumonia. In fact, her recipe for a sure-cure cold remedy is aspirin and exercise. "I'll take two aspirin, then head on out for a walk, and I always feel better by the time I'm done," she says.

Vicks VapoRub has been around long enough for 62-year-old Thelma, of Columbia, South Carolina, to recall submitting to its vaporous qualities as a child. "When I had chest congestion, my mother would put it on my chest and throat and then wrap an old flannel rag around my throat," she recalls. It did warm up her skin, and the smell seemed to help clear her head. "I never did like the smell," she admits. "But I'll still use it once in a while just because it seems to help, and I can't take decongestant pills because I have high blood pressure."

Cold Sores

Send Them Packing—For Good

I've had them since I was a kid, and they've always made me feel like hiding."

That's how one survey taker describes her feelings about cold sores. People know cold sores won't do them in, but some of the 99 people who provided remedies for them could have died from embarrassment for all the trouble this pesky ailment causes. "I actually played hookey from school on the days they were worst," says Cecilia, 34, a Staten Island, New York, mother of two teenage sons.

Also called fever blisters, cold sores crop up around the edges of the lips, on the skin between the mouth and nose, even, sometimes, inside the mouth. They're caused by the herpes simplex virus, which is transmitted by direct contact—kissing someone else who's got a cold sore—and can linger for years in nerve cells in your body, erupting occasionally.

Many people say that outbreaks follow stress, illness, too much sun, onset of menstruation, allergies to foods, even dental procedures. The skin blisters, then breaks down to form a scabby sore that lasts for a week to ten days. Luckily, outbreaks tend to lessen as people age.

People who get cold sores usually can detect a telltale tingling in the spot where an eruption is due. And that's when they act. "You've got to get after them right away," explains George, 45, an electronics repairman from Tulsa, Oklahoma. "Otherwise, nothing does much good."

Here, then, are the home remedies for cold sores from those who took part in our survey.

THEY LICK IT WITH LYSINE

Twenty-three said they rely on an amino acid, L-lysine, to cut down on the number of outbreaks, to abort a pending outbreak or to reduce the severity of a cold sore once it has erupted.

"There's no question that lysine worked for me," says Viola, 75, a mental health therapist from Amarillo, Texas. "I'd been getting cold sores since high school and could count on getting about one a month until, on the recommendation of a coworker, I started using L-lysine." That was two years ago. "I used it several times a week for about a year, and then, because I stopped having cold sores, I stopped using it. It's now been about a year since I last used the L-lysine, and I haven't had one cold sore in that time."

She thinks one reason the lysine worked so well for her was that she took it on an empty stomach. "Since I like to eat first thing in the morning, the only time I have an empty stomach is about 2:00 A.M. So I'd put a lysine tablet and a glass of water on my nightstand, and when I'd wake up in the middle of the night, as I am prone to do, I'd take the pill and then go back to sleep." She took 500 milligrams several times a week.

Doctors who recommend this treatment to their patients suggest larger doses than this. Mark A. McCune, M.D., chief of dermatology at Humana Hospital in Overland Park, Kansas, advises people who have more than three cold sores a year to supplement their daily diets with 2,000 to 3,000 milligrams of lysine and to double the dosage when they feel the tingling that signals the eruption of another cold sore. Or, you can try getting lysine in your food. Good food sources of lysine include dairy products, potatoes and brewer's yeast.

EDITOR'S NOTE: Check with your doctor before you use this supplement. That's especially important if you are pregnant or nursing. Some studies with laboratory animals have shown that excess lysine can interfere with normal growth.

SUNSCREEN IS THEIR SOLUTION

Ten people suggest using a sunscreen regularly to prevent cold sore outbreaks.

"I carry a stick of Blistex lip protectant with me at all times. I keep several around, in my purse, my car and my gym bag," says Stacy, 37, an aerobics instructor from Trenton, New Jersey. "I apply the lip gloss whenever I am going to be outside for a while, making sure it covers the area where I'm prone to get sores. It's cut the number of outbreaks I have to practically zero. I used to get about three a year, and I've only had one sore in the two years I've been using sunscreen." Her doctor suggested she try it.

Sunlight triggers one of every four cases of cold sores. Research shows that applying a sunscreen with a sun protection factor (SPF) of 15 to your lips and other susceptible areas before heading outdoors may be all you need to prevent recurring cases. In studies, researchers at the National Institutes of Health in Bethesda, Maryland, and the University of California Hospital in Los Angeles found that people prone to cold sores who applied sunscreen prior to ultraviolet light exposure got total protection. Those who didn't apply sunscreen got the usual number of new outbreaks.

ACIDOPHILUS RESCUES HER

Several people say they eat live-culture yogurt or take capsules of the friendly bacteria in yogurt, *Lactobacillus acidophilus*, to ward off cold sores.

"*L. acidophilus* capsules stopped the cold sores I'd get on my nose and upper lip after an allergy attack," says Rosemary, of Dayton, Ohio. "I would start taking several a day the minute I felt one developing. Taking them for two or three days kept the sore from erupting."

Lori, a piano teacher living in Oak Brook, Illinois, says she's used yogurt for about 20 years—"more as a preventive than a cure. Before I discovered it, I had cold sores several times a year. Now, as long as I eat a cup of yogurt every other day, I don't get cold sores." The few times she's gone off this regimen, she's gotten a new crop of unsightly blisters.

Yogurt has a long reputation as a healthy food, but until recently there was little in the way of scientific proof that it did anything to promote health. Now there's a bit of evidence that it may help strengthen the immune system, perhaps by providing an antiviral action. A study by French researchers found that people who ate two cups a day of yogurt with live cultures produced four times more gamma interferon—an immune system stimulant—in their blood than folks who ate heat-treated yogurt (which kills the cultures) or who avoided the food altogether.

One woman says her husband is able to stop his severe cold sore breakouts by taking both lysine and *L. acidophilus* at the first inkling of an outbreak. "He's had cold sores his whole life, and this is the only thing that has worked," says Carolyn, of Medford, Oregon. At the first signs of an outbreak, her husband takes two 500-milligram capsules of lysine and two capsules of *L. acidophilus* a day for three or four days. Since he's been using this remedy, he's also had fewer attacks, she says. "He used to have frequent severe attacks, and now he hasn't had one for more than a year. That's a first."

ALOE SUITS HER BETTER

"I have been able to completely prevent cold sores from erupting by rubbing fresh aloe vera juice on the spot as soon as the tingling starts," says Rosemary, of Dayton. Yes, she's the same woman who has used *L. acidophilus* to prevent cold sores.

"They both work equally well for me, but guess which one is cheaper?" she says. She owns an aloe vera plant, which doesn't mind occasionally losing a leaf for a good cause. She simply breaks off a tip of leaf, and rubs the juice on the spot. If she's late in attending to the cold sore, she will bandage a bit of the leaf on the sore spot overnight. "By morning, the tingling sensation is gone," she says. "Several of my friends have tried this, too, and it also works for them."

The gel of this fleshy succulent has long been used for skin problems, and a few studies suggest that compounds in aloe vera gel promote healing.

CREAMS SOOTHE THEIR SORES

Six people suggest over-the-counter products marketed specifically for cold sores, such as Campho-Phenique. These products contain camphor, phenol or menthol, usually in a petroleum base.

"But I'll tell you something that's a lot cheaper and works just as well," says Frank, a postal service worker from Indianapolis. "I have the pharmacist mix up a solution of spirits of camphor. Then, I dab that on the sore with a bit of cotton. It doesn't prevent a sore from erupting, but it stops the pain and dries it up."

Others mentioned a variety of ointments—either petroleum jelly or something containing petroleum jelly.

Petroleum jelly helps keep the cold sore from cracking and bleeding, which can set the stage for infection, experts say. By coating the cold sore, these products may also help prevent spreading the infection to additional places on your face.

THEY FREEZE-DRY THEIR LIPS

Kissing an ice cube can chill out a cold sore, several people contend. "It doesn't always prevent the sore from erupting, but the times I've used it, the ice seems to keep the sore from being so painful and tender," says Anne, 49, a secretary from Asheville, North Carolina. "I'll hold an ice cube on the spot off and on for a few minutes at a time."

Experts say ice may help ease the pain of cold sores by reducing swelling and inflammation.

VITAMIN C STOPS HIS SORES

Only one person suggested taking vitamin C for cold sores, and he thinks it does a pretty good job. Since he's been taking vitamin C regularly, he hasn't had many cold sores.

"I take about 400 milligrams of vitamin C a day, and when I feel a cold sore coming on, I double that amount," says Richard, 62, a real estate investor and construction worker from Ithaca, New York. "I've used it several times, and the vitamin C seems to prevent the sores I do get from becoming very bad."

A study done at the National Naval Center in Bethesda, Maryland, shows that a combination of 200 milligrams of vitamin C and 200 milligrams of citrus bioflavonoids taken three times a day for three days beginning at the first signs of outbreak may abort or greatly reduce the duration of the sores. Bioflavonoids are compounds found in the same citrus fruits that contain vitamin C. They may have some antiviral properties.

THEY'LL TAKE ZINC ANY DAY

Some people consider zinc essential, not just for good health but for a life without bothersome cold sores.

"My husband normally takes a multivitamin, but when he feels a cold sore coming on, he takes extra zinc," explains Evalee, of Mount Pleasant, Iowa. "He gets bad cold sores between his upper lip and nose, and he has used the zinc five or six times now; and it has stopped the sore from erupting. I'm not sure what made him try using it. I guess we read about it somewhere."

Only one study, using a topically applied water-based zinc solution, shows an effect on cold sores. In the study, which was done in Boston, a zinc solution applied every 30 to 60 minutes resulted in disappearance of pain and itching in one to three hours, drying of the blisters with superficial crusting in one to three days, and healing of the scab in two to four days.

EDITOR'S NOTE: If you take oral zinc for cold sores, don't continue high doses for more than a week or so at a time without your doctor's supervision. Amounts of zinc above 15 milligrams or so can interfere with your body's ability to absorb other minerals.

Colic

Common Ways to Calm a Crying Baby

Has your colicky baby turned you into a crybaby? No wonder! This malingering malady has probably been maddening moms—and Mr. Moms—since the first stork touched down with a bill full of swaddling clothes.

You know the drill: As if on cue, your newborn starts crying nearly every day at the same time for what seems like hours. But this is no run-of-the-mill whining session: His face is tense, his tiny fists are clenched, you may have even detected a slight bulge in his belly. What's worse, the howls have been going on for so long that you've started doing some hooting yourself. Although doctors aren't sure exactly what's causing the fuss, most suspect that gas and air trapped in the infant's immature digestive system play a role.

Instead of simply buying a pair of industrial-strength earplugs, our survey takers claim they successfully combat colic with a host of home remedies. So, once you're assured it's colic—and nothing else—bothering your baby, you might want to try some of their approaches.

GINGER HELPED WHAT AILED HER BABY

For nearly 25 years, Mary Ann worked in labor and delivery at North Passavant Hospital in Pennsylvania as a registered nurse, helping tend to colicky—and otherwise sick—kids. At the hospital, Mary Ann dispensed what the doctors ordered. But, at home, she used ginger ale, just like her mother. "You just can't beat it," she says.

After pouring about two ounces into a baby bottle and swishing it around until the fizz was nearly gone, Mary Ann would give the room-temperature brew to one of her four children—and wait for the noisy results. "They loved the taste, so they'd get quiet real quick," she says. "After about 30 minutes, they do an awful lot of burping, but they wouldn't be crying anymore."

Ginger ale can coax gas from a colicky baby, just as it does in adults, says William J. Fanizzi, M.D., senior physician and director of pediatrics for the Broward County Public Health Unit in Fort Lauderdale, Florida, who's treated over 100,000 children during his 35-year career. But be careful how much you give an infant. "What does ginger ale do? You drink some ginger ale, and you burp a little bit—especially if it's bubbly," he explains. "And when you burp, the gas from the ginger ale and some of the gas that's stuck in the stomach will come out, and you'll feel better. It's the same thing with kids. But I wouldn't advise giving ginger ale to a colicky kid more than a few times—they can get accustomed to the sweetness, and we don't want that."

SHE PUT HER BABY OUT TO DRY

You've heard of horsey rides? Judith says she saddled her granddaughter up to a bucking clothes dryer as a last resort when the infant was suffering from colic. "When a baby's been crying for what seems like 12 hours a day for about two months, you're willing to try just about anything," says the 54-year-old child psychologist.

Judith says she put a blanket in a laundry basket, put the baby on the blanket and placed the basket up against the dryer—not on top of or inside the dryer. Then she put the machine on "Tumble" for 20 minutes.

Within a short time, the child quieted down, Judith says. The combination of the noise of the dryer and the heat seemed to be what helped put the child to sleep, she says. "I'm not sure where the idea came from," she says. "I had read just about every baby book I could find. But it works!"

Can your laundry room really double as a colic control center? You bet your fabric softener. "The dryer is vibrating and, as the child vibrates along with it, the vibrations can help the intestine cause peristalsis—contractions that push food and gas through the intestines—providing relief," says Dr. Fanizzi.

And that's not the first home-spun remedy he's heard, either. "Nothing's too bizarre if it's safe and it works. I've heard of people taking their child on a drive in the car after an attack and within a half-hour, the child's better. And then there's the old vacuum remedy, where mom runs the vacuum for a while and the child relaxes. I've also heard people say that white noise from a television or radio—just setting them on a channel that's full of static—will work. I even know of an obstetrician who had a record made of the flow of blood through the vessels of the uterus that he'd play for the baby. And this blood flow, this soothing noise, this swoosh, swoosh, swoosh, would calm the baby down. Repetitive noise and movement, for whatever reason, should be helpful."

She Feeds with Fennel

When Francine's daughter suffered from repeated bouts of colic, she sought the advice of mothers who had been at it much longer than she— all to no avail. "You're at wit's end because the kid's crying for hours and hours on end, and you can't figure out what the problem is," says the 41-year-old Denver resident.

Finally, Francine asked a wise 70-year-old friend of the family for her opinion. Known for her herbal and other natural remedies, the woman suggested brewing some tea from fennel seed.

Using a cup of bottled water she heated on the stove, Francine says she mixed in a teaspoon of seeds and a quarter teaspoon of raw sugar. After letting the mixture cool, Francine strained out the seeds as she poured it into the child's bottle. It was a process she would become familiar with. "Within a half-hour, she was able to burp and expel gas," says Francine. "I'm sure that I used it several times until she outgrew it."

Fennel tea in particular is a favorite colic remedy in Germany, says Varro E. Tyler, Ph.D., professor of pharmacognosy at the School of Pharmacy and Pharmacal Sciences at Purdue University in West Lafayette, Indiana, and author of *The Honest Herbal.* "They've been using it over there for years," he says. Fennel not only helps expel gas but also has been found to have a calming effect, he says.

Peppermint Passes Their Test

Veronica first planted her herb garden because she liked the way the plants look. Soon after, however, she learned her crop included a plant that some use for treating colic: peppermint.

After picking about an ounce of fresh peppermint leaves, the Cupertino, California, bookkeeper says she adds them to a pint of boiling water, steeping them to create a tea. A quarter-cup of lukewarm peppermint tea is usually enough to quell the crankiness in the most colicky kid, says Veronica. "It really calms them down; they're definitely less agitated. Within 20 minutes, they're asleep," she says.

Other survey takers also report success with peppermint. Betty, of North Richland Hills, Texas, says her best friend claims that she successfully treated her child's colic by giving her a stick of peppermint. "It sounds weird, but she says that it works great," says Betty. "She said it seemed to soothe the ache in the child's belly."

Editor's Note: While peppermint will perform its belly-soothing magic on infants, be cautious, says Dr. Tyler. "There's some indication that some infants will gag on the menthol in the peppermint," he says. "That's not so surprising: It happens to me, too. That doesn't mean to avoid it at all costs, heavens no. It means if it doesn't work, try something else."

MAKE HERS A HOT WATER BOTTLE

Growing up in rural northwestern Louisiana, Nettie says her mother was quick to use a rubber hot water bottle to treat common aches and pains. So it's no surprise that, when she left home and had two daughters of her own, an old-fashioned hot water bottle became a part of Nettie's home remedy repertoire—even for colic. "We were country people, and there was no such thing as going to the doctor," says the 61-year-old beauty salon owner. "We had to take care of things ourselves."

After filling up a hot water bottle with warm—not hot—water and laying it either on the child's stomach or back, Nettie would gently rub the area that wasn't covered. "I don't know whether it was the patting or the warmth, but it seemed to soothe them in just a few minutes," she says.

EDITOR'S NOTE: While warmth will soothe a colicky baby, it's better if that warmth comes from mother, says Dr. Fanizzi. "You could burn the baby with a hot water bottle," he says. "But when you nurse the baby or hold the child close to you, the warmth of your stomach and the rest of your body does the same thing as a hot water bottle. So you might just want to hold the baby close for a little while and see if that helps." If you do opt to use a hot water bottle, make very sure that it's warm and not hot.

THEY REPORT SWEET SUCCESS

Putting corn syrup on a baby's pacifier may seem like an odd treatment for colic. But if you wonder whether it works or not, talk to Mary Lou in Chattanooga, Tennessee. "I used it on my son and he's 23 and six-foot-two, so it didn't hurt him any," she says. "Come to think of it, he doesn't even like sweets."

The remedy worked so well at quieting her colicky son that Mary Lou says she kept a small jar of corn syrup in his baby bag and used it until he was two months old. "It seems like he'd settle down as soon as he got the corn syrup into his system," she says.

Dee, of Jackson, Michigan, says a close friend reported success with colic by adding ¼ teaspoon of brown sugar to an eight-ounce bottle of milk. "She thought that it allowed the baby to pass gas," she says. Once again, give sugar to kids sparingly, says Dr. Fanizzi.

BURPING IS HER BOAST

A registered nurse for many years, Valeta was somehow spared from treating her own kids for colic. But she say she thinks she knows what brings it on: cold foods or foods that have a lot of air in them.

Her treatment: helping the baby burp.

"If you can get the baby to burp, that seems to solve the problem," says the 68-year-old Manhattan, Kansas, resident. "You can rub their tummy, you can walk them—any of those things will get them to burp."

Although burping a baby seems to drive air out of its stomach rather than its intestine, it might just help, says Dr. Fanizzi. More important, he says, it may be preventing air from getting into the digestive system in the first place. Breast-fed babies, for example, seem to get less air into their system than those who are bottle-fed, he says.

But above all, Dr. Fanizzi says, parents must be patient with their newborns. "At the most, colic will last for three months, and then it just goes away—and you're going to be with your child a lot longer than that."

Constipation

How to Keep Things Moving

Irregularity? Not among our survey takers. Seems like you could set your watch by their bathroom habits.

When it comes to curing constipation, they draw on an impressive array of remedies—hot prune juice, a strong cup of coffee, bran and beer, sauerkraut juice and a brisk walk, among other things. We even received instructions on tummy massage to move things through. And we got a recipe for what one woman calls goop—a high-fiber concoction guaranteed to get you going when all else has failed. In fact, more than 200 people offered remedies for this common problem. Here are some of the best.

FIBER WINS TOP HONORS

Fiber works so well at preventing constipation it couldn't take anything but first place. What is surprising, however, are all the ways people add fiber to their diets.

Mixing wheat bran into cereals or juices is an easy way to bulk up, and many people do just that. "I simply add a heaping tablespoon to whatever cereal I eat in the morning," explains Pamela, 45, a Houston, Texas, oil company secretary who learned this trick from an obstetrician years ago. "The bran helped a lot when I was pregnant, and I continue to use it because I know that if I do so, I won't have any problems with constipation."

Others turn to cereals and fruit. "I eat a big bowl of oatmeal with bananas and raisins, almonds and stewed apricots, or even apple butter and walnuts, just about every morning. That's kept me regular for years," says Walker, 68, a retired shipbuilder from Portsmouth, New Hampshire. "Of course, I also eat a lot of other high-fiber foods, but this gets me off to a good start."

Claudia gets her fiber from greens. "I come from the South, and down there they'll cook up a mess of greens to cure this problem," says this 49-

year-old musician and arts administrator, who now lives in Hopewell, New Jersey. "We boil turnip, collard or mustard greens and eat the greens. But we also drink the cooking water—called pot likker—and I think it's the pot likker that does the trick, although I couldn't tell you why."

Her favorite high-fiber meal? Cooked greens with pinto or black-eyed peas and cornbread—a tasty treat that reminds her of home.

A soup made of lentils and brown rice, along with carrots, celery and onion, works intestinal wonders for Corrine, of Fort Myers, Florida. "I made this dish once for a friend who was having constipation problems after surgery to insert a pacemaker, and she said it helped her more than any medicine the doctor had given her."

Research shows that both soluble and insoluble fiber play a role in preventing constipation. Wheat bran is mostly insoluble fiber—meaning that it doesn't dissolve in water. It adds bulk to the stool and has been shown to speed up the amount of time it takes food to move through the body.

Oats and fruits, on the other hand, contain both insoluble and soluble fiber. Soluble fiber absorbs water and becomes soft and gelatinous. It provides some bulk, but more importantly, it helps to keep stools moist and soft, aiding passage. This sort of fiber also helps to maintain a proper balance of bacteria in the bowel, which also aids in normal digestion, experts say.

PRUNES PROD THEIR PLUMBING

Prunes and prune juice have long been considered a sure fix for constipation. And our survey takers think highly of this remedy.

"If I haven't gone one day, I'll stew up some prunes that evening, and have a few of them for breakfast the next day," says Alma, 67, a Macungie, Pennsylvania, retired hairdresser. "I always go within a few hours." Other people do likewise. But one cautions: "I do like prunes, and I have to be careful not to eat too many of them at one time, or I get the runs."

THEY DRINK UP TO STAY REGULAR

If you're sure you're getting plenty of fiber, but you still get constipated, it's possible that mild dehydration is your problem. Fiber needs to absorb plenty of water to stay soft enough to move along in the digestive tract. Otherwise it balls up and slows down.

Many of our survey takers suggest both fiber and fluids—oatmeal and orange juice, bran and honey in hot water, even bran and beer. "Yes, I know it sounds strange, but bran and beer works for me, and it certainly isn't an unpleasant way to correct this problem," says Diane, a school bus driver from Wilmington, Delaware. About ¼ cup of bran cereal in the morning and two bottles of beer after work will have her regular by bedtime. "Just having one beer doesn't work. It's the second one that does the trick," she contends.

COFFEE KEEPS HER BOWELS PERKING

Hot coffee first thing in the morning provides a bodywide wake-up call for some people. "I don't drink coffee all the time, but I will have a good strong cup if I'm constipated, and believe me, I better stay near a bathroom, because it works fast," says Jean, 39, a Dayton, Ohio, beauty shop owner.

Experts explain that caffeine has a kick that extends to the intestines, stimulating peristalsis—the muscular contractions that move food along. People who are particularly sensitive to caffeine may even develop cramping and diarrhea if they drink coffee.

To treat constipation, dieticians recommend water and juice over caffeine-containing colas and coffee, because caffeine acts as a diuretic and can actually deplete the body's water supply. They recommend drinking six to eight glasses of water or juice a day.

Some of our participants have found that any sort of hot drink in the morning works for them.

"I used to think I had to have coffee to be able to you-know-what in the morning," explains Thelma, 42, a health insurance company claims adjuster from St. Paul, Minnesota. "But once, when I was sick and nauseated and couldn't stand the taste of coffee, I started drinking herb teas instead. And guess what? They worked just as well for me."

EXERCISE KEEPS THEM RUNNING

Exercise, like fiber, moves things along faster in the bowels. In fact, it works so well that some long-distance runners have to be careful about when and what they eat before a race.

Less vigorous exercisers also report satisfactory—if less dramatic—results. "I was recovering from abdominal surgery, and my doctor encouraged me to walk every day for at least 15 minutes, to help restore normal bowel function," says Norman, 67, a retired foundry worker from Toledo, Ohio. "I did do this faithfully, and I seemed to have fewer problems than other people who've had similar surgery who couldn't or didn't get out of bed and move around."

"I don't think of exercise as something that I do specifically to relieve constipation, but I have noticed that, in the last three years, since I've been walking regularly, that I am much less likely to become constipated," says Renee, 45, a telephone operator from Duluth, Michigan. "I have to sit all day long, so my walk is about the only exercise I can count on each day."

METAMUCIL WINS THE LAXATIVE AWARD

Perhaps because they have so many natural ways to relieve or prevent constipation, our survey participants do not consider laxatives a top choice. One laxative mentioned a few times is Metamucil—an over-the-counter chemical-free powder meant to be mixed with fruit juice or some other drink.

Metamucil is a bulk-forming laxative that contains a water-soluble fiber, psyllium. This fiber dissolves or swells in the intestine, forming a gel that aids the passage of stools and stimulates the muscular contractions that push food through the bowel.

Experts consider this and other psyllium-containing laxatives the first choice for constipation. That's because the laxative acts only in the bowel. It is not absorbed into the body and does not upset the body's fluid or mineral balance as chemical-based laxatives do. It's considered safe for long-term use.

Several people bypass the manufacturer completely and go straight to the source. They buy psyllium seed, available at health-food stores, and use it in a number of ways—in bread, mixed in foods, ground up, or simply chewed along with juice or water.

Claudia, our southern high-fiber cook, has also used psyllium to relieve constipation. "I take a teaspoon or so of seeds, just chew them up and swallow them down with a full glass of water," she explains. "It works by the next day."

Flaxseed has properties similar to psyllium, and it's one of the ingredients in "goop," a gut-reaming mixture developed—and named—by Evelyn, a Nebraska woman who had a section of colon removed five years ago due to blockage. "I grind flaxseed in a coffee grinder and use apples, oranges and grapefruit sent through a blender. I mix three tablespoons of flaxseed and three of the fruit mixture to make a cup of goop. I eat a cup a day."

EDITOR'S NOTE: Regular use of any laxative, even those labeled as natural, can lead to dependency on the product to have a bowel movement and medical problems associated with fluid and electrolyte loss.

THEY GET A LUBE JOB

Several people suggest using castor oil, mineral oil or olive oil to cure or prevent constipation. "I'll sometimes take two tablespoons of mineral oil before retiring for the night," says Edward, 71, of Fall River, Massachusetts. "It usually works sometime during the next day."

These oils soften stools by coating them and thus preventing the water they contain from being absorbed through the intestinal walls. In fact, emulsified mineral oil—which contains a bit of detergent—is sold as a laxative and seems to work better than plain mineral oil, because it is dispersed through the stool.

EDITOR'S NOTE: Experts caution, however, against more than occasional use of lubricant laxatives because they can interfere with absorption of nutrients, including the fat-soluble vitamins A, D, E and K.

And castor oil breaks down to form an additional bowel-irritating ingredient— ricinoleic acid—that does do the trick, but rather too well, experts say. It's considered a harsh laxative that can cause a bout of watery diarrhea, depleting the body of fluids and nutrients.

HE REACHES FOR RHUBARB

"I eat stewed rhubarb, made with some sugar, and eat it while it's still warm, out of a little dessert dish," says Roy, a retired farmer living in Riverton, West Virginia. "I haven't had much need for it, but it's something my grandmother used, and it does work. Around here, most people have a rhubarb plant or two growing at the edge of their garden."

In fact, rhubarb stalks or root is a delicious and effective bowel cleanser, says Ronald L. Hoffman, M.D., director of the Hoffman Center for Holistic Medicine in New York City and author of *Seven Weeks to a Settled Stomach*. He suggests this recipe: Chop three stalks of rhubarb (remove the leaves, which are toxic) and mix with one cup of apple juice, ¼ peeled lemon, and one teaspoon of honey. Put all the ingredients in a blender or food processor and puree until smooth.

You may want to try only a small amount at first, to see how your body responds.

SAUERKRAUT SCOURS THEM OUT

"I've used sauerkraut juice many times to relieve constipation of five or six days' duration, and it has always worked for me," says Jacqueline, 49, a Floral Park, New York, housewife. She picked up on the remedy from her father, who used to drink sauerkraut juice regularly. "He lived to be 86 years old and never had any health problems," she says.

She simply drains the juice—usually about ¾ cup—from a large can of sauerkraut, then drinks it. "For me, it works as well as milk of magnesia. I can count on results in about 1 to 1½ hours." She's not alone. Several other people said sauerkraut juice is an effective laxative.

Sauerkraut juice is very salty and works by drawing fluid into your bowels, causing a flush that works well at alleviating constipation, experts explain. Laxatives such as milk of magnesia work the same way, using an unabsorbable form of magnesium that draws water into the bowel.

EDITOR'S NOTE: This isn't the sort of constipation cure you'd want to use on a regular basis, however. That's because it can upset the balance of electrolytes—sodium, potassium, magnesium, calcium, phosphorus and other minerals—in your body and may lead to health problems.

HERBS GIVE THEM AN EDGE

Several people say they use herbal remedies to relieve constipation. Cascara sagrada and senna were mentioned most often.

Cascara sagrada, also called sacred bark, is known to relieve constipation within eight hours after it's taken. Senna, an ancient herbal remedy, is a powerful laxative found in commercial preparations such as Senokot and Swiss Kriss. It's usually combined with other ingredients to make it milder. Goldenseal is best known for its immunity-boosting properties, but it apparently also acts as a digestive aid.

EDITOR'S NOTE: Experts point out that some herbs can be just as harsh on your bowel as commercial laxatives.

Coughing

Soothing the Savage Hack

Hack attack have you flat on your back? Think of your cough as a cry for help from your bronchial tubes. "Hey, Mack," they're saying, "quit smoking." Or "send something soothing our way, we're dry as dirt."

There are lots of ways to respond to the call of the cough. Whether they're sipping depression-era cough syrup or swallowing red-hot mustard, our survey takers say the best way to beat the hack is counterattack.

THEY LOVE LEMONS

Whether squeezed over a spoonful of honey, sucked, poured into tea or hidden in a cough drop, lemon juice topped the list of our survey takers' cough stoppers. In fact, nearly half cite this sour, yellow citrus for its cough-fighting qualities.

With 4 children, 24 grandchildren and 14 great-grandchildren, Dorothy knows a thing or two about treating a cough. Her remedy of choice: gargling with warm lemon juice and water. "I never bought any cough medicine in my life," says the 77-year-old Sioux City, Iowa, resident. "Lemon really brings the phlegm up."

Dorothy creates her lemon gargle by combining about four ounces of warm water with ¼ cup of fresh-squeezed lemon juice and uses it three to four times a day.

Lemon juice not only stimulates the glands that lubricate your mouth and throat, but also lessens the little-known cough-producing effects of excess stomach acid, says Anthony Yonkers, M.D., professor and chairman of the Department of Otolaryngology–Head and Neck Surgery at the University of Nebraska Medical Center in Omaha. "We've found that about 30 percent or more of the people who have a cough are actually suffering from a form of heartburn. The acid from their stomach will come up into the lower esophagus, causing coughing fits. Lemon juice stimulates the saliva flow. It makes the mouth water and neutralizes the acid."

THEY TOUT TEA

Teas of all types help spell relief for a nagging cough, according to our survey takers.

The folks in Lebanon, Tennessee, drink a ton of iced tea—and Nelle is no exception. But she says she started taking hot tea with honey for a cough a few years ago at her boss's suggestion. "It made my throat feel better, and I quit coughing, too," says the 61-year-old hospital dietary manager. "Now, anytime I have a cough and some tea around, that's what I'll do."

Drinking hot tea will provide at least two things that can help do battle with your cough, says Dr. Yonkers: steam and liquid. Steam loosens thick mucus, and the increased fluid intake keeps your circulation water levels higher, which increases the salivary glands' production, he says.

SLIPPERY ELM SLIDES DOWN EASY

Paul, a Basking Ridge, New Jersey, writer, sampled slippery elm tea at a friend's suggestion when he started to come down with a cough. The drink provided immediate relief, he says, and tasted great.

Slippery elm was a common remedy in colonial America. Mixed with water or milk, it was served as a soothing nutritious food similar to oatmeal and was used to treat sore throat, cough, colds and gastrointestinal ailments. Slippery elm is found in teas and lozenges carried in health-food stores.

PEPPERMINT POWER

With a peppermint farm in the family (her grandsons run it), Fern has long been familiar with the plant's pluses. So when it comes to soothing a cough, it's not hard to guess the preference of this 77-year-old Seattle resident. "I even keep a little bottle of peppermint oil in my purse," she says. "If I start coughing in church, I'll just put a dab on the end of my finger, touch that to my tongue and that's the end of it. It's a little strong, but it will sure stop your coughing." Of course, Fern doesn't have to buy her peppermint oil, but she has seen it stocked in drugstores.

When a cough came along with her husband's flu recently, Fern says she heated a cup of water in the microwave, put in two drops of peppermint oil and then had her husband breathe the vapors. "The aroma really seem to open up the congestion that comes with some coughs," she says. "It's very soothing."

In a pinch, Nelle, our Tennessee tea-timer, also calls on peppermint candy as an emergency cough-buster. "Once, I was coughing my head off and I couldn't find anything around the house that would help it. So I thought, 'Maybe I'll try a piece of peppermint,' and I popped that in my mouth. Sure enough, it worked. Now I keep some peppermint candy in my purse all the time just in case."

EDITOR'S NOTE: Pure peppermint oil can be toxic. So don't take more than six drops. Some experts say peppermint tea should not be given to infants and young children because they may experience a choking sensation from the menthol. "That's not so surprising; it happens to me, too," says Varro E. Tyler, Ph.D., professor of pharmacognosy at the School of Pharmacy and Pharmacal Sciences at Purdue University in West Lafayette, Indiana, and author of The Honest Herbal. *"That doesn't mean to avoid it at all costs, heavens no. It means if it doesn't work, try something else."*

COUGH DROPS DROP THEIR COUGHS

In her job in the research and development department of a medical and dental equipment manufacturer, Laura is surrounded by the latest in high-tech hardware. But she definitely prefers a low-tech solution when she's suffering from a cough: ricola herbal cough drops.

"The first time I saw them was when I was in a health-food store," says the 54-year-old Rochester, New York, resident. "But once I tried them, I found that I didn't need to use anything else." Sugary cough drops tend to help clog Laura's throat, making her cough worse, she says.

Horehound, eucalyptus, and Halls cough drops also get votes from our survey takers. "If we're traveling, we keep horehound drops in the car just in case," says one person.

Evelyn, of Greenville, South Carolina, prefers herbal cough drops not only for what they do but for what they don't do to her. "I have allergic reactions to lots of drugs, so I don't take them if I don't have to," she says. "Why kill a mouse with an elephant gun?"

"Herbal cough drops are laden with benefits," says Steven Rayle, M.D., staff physician at St. Mary's Hospital in Tucson, Arizona. "Many of these things can soothe and settle and help bring increased blood flow to the bronchial linings."

Cough drops work so well at relieving a minor cough that the Omaha Symphony in Nebraska installed a large box containing free Halls cough drops in the lobby, says Dr. Yonkers. "If you have a mild cough, you can suck on one of the cough drops during the symphony and keep the annoying coughs reduced significantly."

THEY'RE SWEET ON ONIONS AND SUGAR

Judging from our survey takers, a common depression-era cough remedy—onions and sugar—may have made as deep an impression as that steep economic downturn.

A pharmacist's assistant for 34 years, Virginia says she still hasn't found a better cough remedy. "My mother kept five kids from coughing with that," says the 65-year-old Ramsey, Illinois, resident. "It doesn't taste too great, but it's effective."

Virginia says she puts an entire finely chopped onion in a bowl, covers it with half a cup of white sugar, and allows the mixture to sit overnight. By morning, the sugar has absorbed much of the liquid from the onion, creating a clear syrup, she says. One tablespoon of syrup every four or five hours seems to be enough to tame the toughest cough. "My children took a dim view of it, but it works," she says.

Rather than send his children ten miles on foot to reach the nearest doctor when one of them had a severe cough, Norma's father brewed up onions and sugar just like she does today. The only difference: Her dad used a wood stove to cook the concoction, while Norma says her range or microwave works just fine.

After slicing two medium onions and putting them in a pan, Norma says she sprinkles sugar over them and places them on low heat. About a half-hour later, her cough is all but cooked. "The juice seeps out and blends with the sugar to create a good cough syrup," says the 66-year-old Spanish Fork, Utah, resident. "One spoonful every couple of hours is usually enough to help quite a bit."

While science has yet to pinpoint the curative powers of onions, we know they exist, says Dr. Yonkers. "An onion or the stimulating effect of honey or sugar tends to make your salivary glands secrete, probably lubricating your mouth and throat, and minimizing the coughing sensation," he explains.

In fact, German scientists have actually identified several substances in onions that produce an anti-inflammatory effect dramatic enough to head off an asthma attack.

They'll Drink to That

Whiskey—combined with ingredients like lemon, honey, even peppermint and rock candy—proved a big favorite with our survey takers . . . as a cough remedy, that is. A couple of people recommend downing a whole shot of whiskey, but others report that even a tiny amount does the job.

Barbara, a 57-year-old Gulfport, Mississippi, mother of five, sings the merits of sugar—seasoned with a few drops of whiskey—for beating a cough. "When we were kids, they didn't have all the cough syrup that they have out now," she says. "This was our cough medicine."

Any time she, her husband or her children suffer from a cough, Barbara says she loads a teaspoon with white sugar and drips on a few splotches of whiskey—just like her Mom used to do. Almost immediately after swallowing it, she says, the hacking stops. "The whiskey odor seems to clear the sinuses and any phlegm out and the sugar makes it taste better," says Barbara.

Taken in small doses, whiskey can kill bacteria and act as a counter-irritant throughout the esophagus—perhaps explaining why alcohol is used in many commercial over-the-counter cough and cold preparations, says Dr. Rayle. "If you drink whiskey, you'll feel a burning all the way down. That would be a counterirritant that essentially gets the nervous system's attention away from the cough."

UNIQUE GARGLE GIVES HER RELIEF

Rose's home cough remedy came straight from a doctor—but it's not the kind of cure you'd expect. Rather than recommending pills or prescription cough medicine when she was hacking from strep throat, he had the hospital staff tap a bottle of dark Karo syrup.

"Each hour that first day they'd bring me a glass of hot water with three tablespoons of dark Karo syrup mixed in to gargle with," says the 57-year-old San Benito, Texas, resident. "My doctor said, 'I could give you a lot of medicines, but this works just as well.' "

A few minutes after her first sip, Rose knew what the doctor meant. "It worked almost immediately, and by the end of the hour I was ready for more," she recalls. Years later, Rose says she still hasn't used anything else for a cough.

Although he's never heard of this treatment, Karo syrup would help stimulate the salivary glands, says Dr. Yonkers.

SHE PUTS THE CHURN TO HER COUGH

Three weeks into a cough that her doctor thought might be turning into walking pneumonia, Helen gave up on her third prescription cough medicine. Instead, she opted for the same cough remedy that her grandmother used when Helen was a child: milk and butter. Six days later, she says, her cough was gone. "I know these old-fashioned things sound funny, but they are worth a try," says the 76-year-old Saddle Brook, New Jersey, resident. "Nothing else helped."

After filling a cup with warm milk and then adding two teaspoons of sweet butter, Helen says she drinks the mixture while it's still warm. Within a few days of drinking two to three cups of whole milk a day, her cough is generally gone, she says. Skim milk does not seem to have enough fat to coat the throat and ease coughing. "The most important time is night, because it relaxes and soothes throat muscles," she says.

While this remedy may be effective for a dry cough, it probably should not be used for what's called a productive cough, says Dr. Rayle. "You have to differentiate. In general, milk tends to produce mucus. If a person has a productive cough, that is, a lot of mucus, then he's going to want to stay away from milk and butter and other dairy products. On the other hand, some coughs are completely dry, and except for a little bit in the morning, they have relatively little mucus. In that case, it might work."

SHE SEEKS A CHINESE SOLUTION

Although Gleena drinks tea and lemon juice and takes vitamin C supplements to help end a cough, this 76-year-old great-great-grandmother says she also eats hot Chinese mustard. "When you get to be my age, a cough can settle in if you're not careful," she says.

Rather than simply swallowing the mustard by itself, Gleena says she works a teaspoon through a vegetable stir-fry that she eats once a day.

"It's not as severe a hit as you might take if you spread some hot mustard on some barbecued pork, but it's the same effect," she says. In a short time, the hot mustard seems to help break up the congestion that often accompanies a cough, she says.

Is Chinese mustard an ancient Chinese secret for fighting a cough? You bet your chopsticks. In his book *Natural Health, Natural Medicine*, Andrew Weil, M.D., associate director of the Division of Social Perspectives in Medicine at the University of Arizona College of Medicine/Arizona Health Sciences Center in Tucson, agrees that "freshly prepared horseradish, hot mustard and wasabi (Japanese horseradish) all help to liquefy bronchial secretions. Eat as much as you can tolerate."

Dandruff

Turning Off the Snowstorm

You might think dandruff is a problem that really upsets only teenagers angling for a hot date. Not so, according to our survey takers. People want to look their best at work and for their spouses, they tell us, and a flurry of white flakes takes the sparkle off even the best-groomed appearance.

For run-of-the-mill dandruff, our survey participants offer these remedies.

THEY STAY SQUEAKY CLEAN

"I wash my hair every day using a gentle shampoo recommended by my hairdresser," says Susan, 44, an elementary school teacher from Worcester, Massachusetts. "This controls my flaking enough so that I don't have to use a special shampoo or anything else for my dandruff."

In fact, a number of survey takers suggest washing every day with a shampoo that doesn't dry out your scalp. And they may be onto something.

Experts say that regular shampooing breaks up the larger-than-normal flakes of skin from dandruff, making them less noticeable. And it helps to prevent the buildup of hair spray, mousse and styling gels, which can cause flakiness and set the stage for scalp itchiness.

DANDRUFF SHAMPOOS SHAKE FLAKES

A wide array of dandruff shampoos are popular with our survey takers. And they suggest shopping around until you find one that works for you. It appears that when one dandruff shampoo fails, another with a different active ingredient just might do the trick.

"My husband had plain old dandruff, but it was a stubborn case," explains a Belfair, Washington, woman. "He'd tried a few common dandruff shampoos, but they didn't help much. His doctor suggested he try T-Gel, a coal-tar product made by Neutrogena, and with just a few uses he could really see a difference."

Coal tars may have been used since ancient times for hard-to-beat dandruff. They appear to work by dispersing flakes and by reducing the number and size of flakes. If you've been avoiding coal-tar products because of the unpleasant smell, be aware that some formulas have a more pleasant aroma.

If you find your dandruff shampoo isn't doing the job, make sure you leave it on for a full five minutes, says Patricia Farris, M.D., clinical assistant professor of dermatology at Tulane University School of Medicine and Medical Center in New Orleans. "If you leave it on for less time, you're undermining the shampoo's effectiveness," she says.

SHE STRIKES OIL

"I wash my hair, then massage in a few ounces of warm olive oil and wrap my hair in a towel overnight," says Dorothy, 82, of Pensacola, Florida. "In the morning, I wash out the oil and dry my hair."

Although excess scalp oil can cause problems, an occasional warm-oil treatment may help loosen and soften dandruff scales, says New York City hair stylist, Louis Gignac, owner of Louis-Guy D Salon. It also treats the dry scalp that causes the flakes in the first place.

You may want to apply the oil, then brush vigorously with a natural-bristle hairbrush for a few minutes to loosen flakes before you wash, suggests Gignac.

EDITOR'S NOTE: Excess oil can aggravate dandruff. It's okay to give this tip a try, but pay close attention to whether it actually helps or, in fact, temporarily worsens your condition.

VINEGAR RINSES AWAY HER FLAKES

Here's a remedy for dandruff that one woman says smells as good as it works.

She brews up a batch of apple cider vinegar and mint. "I read about this years ago, and both my husband and I have been using it ever since," says Mary, of Rancho Cordova, California. To make this rinse, bring one cup each of apple cider vinegar and water and a handful of mint to a boil. Remove it from the stove and let it stand overnight. Then strain the solution and put it into a container. To use it, simply wet your fingertips with the liquid and rub it into your scalp, she says. "You don't have to rinse it out," she explains. "Just let it dry."

Vinegar and other mildly acidic solutions, such as lemon juice, may help fight dandruff by helping to remove flakes, experts say.

MOUTHWASH BANISHES HER FLAKES

Some commercial antidandruff products contain antimicrobial ingredients. So does Listerine mouthwash, and that's what one of our survey takers chooses to use for her dandruff problem.

"I haven't had to use this for years, but I did use Listerine, and it worked," says June, an office worker from Dover, Delaware. "I'd saturate a cotton ball with the mouthwash, wet my entire scalp, massage it, and then wait an hour or so before I washed my hair. I did this about three times a week for a few weeks, and my dandruff problem was cured."

An ingredient in this mouthwash, thymol, obtained from thyme oil, has antiseptic properties that can help alleviate dandruff, says Gignac. You can make your own thyme rinse by boiling four heaping tablespoons of dried thyme in two cups of water for ten minutes. Strain the brew and allow it to cool. Pour half the mixture over clean, damp hair, making sure the liquid covers the scalp. Massage in gently. Do not rinse. Save the remainder for another day.

EDITOR'S NOTE: If you have a severe case of dandruff, it's best not to use this tip. Listerine could prove irritating if it comes in contact with any open cuts.

Denture Problems

Making Sure That Teeth Don't Bite Back

Your pearly whites may have arrived at the Pearly Gates ahead of you, but that's no reason to stop smiling. The people who responded to our survey don't let denture problems—like staining or sores—bring them down. Instead, they say they tap some common kitchen items—such as salt and baking soda—to take the bite out of denture problems.

But before self-treating your denture problems, make sure your woes aren't being caused by a need for a new fit. Because the inside of your mouth can change substantially in a short time, your dentures should be checked at least once a year. "The bone can become more dense or change its shape, causing the tissues to do the same," explains Dan L. Watt, D.D.S., a dentist in Reston, Virginia, and chairman of the International Dental Health Foundation, also in Reston.

You can get a good idea whether your dentures fit on your own, however. Look for these signs of a good fit: Your upper denture stays in place when you open your mouth wide, and your bottom denture stays in place when you chew most foods. "Some people would like to use eating corn on the cob as the criterion, but a lot of people don't have enough bone to support the denture well enough to chew corn on the cob," he says.

THEY'RE SWEET ON SALT WATER

Warm salt water is the gum-soothing choice of several survey takers with mouth sores from dentures. In fact, salt water works so well for one 69-year-old woman, she says she rinses her mouth with it three to four times a day.

Of all the treatments for mouth soreness caused by dentures, a saltwater rinse may actually be the best, says Dr. Watt. "Salt water actually draws fluid out of those tissues, reducing swelling, increasing circulation, and as a result, reducing soreness," he says.

Dr. Watt recommends mixing a tablespoon of salt in about six ounces of water to create a briny solution that can be swished in your mouth for about a minute twice a day. Be sure to rinse your mouth with regular water afterward, he says.

SHE PUTS PAIN AWAY WITH PAINALAY

Over the past 43 years, eight American presidents have come and gone, but Violetta, a 70-year-old resident of Topeka, Kansas, is still using the same over-the-counter liquid called Painalay for most of her denture problems.

When loose dentures cause gum soreness, Violetta says she puts some Painalay on a cotton swab and dabs it on her gums. "I'm Scotch, so I don't like to waste any of it," she says. "By the next morning, the soreness is usually gone."

But Painalay wasn't the only over-the-counter medication mentioned by our respondents: Anbesol, Listerine and hydrogen peroxide all received votes.

Over-the-counter products will reduce pain, but the need for repeated use may mean you need new dentures, says Dr. Watt. "Those are all short-term palliative remedies that can help you if you have a sore or until you can get to the dentist. Most times, however, dentures will not cause large sores unless they don't fit."

EDITOR'S NOTE: *Hydrogen peroxide should not be used to heal mouth sores. "It kills too many good bacteria and could allow yeast and fungi to grow," says Dr. Watt. "We need friendly bacteria in our mouths to help fight the bad bacteria."*

BAKING SODA POPS THEIR CORK

Baking soda tops the list of suggested cleaners for stained dentures. In fact, one 84-year-old woman is so fond of baking soda that she says she won't use anything else.

While baking soda is great for removing tea, blueberry and other stains from dentures, bleach is better for removing odors, says Dr. Watt. "If your primary goal is to remove stains, baking soda is better," he says. "If your primary goal is to detoxify and deodorize dentures, then bleach is the best choice. Some people have much more odoriferous mouths than others, and, for them, baking soda doesn't quite get the job done. Bleach will take away most of the protein and other things that get stuck in dentures and cause odor."

After filling a denture pan with water, Dr. Watt says to add a teaspoon of bleach and set the dentures inside. Be careful with the bleach, however; too much will actually remove the pink coloring of the dentures, he says. Also: Be sure to rinse the dentures thoroughly in water before putting them back in your mouth.

HER FINGERS DO THE TRICK

One woman says massaging her gums with her fingers helps relieve soreness caused by denture problems.

"Massaging will increase circulation and help remove some of the swollen tissues, but if you need finger massage often, you may need to have your dentures checked," says Dr. Watt. "Probably the dentures don't fit very well and you are getting more swelling than you should."

Depression

Recipes to Chase the Blues

There's no doubt life has its ups and downs. Our survey takers understand that. These are spunky people who have lots of little ways to chase away their personal rain clouds—from visiting friends who are worse off to practicing a plaintive violin solo, from taking a solitary walk through the woods to indulging in a garage sale shopping spree.

They make it clear that what cheers up one person may be the exact opposite of what works for someone else. "Hard work" is an upstate New York man's way of pulling out of the dumps. A Texas woman, on the other hand, prefers being pampered by her hairdresser.

Serious depression—the kind that lingers for days and prevents you from functioning—requires professional help. But here are a number of suggestions for pulling out of a common case of the blues.

THEY SHAKE A LEG

The number one depression antidote? More than one-third of survey participants recommend exercise as a good way to blast through the blues, and several emphasize the importance of exercising outdoors—rain or shine, hot or cold—to suck in some fresh air, embrace the elements and commune with Mother Nature.

"I'm prone to come home from work, sit down in front of the TV and eat all night long, which isn't productive and just makes me feel bad," says Pat, of Clear Lake, Texas, a drafting supervisor for an oil refinery. "To counteract that, I'll take a walk, not to work up a sweat but to relax and calm down. I'll stroll around the neighborhood, looking at people's gardens. This always gives me a boost of energy, so that when I get back home I'm ready to go tackle some project."

"I started walking because of heart problems, but I found that it really improved my mood," says Shirley, 57, of Cordova, California. "I feel like I am doing something good for myself, for starters, but simply being physically active made me feel more alert and relaxed."

How might exercise block the blues? Well, medical researchers say that it increases norepinephrine, serotonin and dopamine. These brain chemicals, which transmit messages between nerves, are thought to be low in depressed people. Regular aerobic exercise also boosts endorphins—naturally occurring feel-good substances produced in the brain. And it might simply boost self-esteem.

THEY BET ON THEIR PETS

If you don't have enough get-up-and-go to get out the door, you might do with a little encouragement of the canine sort, says one California woman.

"Having a dog that adores you is the best antidepressant I know of," she says. Several other people also rely on their pets for an enthusiastic rousing. "How could I not get up in the morning, when this creature is jumping all over me in the bed?" one explains.

HARD WORK IS HIS ANTIDOTE

"I like exercise as much as the next person, but I figure there are more productive things I could be doing," says Richard, 62, an upstate New York construction worker and building contractor. "I can get a good workout hammering nails or cutting trees and have something to show for it when I'm done."

The trick to using work as a mood elevator, he says, is to "find something you are really interested in and enjoy—not busy work—and concentrate on it. It lets you loose emotionally, and as far as I'm concerned, that's the best therapy there is."

HOBBIES HELP THEM

On the other hand, you may need something that takes your mind off work. Several people mention hobbies as pleasant ways to distract themselves from depression—everything from doing crossword puzzles to gardening and feeding the birds.

"There's not much mystery to it. It takes your mind away from unproductive thinking and allows you to create something," explains Frank, 45, an Indianapolis postal worker who enjoys crocheting and painting.

"I get lost in books," says Margie, 71, of Irving, Texas. "I often read four or five hours a day, and I take books along with me if I'm going someplace where I will probably have to wait. I even read in the car. I'll read just about anything, but I especially enjoy travel books. I can't afford to travel much, but at least I can fantasize, and that takes my mind off my troubles."

PAMPERING PEPS HER UP

"Treat yourself like you matter." That advice from several survey participants takes many forms, including eating better, resting and saying no when overwhelmed by requests.

"I tend to get depressed when I am overworked, because I tend to neglect myself," explains Pat, of Texas. "I'll go to the hairdresser and have my hair done. I like the attention I get, having people fuss over me, and I look better when I'm done, so I feel better."

HE TAKES A DOSE OF MUSICAL MEDICINE

The power of music to transform moods is common knowledge. Several of our survey participants say they use music to lift their spirits, boost their energy or soothe their frazzled nerves.

"I lost my wife about seven years ago, and that floored me," says Stan, 77, a Lebanon, Oregon, jack-of-all-trades. "It took me three or four years to get over it, and I wouldn't say I am fully over it. I simply didn't know what to do. If it wasn't for television, I would have gone crazy. Finally, I dug out my old violin, refurbished it and started practicing. I now spend two or three hours a day doing that. It took a lot of perseverance at first. I sounded like I did when I first picked up the instrument—awful—but I kept at it, and now, I feel I sound better than I did when I was young. It has inspired me."

Other people listen to music—everything from oldies-but-goodies to classical and New Age. Experts say that slow, quiet, nonvocal music generally lowers heart rate and respiration, while the faster variety heightens alertness and arousal. Exactly how music affects us remains a mystery. But at least part of the thrill of music may come from the release of endorphins—those opiate-like substances that induce euphoria.

THEY GOTTA HAVE FRIENDS

What's your security in a storm? For many of the people we talked to, it's friends—people who will listen, love, help you to laugh at yourself and the world, and, when asked, offer a bit of wise advice.

"Although I can always count on the members of my family to stick by me, they tend to react to problems the same way I do and to have the same fears and worries," explains a 43-year-old New York woman. "If I talk with my mother about something that's troubling me, for instance, I often end up feeling worse, because she is so anxious about things. That's why I turn to my good friends. They have a different perspective on things; they are not so quick to judge or to offer unwanted advice. They know how to listen, and that's why they are my friends. There is no substitute for the help they offer, and I try to do the same for them."

Experts say that talking about upsetting or traumatic experiences, as difficult and emotionally distressing as it may be, can lead to improved mental health.

Realize that it takes time and effort to build supportive relationships, then get to work, suggests Ellen McGrath, Ph.D., chairperson of the American Psychological Association's National Task Force on Women and Depression and author of *When Feeling Bad Is Good.* "Do everything and anything you can to develop the skills it takes to have quality relationships," she says. That includes learning communication skills, improving self-esteem and taking time to be with people.

SHE ADVISES BEING A FRIEND

Remember that old adage, "A friend in need is a friend indeed"? That's a saying that Judi, 52, a school food services manager from Goodland, Kansas, has taken to heart.

"I believe that if you sit at home by yourself, you feel even more depressed, while if you do things for people who need help, you feel better about yourself," she says.

So she spends time with an older friend who has health problems. "She is pretty much housebound unless someone comes to help her get out, so that's what I do," Judi says. "We will go shopping for groceries, or just do something to get out. She likes to tell me about her problems, and I don't mind listening, because it helps me put my life into perspective. I feel like my own troubles aren't so bad, after all. I never get down listening to other people's problems."

Experts point out that altruism—doing unto others—may actually lead to a longer life. And its opposite—hostility—has been linked to heart disease.

LAUGHS LIGHTEN THEIR LOAD

How many depressed people does it take to change a lightbulb? A hundred and one. One to change it and 100 to worry about doing it right.

Our survey participants seek out humor wherever it can be found. Silly cartoons, Steve Martin movies and old "Saturday Night Live" reruns were all mentioned as sure chuckle inducers. And one woman's suggestion— "surround yourself with people with a sense of humor"—has helped her to look on the light side of life.

"I'm the administrative director of a day care center, and we have to deal with parents, teachers, and state officials, not to mention children, every day," says Joan, 56, of San Jose, California. "I think I'm pretty good at laughing at things, and I like to be around people who are the same way. If you can't laugh when a child spills ketchup on you, you're in pretty bad shape."

SHE SPICES UP HER LIFE

Is there such a thing as mood food? Several people mention carbohydrates or caffeine as a way to favorably alter their brain chemistry. And one woman swears that hot chili peppers cheer her up.

"If I'm feeling down, I go out for a good shot of hot peppers or hot salsa with corn chips," says Merry, 42, of Pensacola, Florida. "In fact, my husband and I have been doing this for years, and it works for both of us. We'll eat hot Chinese food—the place we go leaves in the hot peppers for us—or Mexican food. I feel like my mood is elevated shortly after eating the food, and that feeling lasts for a few days."

Compounds from hot chili peppers are used topically to reduce pain. It's possible eating chili peppers intensifies people's perception of taste, and like other depression relievers, it, too, triggers the body's release of feel-good chemicals, or neurotransmitters.

POSITIVE SELF-TALK TURNS HER AROUND

Are you your own worst critic? Listen in on your thoughts, and you may hear a lot of negativity that, unconsciously, may be darkening your mood: "I can't do that." "I shouldn't have said that." "I'll never be able to get that done."

Becoming aware of these thoughts and then replacing them with the kinds of thoughts that allow you to get on with your life is a form of psychological therapy called cognitive (thinking) therapy or restructuring. It's what Ruth, 49, of Granger, Indiana, turned to when it seemed like she was at her wit's end.

"I had a lot of stuff going on that I didn't think I could handle," she says. "My husband died, I had two teenage boys, I was trying to finish a master's degree in social work, and I had financial problems. I could hear myself saying, 'I can't handle this.' I'd read about cognitive therapy and started to turn in on my thoughts and to deliberately replace them with others. I'd think something like 'Okay, this is a difficult situation, but there are things that I can do about it. Here's what they are . . . ' Then, I would write them down. Staying conscious of what I was thinking helped me to stop being so discouraged and fearful. It helped me to figure out what I needed to do and then do it."

Diabetes

Keeping Blood Sugar under Control

et's get something straight from the very first sentence: If you've been diagnosed with diabetes, you need to be under a doctor's care. This is important no matter what kind of diabetes you have—whether you are insulin-dependent (called Type I) or have the adult-onset version (Type II).

That said, however, there are many doctor-recommended approaches for improving the way your body handles the sugar in your blood. These approaches, which you can institute yourself at home, include losing weight, exercising and eating more fiber and less fat and sugar.

Our survey takers are well aware of all these medically approved methods of keeping their condition under control. And they've come up with all kinds of hints and tips to smooth the way. All of them say they feel healthier since starting their antidiabetes regimen.

DIET DOES IT FOR THEM

Eating right is by far the favorite method named by our survey takers for getting their diabetes under control.

A former chocaholic, Dorothea's dietary victory over diabetes received a seal of approval from no less than her doctor. "He told me that if everyone did like me, he wouldn't have any customers. He said, 'You still have diabetes, but you've conquered it,' " says the 76-year-old Gainesville, Florida, professional dog groomer.

Dorothea found herself with a case of Type II diabetes. But rather than taking medication, she asked her doctor if dietary changes would do the trick. He gave her six months to try working with just her diet. The dietary changes that she instituted did, in fact, bring the condition under control without medication. That was 20 years ago, she says, and she's still eating a carefully planned menu of several small, healthful meals a day.

Dorothea's six-meal-a-day schedule goes something like this: for break-

᪑ᴥᴥ

156

fast, cereal and whole-wheat toast and fruit; a midmorning snack of low-sugar, low-fat cookies and a small glass of nonfat milk; a turkey sandwich and a piece of fruit for lunch; a midafternoon snack of nonfat yogurt; for dinner, boiled cabbage with potatoes and ham; and half a cantaloupe for an evening snack.

"All my meat has to be baked, boiled or broiled," she says. Among vegetables, mixed and green beans are her favorites.

And as for chocolate: "Once I couldn't pass any of it by—now I can't stomach it. If I get the least bit of sugar, just a taste of it, I get sick to my stomach."

Don't be surprised at Dorothea's progress. Studies show that diets high in complex carbohydrates—whole grains, fruits and vegetables—help improve blood sugar control.

Beverly was insulin-dependent for eight years before failing eyesight frightened her into enrolling in a class taught at a local hospital to learn more about her condition. (Poorly controlled diabetes can lead to impaired vision and even blindness.) When graduation day came, the Jacksonville, Florida, resident got more than a diploma—she acquired a road map to a more healthful life. "I really got into it," she says.

Today Beverly faithfully eats six small meals a day, avoids fat and exercises regularly. So far, she's lost 25 pounds. "I loved margarine, mayonnaise, fried food, but I just can't have them anymore," she says. Beverly even shuns lean beef because she's noticed her blood sugar goes up dramatically after eating foods like steak or hamburger. When she does eat meat, she chooses buffalo, reportedly extra low in fat.

Whether burgers immediately boost blood sugar may be debatable, but researchers have found that foresaking meat may help people avoid the devastation of diabetes.

Overall, both Dorothea and Beverly are incorporating sound strategies that have been found to reduce diabetic symptoms or prevent them altogether, says Byron Hoogwerf, M.D., staff endocrinologist at the Cleveland Clinic Foundation in Cleveland. "The most important thing to remember is that 80 percent of those who have Type II diabetes are obese. But something about losing weight reduces blood sugar. And you don't even have to get to a 'normal' body weight. Even losing some weight is beneficial. Fifteen pounds in some people can have a profound effect on blood sugar."

And while eating more meals seems to help level out volatile blood sugar in those suffering from Type II diabetes, cutting fat may be the best way to trim extra pounds, he says. "If I've got two minutes with a patient, I say you have to cut the fat and start here: red meat, cheese, dairy products and many snack foods. And, really, you can't eat out as much—there's too much fat in restaurant food."

EXERCISE GETS THEIR ENDORSEMENT

Sore, swollen ankles may not seem like a benefit—but they may have been one of the best things to happen to Alleyne's health in over a decade. A visit to the doctor to discover the cause of the swelling led to a diagnosis of Type II diabetes. And that, in turn, motivated the Clifton, Texas, resident to lose 51 pounds—and get her condition under control. "The doctor said, 'You've got diabetes, but I've got news for you. You can do something about it,' " she recalls.

After her diagnosis, Alleyne attended a six-week course at a local hospital that described how to reduce her diabetic symptoms through exercise and diet. And while exercise is difficult for her—the retired 71-year-old has a nerve problem in her leg that makes walking painful—Alleyne spends several hours a week sweating over her garden. And that's exercise by any measure.

Remember Beverly? She boosted her exercise program (she already walks a half-hour in the evening with her husband) by buying a combination ski/rowing machine. "I got tired of my exercise bike, so I gave it to my daughter," she says.

To speed weight loss and decrease diabetic symptoms, nothing beats working up a sweat, says Dr. Hoogwerf. "If you look at successful weight reduction, there are several things that are important," he says. "Key features are keeping accurate food records—so you can tell how much fat you are eating—and a regular exercise program, at least 30 minutes every other day."

HERB TEAS EASE THEIR SYMPTOMS

Laura still hasn't told her doctor about the sage tea she drinks to help bring her blood sugar back to normal. But she didn't mind telling us. "You know how doctors are—they don't want you taking anything that they haven't given you," says the 67-year-old retired medical attendant.

After suffering from Type II diabetes for seven years, the Detroit resident read about the benefits of sage tea and decided to give it a try. The hard part was finding some: Sage tea sells out as quickly as it arrives at her local health-food store.

Laura says she brews enough tea for a day by spooning three tablespoons of leaves into a Thermos and adding three cups of hot water. The amount she drinks depends on her blood sugar level. If it registers over 200, she'll probably have three cups that day; midway, probably just one. Less than 100? She'll skip the tea altogether.

A year after she made her first one-pound purchase, Laura is a bigger believer in sage tea than ever. That's because her doctor has cut her daily dose of prescription diabetes medication in half since she began taking the tea. "You still have to eat right, but that sage tea will bring your blood sugar down," she says.

Although sage tea may be associated with feeling better in dealing with diabetes, there's no overwhelming proof that it directly affects blood sugar, says Dr. Hoogwerf.

Touted through the ages as a successful treatment for more than 60 health problems, sage tea was found in at least one study to be effective at reducing the blood sugar of those suffering from diabetes.

SHE SINGS THE PRAISES OF GINSENG

Marilyn became a believer in the healing power of vitamin and herb supplements several years ago when they helped her husband recover from a serious liver problem.

As a result, Marilyn is constantly on the lookout for the latest health information. So when the Oneida, New York, resident read that ginseng would prevent her blood sugar from climbing, she decided to give it a try. "They say there is an herb for everything," she says. "This one really keeps my blood sugar down."

Marilyn purchases ginseng capsules at her local health-food store and takes one to three a day.

Ginseng has been prized for centuries for its role in maintaining health. What's more, experts have documented that ginseng is "useful" in helping to control diabetes, according to Varro E. Tyler, Ph.D., a professor of pharmacognosy in the School of Pharmacy and Pharmacal Sciences at Purdue University in West Lafayette, Indiana, and author of *The Honest Herbal.*

THEY GIVE B VITAMINS STRAIGHT A'S

With her ten-year-old son experiencing some of the symptoms of diabetes—like excessive thirst and urination—and a history of the disease in the family, Regina wasn't taking any chances.

The St. Augustine, Florida, mother of three learned of a health practitioner who prescribed natural remedies for many illnesses and set up an appointment. After examining her son Luke, the practitioner recommended a single 50-milligram vitamin B_6 tablet each day.

The result a year later, according to Regina: "I really feel like it has staved off diabetes. Now he's really healthy."

Gone are the child's excessive thirst and need to go to the bathroom, says Regina. "We've always tried to practice preventive medicine, and it's paid off," she says.

Violeta, a 43-year-old from McMinnville, Oregon, says she uses brewer's yeast—a supplement rich in B vitamins—to manage her blood sugar levels.

"It was really bad at one point," she says. "I was having headaches, I was always in a bad mood and my body felt tired."

After reading books about diabetes and hypoglycemia (low blood sugar), Violeta says she started taking two tablespoons of brewer's yeast mixed with grapefruit juice between meals three times a day. She also changed her diet to exclude refined foods, replacing them with whole grains and vegetables. "I'm in perfect health now. I've never been better," she says.

There is some evidence to suggest that people who suffer from diabetes may benefit from B vitamins, but more research is needed, says Dr. Hoogwerf. "I don't think there's any clear evidence that B vitamins necessarily improve blood sugar control. My bias is that, when people start working at things and become concerned about their health, they initiate other changes that may have benefits along with taking vitamins, like improving their diet, exercising and changing their lifestyle," he says.

Scientific studies have shown that vitamin B_6 may be beneficial in treating diabetes and its complications. Some people with diabetes are B_6-deficient, and for them B_6 supplements may be helpful.

Brewer's yeast contains such nutrients as thiamine, riboflavin, biotin, folic acid, selenium, and chromium and is sold in health-food stores.

EDITOR'S NOTE: For all its purported merits, experts say that taking more than 50 milligrams of vitamin B_6 daily can be toxic and can cause nerve damage. If you'd like to try B_6 supplements, discuss it with your doctor.

Diaper Rash
Protecting Tender Bottoms

Diapers certainly are one of civilization's praiseworthy inventions, and if you doubt that for a single moment, imagine life without them. Yes, diapers are worth it, even if it means putting up with an occasional sore bottom.

Diaper rash starts out as red, irritated skin, but it can turn nasty, causing the skin to break down if it's not treated promptly. It occurs when a baby's tender bottom remains in contact with urine or feces for too long.

Diaper rash can be averted, but it requires some diligence. "You really have to stay on top of it, especially if a child has diarrhea or strong urine," says Connie, of Voluntown, Connecticut. She should know. "When my children were young, I took care of them and other people's children during the day, and I once had five babies, all in diapers, to care for. I spent most of my time changing diapers."

Here's what she and others say puts diaper rash on the run.

THEY BARE THOSE BUNS

What's rarer than dandelions in December? A newborn nudist with diaper rash.

Fresh air and sunshine help heal diaper rash, while wet diapers encased in plastic pants set the stage for a full-blown case, experts say.

A number of people recommend laying the baby on a diaper and letting its bottom air-dry for a time before rediapering.

"We call this an air bath, and babies just love it," says Becky Luttkus, head instructor at the National Academy of Nannies in Denver. "It really is a good way to prevent or cure diaper rash, and it even helps to clear up yeast infections, which are often the cause of stubborn cases of diaper rash."

To prevent baby's skin from becoming so dry that it cracks, smooth on a bit of moisturizer or diaper rash cream before airing, suggests Al Lane, M.D., associate professor of dermatology and pediatrics at Stanford University Med-

ical Center in Stanford, California. "You want the skin to retain some moisture, but you don't want it exposed to excess moisture," he explains.

BLOW-DRYER WORKS WONDERS

Not all parents have the time or the place for an air bath, but some
moms have employed this quick and handy alternative—blow-dry baby's
bottom.

"I use the blow-dryer on myself sometimes to get really dry, and it works
well; so I figured, why not use it on the baby, too?" says Terri, 34, a first-time
mother from Towson, Maryland. "She likes it, I'm careful, and it seems to
help prevent diaper rash. I imagine it would be especially helpful if the
baby's bottom is too sore to dry well with a towel."

*EDITOR'S NOTE: Safe blow-drying depends on a low temperature setting, keeping
the blower at least ten inches away from baby's skin, and keeping the air moving back
and forth. "And I'd apply some moisturizing or diaper rash cream to keep the skin
soft and flexible," adds Dr. Lane.*

THEY LAY IT ON THICK

Ointments that shield a baby's petal-soft skin from urine and feces can
help clear up a case of diaper rash, but experts caution that they are not a
substitute for promptly changing a soiled diaper.

"I've never found anything better than Desitin Ointment put on directly after washing and drying," says Connie. "I've used it to help clear up
some bad cases of diaper rash." Desitin is 40 percent zinc oxide—a thick
paste with weak antiseptic properties, which also acts as a physical barrier to
irritants and absorbs moisture.

White petroleum jelly and A and D Ointment, which contains fish liver oil
and petroleum jelly, also got a few votes. "I learned about A and D Ointment
when I worked in a hospital nursery as a nurse," says Diane, 59, of Williamsburg, Pennsylvania. "It cleared up diaper rash faster than anything else we
tried, so I was sold on it. I also used it on my six babies with good results."

Dr. Lane is partial to a particular product himself. "I recommend
Aquaphor Natural Healing Ointment, a petroleum-based moisturizer that
is less gooey than most diaper rash ointments." This fragrance- and preservative-free cream from Beiersdorf of Norwalk, Connecticut, is recommended for dry, cracked skin and minor burns.

*EDITOR'S NOTE: Creams you'll want to avoid using on diaper rash are those that
contain steroids. Used regularly, these creams can inhibit tissue growth, which can
increase the likelihood of skin irritation and other problems, Dr. Lane explains.*

ANTIYEAST CREAMS MAY HELP

Some of our survey takers recommend Gyne-Lotrimin as a home remedy for diaper rash. Gyne-Lotrimin is an over-the-counter cream normally used to treat vaginal yeast infections, not diaper rash.

Both Luttkus and Dr. Lane give a thumbs-up to Gyne-Lotrimin or other yeast-fighting creams in cases when diaper rash has been diagnosed as being caused by a topical yeast infection.

"This is most likely to occur in children who are being treated with antibiotics, often for ear infections, and it's often the cause of stubborn cases of diaper rash that persist for more than five days despite normal treatment," Luttkus says. Red, raised bumps distinguish a yeast-caused rash from regular diaper rash.

POWDERS GET SOME VOTES

Plain old cornstarch wins its fair share of votes when it comes to preventing diaper rash and comes out on top among powders. "Clean thoroughly, dry, and then apply cornstarch," directs one survey taker. "Cornstarch is a lot cheaper than baby powder and works just as well," says another.

Both our experts, however, say they believe creams are far superior to powders when it comes to preventing or curing diaper rash.

"Powder is useless at protecting the skin as soon as it absorbs some moisture, and it does that within a few minutes of being applied," explains Luttkus. In fact, studies by British researchers show that talcum powders do nothing to treat diaper rash.

EDITOR'S NOTE: Experts worry that babies who are dusted regularly will inhale particles from the powder, which could lead to congestion or lung problems. "And babies have died from breathing in powder when they pick up a bottle of the stuff and put it to their mouths," Dr. Lane says.

"We tell nannies that if Mom or Grandma insists on powder, to sprinkle just a bit in their hand first, then rub it on the baby," Luttkus says. Parents like their babies to smell like babies; that is, like baby powder, she explains. "A little cologne that smells like baby powder would be safer."

CHOICE OF DIAPERS CAN MAKE A DIFFERENCE

"If you can, double-diaper with cloth and leave off the rubber pants," suggests one woman. "Cloth diapers work just fine if you change them as soon as they're soiled," adds another. It seems disposable diapers just weren't popular with our survey takers.

Dr. Lane, however, points out that, in one study, superabsorbent disposable diapers, which contain absorbent gelling material, came out on top, resulting in less diaper rash compared with cloth or regular disposable diapers. So if you're battling a severe case of diaper rash, you may want to switch to superabsorbent disposables for the duration.

VINEGAR RINSE REDUCES RASH

"If you're old-fashioned and use cloth diapers, add ¼ cup or so of white vinegar to the final rinse," suggests a Rochester, Minnesota, grandmother who's cared for four children and nine grandchildren. "It's no substitute for cleanliness, but it's one more thing you can do to prevent diaper rash." Several other people also said a vinegar rinse helps to nip diaper rash in the bud.

In fact, professional diaper services carefully control the acidity of their wash solutions, Dr. Lane says. Rinsing the diapers in a slightly acidic solution helps to destroy any lingering bacteria.

Diarrhea

Fighting the Intestinal Flood

W hen Paul urges Timothy in the Bible to "use a little wine because of your stomach," he may well be recommending an
early diarrhea preventive. At least that's what some biblical scholars think.
They suggest that Paul wanted Timothy to switch from drinking plain water
during his missionary journey in China to a beverage less inclined to contain the bacteria that causes diarrhea.

People are still taking wine and fruit juices to treat this troubling intestinal disorder. Our survey takers recommend both blackberry "wine"
and apple juice for relief.

Though created by such diverse causes as parasitic or bacterial infection, excess magnesium (found in some antacids), antibiotics, and the inability to digest milk products, diarrhea is often nothing more than
increased water in the stool. But rather than get caught in the proverbial
flood, our survey takers say they've learned to treat diarrhea on their own.
Here's how they do it.

THEY FIND FRUITS INTESTINALLY FRIENDLY

Wild blackberries have tamed the upset tummies of four generations of
Valerie's Baxter Springs, Kansas, clan. "If you had diarrhea at Grandpa's
house, he would get some blackberries out of the freezer and either give
you three or four tablespoons of juice or a bowl of them with some sugar on
it," says the 34-year-old housewife. In fact, blackberries worked so well for
Valerie that a sudden case had her rummaging through her mother's
freezer for relief last summer. "Usually one serving does it," she says.

Miriam, of Dayton, Ohio, says she finds blackberries better at stopping
diarrhea than either yogurt or acidophilus (the culture found in yogurt
that comes in tablet form), two other common home remedies. "After undergoing intestinal surgery and taking antibiotics for an infection, I developed chronic diarrhea," she remembers. "I took yogurt and acidophilus

capsules to restore the beneficial bacteria in my intestines and that helped somewhat, but I was still running to the bathroom. I remembered hearing people say that blackberry wine could stop diarrhea. Since I don't like wine, I decided to try blackberries. I ate blackberries that I bought frozen, and this seemed to control the diarrhea."

Ervin, of Unityville, Pennsylvania, shares this recipe for blackberry wine, passed down, his wife thinks, from his mother: "Take four quarts of wild blackberries for each gallon. Crush the berries. Pour in a gallon of boiling water. Let it stand for 24 hours, add three pounds of sugar to each gallon, then strain the juice from the berries. Wait until the formula starts bubbling, then bottle it."

Apples also rate as a favorite fruit remedy. "In severe cases, I start with apple juice and chicken broth," says one. Says another: "For my young children, I peel and grate an apple and let it stand on the plate until it turns brown." (No mention on how she gets her children to eat brown apple mash, however.) Others say simply that they eat an entire apple with the skin on.

Old-fashioned fruit remedies may have actually inspired today's over-the-counter antidiarrheal preparations, says William B. Ruderman, M.D., chairman of the Department of Gastroenterology at the Cleveland Clinic Florida in Fort Lauderdale. "Remember that a lot of medications have been developed based on remedies that people have used over the years. Kaopectate, an over-the-counter antidiarrheal, contains pectin, which is found in fruits like apples and blackberries and seems to be very useful in treating diarrhea."

From the same plant family, both apples and blackberries have a tradition of use for diarrhea dating back at least as far as ancient Rome. Pectin, a water-soluble fiber which can bind bile acids and cholesterol in the intestines, is found in many fruits, vegetables and seeds. Blackberry leaves also contain tannins, which could serve as an intestinal astringent.

THIS BUNCH LIKES BANANAS

Brenda had never tried bananas for diarrhea until her pediatrician recommended them for her son Blake. Now, she won't use anything else. "He doesn't believe in putting chemicals into babies," says the 30-year-old Goldendale, Washington, resident. "He only tries the most natural remedies first."

Because Blake is a bit on the stubborn side, Brenda simply handed over a couple of bananas to her 18-month-old. By the end of the day, he'd eaten the bananas and his diarrhea was gone, she says. "It's hard to know whether it was the banana working or just his body, but it was gone," she says.

Slipping bananas into your diet when you have diarrhea adds important fiber and potassium, says Dr. Ruderman. While fiber helps sop up excess water, helping firm your stool, potassium is a chemical essential for metabolism, he explains. Some who suffer from diarrhea can develop low levels of potassium, which bananas can help replace.

EDITOR'S NOTE: Adding fiber to your diet to help fight diarrhea can be dangerous if the diarrhea is accompanied by vomiting. If you have both these symptoms, it's best to see your doctor before trying any home remedy.

HER KEY IS YOGURT

A professional piano teacher, Lori knows a sour note when she hears one. So when her stomach starts rumbling from a case of diarrhea, the 47-year-old Oak Brook, Illinois, resident reaches for a cup of nonfat yogurt. "It seems to settle my stomach," she says. "In fact, it's probably the only thing I can handle when I have something like a stomach flu."

Andrew Weil, M.D., associate director of the Division of Social Perspectives in Medicine at the University of Arizona College of Medicine/Arizona Health Sciences Center in Tucson and author of *Natural Health, Natural Medicine,* says he takes acidophilus tablets with meals when he travels to help prevent getting traveler's diarrhea. Thought to help control the balance between friendly bacteria and bad bacteria in the digestive tract, acidophilus can also be found in yogurt. Check the label before you buy to make sure your yogurt contains live acidophilus cultures. Acidophilus tablets are available at most health-food stores.

SHE DOES DOUBLE DAIRY

Unable—and perhaps unwilling—to write a prescription for her son's diarrhea, Gloria's osteopath gave her something even better: a home remedy made from cottage cheese and sour cream that she says she's used successfully for 40 years.

"It worked like a charm and we really haven't used anything else since," she says. "One of the best things about it is that you have nothing to lose— it can't do you any harm."

The Melbourne, Florida, resident says she simply combines two tablespoons of cottage cheese in a dish with two teaspoons of sour cream and eats the mixture three or more times a day for as long as she has the problem. "I wouldn't say I can take it just once and that's the end of it," she says. "How much I eat depends on the severity of the problem."

The double dairy approach is new to Dr. Ruderman. "I'm not aware of this particular remedy, nor any medical reason for it to be effective as a cure," he says. While its benefits are uncertain, Dr. Ruderman says there is no reason you shouldn't use it if it makes you feel better. For people with lactose intolerance, however, eating dairy foods may actually make the diarrhea worse.

BLAND IS BEST

Experts say a bland diet is among the best remedies for an acute attack of diarrhea, and many of our survey takers agree.

To cure her son of a bout of diarrhea, Shirley's 75-year-old Czechoslovakian grandmother suggested pouring a few cups of rice into a pot of water and allowing the rice to soak until the water became milky. The 57-year-old eighth-grade English teacher strained out the rice and let her son drink the rice water. "By the next morning, he was holding his food," she remembers.

Alice, of Portland, Oregon, conducts estate sales on the weekend, helping folks dispose of unwanted personal belongings. But no one has to sell her on homemade potato soup's potential for stopping diarrhea. Alice says her mother would mix up a batch and serve it to her if she came down with a case when she was a child. "Way back when, they didn't have access to drugstores," says the 68-year-old. "By trial and error, they had to think of their own remedies."

Alice says her mother's potato soup recipe is fairly simple: "She'd slice up a potato real thin, cover the slices with water, add a little salt and pepper, and cook until the potatoes were real soft. Then you'd eat a cup or two for lunch and dinner and within a day, you'd be feeling better."

Doris, a 73-year-old Northport, New York, resident eats plain toast to treat diarrhea. "My father was a doctor and my mother was a nurse, and for bilious attacks, as he called them, that's what he recommended," she says.

Doris says she substitutes two pieces of dry toast and a cup of tea for meals and drinks a lot of water to avoid becoming dehydrated. As her symptoms subside, she adds other soft foods like scrambled eggs, grits and oatmeal to her diet.

Rice and rice milk, potatoes and plain toast all have something in common. They are all excellent choices for a bland diet, which can be helpful in combating diarrhea, says Dr. Ruderman. "With an attack of diarrhea, I tell my patients to start with drinking only clear liquids. If they see improvement, then I tell them they can start eating bland foods," he explains.

"It's difficult to say why this type of diet helps you when you're suffering from diarrhea, but we know that a bland diet of complex carbohydrates has less fat, it's easier to digest and it may be more readily absorbed. So it's less taxing on an already stressed digestive system," he says.

In fact, the United Nation's World Health Organization recommends serving rice flour dissolved in water to infants suffering from diarrhea and malnutrition in developing countries.

If you want to go whole hog on bland foods until your diarrhea quits, Dr. Ruderman recommends sticking with the "BRAT" diet—bananas, rice, apples and toast and progressing to a broader diet as you improve.

CHARCOAL CHASES HER DIARRHEA AWAY

You probably won't find "Burned Toast" next to "Tension Tamer" or "Raspberry Patch" in the tea aisle of your local health-food store, but according to Denage, of Colora, Maryland, that might not be a bad idea. The 45-year-old former U.S. Army engineering technician says drinking a mixture of burned toast and water works for stopping diarrhea every time. "It's quick, easy and cheap," she says. "I'm not kidding, it usually works within an hour."

To make the tea, Denage purposely burns a piece of white toast and then scrapes the charred surface into a cup. She then adds hot water and lets the mixture sit for about five minutes before drinking it. She does not drink the crumbs, however.

Denage says she learned about the remedy from her Aunt Edna. And where did Aunt Edna learn about it? She finally tried burnt toast tea after her husband used it successfully for years. "She didn't believe it until she got desperate and actually tried it," says Denage.

Charcoal is known to be adsorbent, meaning that if bacterial toxins are the cause of the diarrhea, they could be attracted and held by the charcoal, says Varro E. Tyler, Ph.D., professor of pharmacognosy at the School of Pharmacy and Pharmacal Sciences at Purdue University in West Lafayette, Indiana, and author of *The Honest Herbal.* This would make the toxins less active. While Dr. Tyler doesn't feel that scraping toast would provide an adequate dose of charcoal, it certainly wouldn't hurt and may even be modestly helpful.

Diverticulosis

Keeping Those Pockets Cleaned Out

Refined table manners are one thing, but when you're eating refined foods, your colon may not display its best party manners. In fact, it may become downright difficult.

Eating mostly refined or highly processed foods, which contain little fiber, puts so much pressure on the muscular walls of your colon (as you try to pass hard, dry stools) that they can develop little pouches, called diverticula. This can result in gas, cramping, severe indigestion and alternating diarrhea and constipation.

"I tell people to compare their bowel to a tube of toothpaste," says Stephen B. Hanauer, M.D., professor of gastroenterology at the University of Chicago Medical Center. "When the tube is full, it requires almost no pressure to get the toothpaste to come out. But when the tube is almost empty, you've really got to squeeze."

If feces get stuck in these pouches, internal bleeding and serious infection can occur. This condition, called diverticul*itis*—meaning inflammation—requires prompt medical attention and, sometimes, no solid food at all for a few days. So if you have diverticulosis that seems to have gotten worse and if you have pain and tenderness in the lower left side of your abdomen, see a doctor without delay.

Our survey takers are big fans of fiber. Some of them learned the hard way, however, what it takes to head off a bout of diverticulosis.

THEY FEAST ON FIBER

"Fiber, fiber, fiber—psyllium and bran. Both soluble and insoluble." You could pay a doctor $50 for those choice words of advice, or if you live in Clayton, Georgia, you might get it for free over the fence if you live near Jo, 81, a retired registered nurse and Peace Corps volunteer.

"I had an attack of this years ago," she says. "I read up on it, and as a result, started eating more fiber." One way she assures she gets enough each day is by downing a sort of fiber cocktail, composed of a cup of orange juice and a rounded teaspoon each of wheat bran, oat bran and Metamucil—an over-the-counter bulk laxative that contains both soluble and insoluble fiber.

The soluble fiber—the kind found in apples and other fruits—keeps stools soft and moist, aiding smooth passage. The insoluble fiber—found in whole grains—adds bulk and so decreases pressure on the colon walls, explains Dr. Hanauer.

"I guarantee you won't be bothered with diverticulosis if you do this every day," Jo says. She believes this regimen also helps protect her from colon cancer. "Both my mother and father had colon cancer, and I am determined not to get it," she says.

Most people get only about 16 grams of fiber a day, about half the amount they should eat, says Marvin Schuster, M.D., chief of the department of digestive diseases at Francis Scott Key Medical Center in Baltimore. (For example, an apple offers 3 grams of fiber, a whole-grain cereal 4 to 6 grams.) Cooked, dried beans, whole grains, and most fruits and vegetables are good fiber sources. Increase your intake gradually over a period of six to eight weeks to minimize gas and bloating, experts advise.

They Steer Clear of Seeds

Remember those little pouches? Well, it seems that foods that contain seeds or hard particles can be particularly irritating to those areas, sometimes becoming lodged in the pouches. Our survey takers say they avoid popcorn, corn, peanuts, poppy and sesame seeds, figs and blackberries.

"It's true that people often say they avoid all sorts of seeds, but there's no proof that the little seeds, such as poppy, fig or sesame seeds, contribute to diverticulosis," Dr. Hanauer says. "I'd be more likely to recommend people avoid larger particles, such as peanuts, corn and sunflower and pumpkin seeds, along with grape or watermelon seeds."

These foods are usually not chewed completely, and so large particles from them move through the bowel without ever being digested. Instead of nuts or seeds, people can safely eat nut or seed butters, he adds.

Fluids Help Fiber Work Wonders

With all the fiber they're packing away, our survey takers know that drinking plenty of fluids is a necessity. Fluids keep the fiber soft and slippery, so it passes through with less assist from the colon walls. "I drink at least eight to ten glasses of water a day," reports one woman. "Lots of raw bran and water works for me," states another.

"I normally rely on cooked cereals, fruits and vegetables for my fiber, but if I'm eating something dry, like rye crackers or whole wheat bread, I'll drink something along with it," says Nancy, 56, a Chapel Hill, North Carolina, middle school teacher who suffers from both diverticulosis and hemorrhoids.

LAXATIVES HELP SOME

Several survey takers say they use laxatives to treat diverticulosis, including bulk laxatives such as Metamucil; stool softeners, which work by maintaining moisture in stools; and stimulant laxatives, such as senna, which work by increasing bowel contractions. One woman even says her mother takes coffee enemas to relieve symptoms of diverticulosis.

"My doctor told me to take a stool softener if I became constipated, but to try to prevent becoming constipated by eating bran," explains Anna, 61, a Tallahassee, Florida, retired schoolteacher who has had diverticulosis for six years. She says the stool softener does work and has prevented painful episodes.

Bulk laxatives are safe for continual use, Dr. Hanauer says. "I don't commonly use a stool softener, however, except in the case of constipation," he adds. And stimulant laxatives or enemas should be reserved for only occasional use, since regular use can make the bowel dependent on them, he says.

EDITOR'S NOTE: Products marketed as herbal or natural laxatives, such as senna and cascara sagrada, can be just as strong and irritating to the bowel as over-the-counter drugs. You should not take laxatives on a regular basis, unless your doctor tells you to, as you can become dependent on them.

Dizziness

Stop the Spinning

Getting dizzy when you were a kid wasn't just a cheap thrill. It was an afternoon-long extravaganza of goofiness, whirling around the backyard with your best friend until you both collapsed in a giggling heap.

For most adults, however, dizziness is anything but fun—it's an upsetting and often dangerous sign that something is wrong with a portion of the body's balance center.

Some episodes of dizziness can be avoided simply by remaining motionless with your eyes focused on a steady point or changing your medications. Other causes are more difficult to treat and may require a visit to your doctor, says Jim Buskirk, director of physical therapy at the Dizziness and Balance Center in Wilmette, Illinois. One example: an ear infection that knocks your body's balance control center—located in your inner ear—off-kilter.

If you're experiencing dizziness and can't pinpoint the cause, it's best to see your doctor. Otherwise, consider what our survey takers say brings their internal spinning to a stop.

SHE TOUTS BIOFLAVONOIDS

It had become Margaret's morning ritual: After waking up, she'd sit on the edge of her bed, waiting for her head to stop swirling before she dared take a step.

The feeling was unsettling all right, but as far as her doctor was concerned, Margaret was going to have to learn to live with it. She'd experience dizziness as long as she had low blood pressure—and that was that.

Then one day, the Fall River, Massachusetts, resident picked up a health magazine and began to read. In a letter to the editor, a woman who claimed she'd spent thousands of dollars trying to find a cure for her dizziness reported success after taking bioflavonoid capsules, made from the nutrients found in the white peel of citrus fruits.

Margaret was thrilled—but she had no idea what bioflavonoids were. "I had to write down the name on a piece of paper because I had never heard of them before. I didn't even know how to pronounce the word," she says.

After a visit to her local health-food store—"I basically ran there"—Margaret began taking two 1,000-milligram tablets a day, as recommended on the bottle. Within two days, her morning dizziness was gone, she says.

That was nearly 15 years ago. Margaret hasn't had a dizzy spell since. Is it the bioflavonoids? "Are you kidding—I wouldn't go without them," she says.

And what do the experts say? Low blood pressure has been linked to dizziness, says Buskirk, but whether bioflavonoids can improve circulation is far less certain.

"Low blood pressure would cause her to feel light-headed and off-balance because she would not get enough blood flow to the head," he says. "Whether the bioflavonoids helped in this case or not is another matter. In my opinion, it was probably coincidental."

EDITOR'S NOTE: Although championed by a Hungarian researcher who won a Nobel Prize for discovering vitamin C, bioflavonoids have a checkered history in the United States. Once prescribed by doctors here to treat circulatory problems, bioflavonoids were abruptly withdrawn from the pharmaceutical market by the U.S. Food and Drug Administration (FDA) in 1968. The FDA felt there was insufficient evidence that the nutrient was effective. Doctors in other countries continue to use bioflavonoids to treat circulatory problems like varicose veins and night cramps. Found in fruits, vegetables, nuts and seeds, bioflavonoids are still sold as supplements in U.S. health-food stores.

HER EYES HAVE IT

How severe was Daphne's dizziness? For nearly six weeks, just rolling over in bed made her feel like she was riding a merry-go-round. "I had to hang on to the headboard for fear my body was going to fly out in the room," she says.

Daphne's doctor says her dizziness was caused by an inner ear infection, and he gave her a prescription to combat the dizziness while she waited for the virus to end. Instead of taking the medication, however, she taught herself how to end her dizzy spells. "This is just something that I worked up on my own because I don't like taking a lot of drugs," says the retired, 63-year-old Dorland, Texas, secretary. "If I kept my eyes straight ahead and my head perfectly straight and balanced for maybe a minute or two and really concentrated, the dizziness would go away."

Daphne couldn't find a better remedy for her condition if she went to a specialist, says Buskirk. "That's what we typically teach people to do to stop an acute dizziness attack—to stare straight ahead. When she keeps her eyes still and focuses on a point straight ahead, she's shutting off the inner ear balance system. But this is only blocking the symptom," Buskirk says. "Long-term cure requires a doctor's care." For temporary problems, like if you're out on the waves in a boat or in a car when dizziness strikes, staring at the horizon works just as well.

The same theory applies for those moments when too many cocktails have launched you into orbit—usually after lying down. Simply putting your feet on the floor is a giant step away from dizziness. "Alcohol is toxic to the inner ear balance system—it knocks it out," says Buskirk. "Putting your feet on the floor when you're in that condition, however, takes over for your inner ear balance system and helps gives you an awareness of where you are."

DEEP BREATHING DOES IT FOR HER

Lucille says she became so used to her bedroom spinning every few months that sometimes she would literally roll over, go back to sleep and take the day off. "Even standing up and turning around too quickly was enough to cause the problem sometimes," she says.

Although Lucille was taking medication that could have caused her dizziness, the Lawrence, Kansas, resident learned that taking occasional deep breaths helped get her through the experience. "I think getting more oxygen has a positive effect," says the 86-year-old.

Staying still probably helped more in this case, says Buskirk, but the deep breathing might also have been beneficial. "If you have any type of balance system problem, when you start to feel dizzy and light-headed and like you're going to start spinning, you become very anxious and panic. So anything you can do to relax yourself—like deep breathing a few times—would be to your benefit."

GINGER GIVES HER RELIEF

Six strokes left Edith suffering from intense vertigo, nausea, vomiting and low blood pressure . . . and with little hope. But the Desert Hot Springs, California, resident says daily servings of ground ginger helped turn her life around.

"I could only take about ten steps at a time. Then I read a small article about ginger helping motion sickness. I figured, 'What do I have to lose? I'm already dizzy and nauseated all the time.' So I started taking one table-spoon of ground ginger in hot water, like tea, once a day. You have no idea what wonderful relief! I am now able to sit and walk around the house and read voraciously. There must be something in the ginger."

Edith is actually onto something. Medical researchers have found that ginger in any form—tea, candy, capsules, powdered, even ginger ale—can help alleviate the symptoms of motion sickness, including dizziness.

A PILL A DAY . . .

Every summer, Sammy and his wife hitch up their travel trailer for the 50-mile drive to Roaring Springs, Texas, and the annual family reunion. But before he goes, Sammy makes sure he's got a bottle of an over-the-counter antinausea medication called Emetrol on board. "When I'm sleeping in that trailer at night and the wind starts blowing, and it starts moving around, I get dizzy," he says. To make sure that doesn't happen, Sammy says he takes a teaspoon or two of Emetrol liquid a day before the trip and continues until he gets home.

He's also found Emetrol effective at preventing dizziness if he goes boating or has to ride in an elevator. "I don't remember if someone suggested it, but I've been using it for many years," he says.

Another survey taker reported using Dramamine—a common over-the-counter motion sickness medication—to treat dizziness.

If he had to choose between Dramamine and Emetrol to treat dizziness, Sidney N. Busis, M.D., clinical professor of otolaryngology at the University of Pittsburgh School of Medicine, says he'd pick Dramamine.

"Emetrol has been around for years, primarily for vomiting. But if it works, fine," says Dr. Busis. "Dramamine, Marezine, all the over-the-counter medications like that, do a much better job of suppressing the balance system which, if malfunctioning, can cause dizziness. Of course, the best of all is to find the source of the problem and deal with that."

Dry Eyes

Getting Back Those Tears

Tears aren't just an annoying sign that you're a softie. They're an important part of your body's defense system. The film of moisture that covers your eyeball each time you blink, or that floods your eyes when they're exposed to irritants, helps to cleanse and protect your eyes. Tears even contain the same infection-fighting immune cells that are found in your blood.

Even the slightest breeze or waft of cigarette smoke can be searingly painful when your eyes lack the ability to wash away airborne irritants. Dry eyes are more likely to become infected, too, since any irritants or bacteria that land in the eyes tend to stay put, rather than being washed away or destroyed.

Here's what our survey takers say works best when their eyes are dry. Do note, though, that if you have pain or blurred vision along with dryness, it's time to see your eye doctor—the sooner the better.

ARTIFICIAL TEARS KEEP THEM MOIST

"I use a brand of lubricating eyedrops, called Tears Plus, three or four times a day, whether I think I need them or not," says Ceil, 74, whose dry eyes problem began when she moved from the humid Northeast to Albuquerque, New Mexico, some years ago. "I use the drops in the morning and at night and sometimes during the day if I'm reading or watching television and my eyes start to feel dry. It keeps them from getting uncomfortable."

Choosing the right kind of drops for dry eyes is important, experts point out. Stay away from those containing tetrahydrozoline, a drug that clears up redness by causing little blood vessels to constrict. "They can be irritating to dry eyes," cautions Eric Donnenfeld, M.D., associate professor of ophthalmology at North Shore University/Cornell Medical Center in Manhasset, New York. Instead, he says, choose over-the-counter eyedrops that contain a mixture of saline (a salt solution) and some type of film-forming substance, such as polyvinyl alcohol or synthetic cellulose.

People with severe dry eyes should also use only preservative-free eye-drops, he adds, since preservatives can also irritate eyes. "I suggest people try three or four different formulations of eyedrops and then stick with those that work best for them," says Dr. Donnenfeld.

NIGHTTIME OINTMENTS KEEP ORBITS OILED

Some people who rely on artificial tears during the day switch to a heavier-duty eye-moisturizing method at night—an ointment that contains oils, lanolin or polyethylene glycol (a synthetic substance similar to lanolin).

"I don't like to use the ointment during the day, because it tends to blur my vision for a while, but at night, I'll often put some in," says Marion, 45, a commercial artist from Tarrytown, New York. "It makes for more comfortable sleeping, and my eyes seem to feel better in the morning."

These nonprescription ointments are good for moderate to severely dry eyes, Dr. Donnenfeld says.

EDITOR'S NOTE: Artificial tears and moisturizing ointments are okay to use, but if you find yourself reaching for them often, you need to see an eye doctor, says Dr. Donnenfeld. A number of physical conditions can make your peepers feel like they're stranded in the Sahara, as can decongestants, tranquilizers, antihistamines and drugs for high blood pressure. Getting rid of dry eye may be as simple as switching your medications. If you suspect your medications may be causing a problem, discuss it with your physician before making any changes on your own.

COMPRESSES HELP MOISTURIZE

"When my eyes are really bad, I lie down with a warm washcloth across them for about ten minutes, three times a day," says Ruth, 60, a retired real estate firm owner from Barrington, Illinois. "It makes my eyes feel better."

Heat helps to open clogged oil glands in the eyelids, which, like tears, lubricate eyes, Dr. Donnenfeld says.

Some people also said they use cool compresses and find them equally helpful.

"Especially during the summertime, when the heat and dust is bothering me, rinsing my face and eyes with cool water, cupped in my hands, then using a cool, wet compress relieves my dry eyes," says Edith, 58, a former ranch owner from Lubbock, Texas.

"Cool is good when your eyes are red and irritated from dust or allergic reactions," Dr. Donnenfeld says. Allergy-aggravated eyes are more likely to water, but it's possible that they will become dry, he explains.

SHADES SCREEN HER EYES

"I don't go anywhere on a sunny day without my sunglasses," says Pamela, 40, an outdoors enthusiast who's had a problem with dry eyes for the last two years. The glasses protect her dry eyes from direct breezes, which can evaporate moisture on the surface of the eyeball.

"Any kind of glasses are helpful, but the wraparound kind really work the best," Dr. Donnenfeld says. Glacier glasses, which have leather shields on the sides, provide even better protection.

In addition to wearing glasses, you can minimize eye dryness by making sure you point automobile air vents away from your eyes and keep a humidifier in your bedroom, especially during the dry winter months, Dr. Donnenfeld adds.

THEY SCRUB THEIR PEEPERS

About half of the people who suffer from dry eyes have "crusty" eyes when they wake up or at other times of the day. This condition, called blepharitis, is actually an inflammation of the glands and lash follicles along the margins of the eyelids. It's thought to be caused by a bacterial infection, and severe cases are treated with antibiotics. "People with certain kinds of acne or dandruff are most likely to develop this problem," Dr. Donnenfeld says.

Washing the eyelids helps to keep this condition under control, and that's exactly what our survey takers recommend.

"I simply rinse my eyes out with warm water, and if they're really bad, I'll use some eyedrops," says Eileen, of Faukville, Wisconsin, a custom cookie-cutter maker whose dry eyes are a result of an immune problem.

"I wash my eyelids each morning, using a special soap that's made just for this purpose," explains Ruth. "I wash my face first, then simply use my fingertips to wash my eyelids."

Saline solution, baby shampoo, even diluted dandruff shampoo (if you're careful not to get it into your eyes!) can all be used to clean eyelids, experts say.

Dry Mouth

Methods for Wetting the Whistle

Adry mouth feels thick and tacky—like you've been chewing on cotton. If you have a dry mouth, it's hard to swallow, to talk properly, and especially, to plant a big wet one on a waiting cheek. And since saliva helps wash away bacteria, a dry mouth sets the stage for dental decay.

"In my experience, no one seems to care much if you have this problem," laments a California woman. "They just tell you how lucky you are you don't have something more serious, then go on to tell you about all their health problems!"

A dry mouth can simply be the result of aging. "Saliva volume decreases as we age, and saliva also tends to become thicker," explains Michael Benninger, M.D., chairman of the Speech, Voice and Swallowing Committee of the American Academy of Otolaryngology, Nose and Throat Surgery, and chairman of the Department of Otolaryngology, Head and Neck Surgery, at Henry Ford Hospital in Detroit.

Dry mouth problems can also result from radiation treatments for head or neck cancer or from Sjögren's disease—an immune system disorder that damages glands, including those that produce saliva and tears.

There's no good substitute for the real thing, but our inventive survey takers have found a number of ways to make "life without spit" worth a lick. Here's what they say works.

SOME SIP ALL DAY

Of course, it makes sense to drink water to keep your mouth moist, and that's exactly what many people suggest. "My mouth tends to get dry at night, and so, I keep a glass of water by the bed," says Althea, 67, a Brockton, Massachusetts, grandmother. When she wakes up with her tongue plastered to the roof of her mouth, she unglues it with a few judicious sips. "Wintertime is worst," she says.

"My mouth tends to get dry while I'm exercising, so I keep a squeeze water bottle with me and drink from that," says Renee, 46, a Cedar Rapids, Iowa, home-care nurse who enjoys hiking and biking. "The squeeze bottle is handy because I can stick it in a fanny pack or on my bike, even take it with me in the car. It won't spill if it's knocked over."

Frequent sips help some people reach their daily quota for water intake. Several people view that daily quota as essential. "I try to drink eight glasses of water a day," says Sarah, a Knoxville, Tennessee, seamstress who says she got into this habit while attempting to diet. "It's supposed to help you feel full and flush out the fat, but in fact, I think it's just keeping my mouth busy," she says.

In fact, this commonsense suggestion is about the best advice there is for dry mouth, Dr. Benninger says. "Mild dehydration is a common cause of dry mouth, because even mild dehydration can cut down on saliva production," he says. Having an optimum amount of water in your body gives your salivary glands maximum secretory power.

"Rather than counting glasses of water, I recommend you check the color of your urine," Dr. Benninger suggests. "It should be clear or very light yellow. If it is dark yellow, you are dehydrated and need to drink more. Once your urine is clear, there is no need for additional water."

Don't count on alcohol or caffeine-containing beverages such as coffee or tea to boost your body's moisture content, either. "These drinks act as diuretics. Ultimately, they draw fluid from your body, making it drier," he says.

SOUR CANDIES MAKE MOUTHS WATER

A number of our survey participants say they rely on sour-flavored candies such as lemon drops to keep their salivary glands active. "My doctor suggested I use sugar-free lemon drops to help keep my mouth moist, and I find they do work," explains Viola, 72, a Dayton, Ohio, retired bookkeeper who figures she goes through about six lemon drops a day. Her dry mouth problems seemed to begin around menopause and slowly got worse.

"Stimulating saliva flow is another good way to treat dry mouth, and there's no doubt that lemon is a powerful stimulant," Dr. Benninger says. He also recommends adding a bit of lemon juice to the water you may be sipping or enjoying an herbal tea with lemon.

SHE SUCKS A PEBBLE

Lemon drops weren't easy to come by when Edith, 53, a Louisville, Kentucky, accountant, was a child. "We'd be playing out in the woods or working in the fields and might not have a source for good water, either," she says. Solution? An old American Indian remedy. "I'd put a small, smooth, clean pebble in my mouth and suck on that. It does get the saliva flowing and temporarily alleviates your sense of thirst," she says.

"Yes, sucking on a pebble will increase saliva flow," Dr. Benninger agrees. "Even if you have a chronic disease that is causing this problem, anything that stimulates the saliva flow will improve things."

PROPER BREATHING BRINGS RELIEF

There's nothing like a steady breeze to dry your sheets—or your tongue.

While breathing through your nose actually moisturizes and filters the air that enters your lungs, breathing through your mouth is terribly drying, not just on your mouth but on your throat and lungs as well. Several people say they take antihistamines or decongestants to keep their noses open so they can breathe.

"I tend to breathe through my mouth at night," says Wilbert, 67, an assistant shoe store manager from San Pedro, California. "I don't take a decongestant every night, but I take one when my nose gets really closed up." Wilbert believes he has several good reasons to have trouble with his nose. He lives in a very polluted area just south of Los Angeles, he has allergies, and he's had his nose rearranged by a mugger.

EDITOR'S NOTE: Antihistamines and, to a lesser extent, decongestants can cause mouth dryness, Dr. Benninger says. To minimize this side effect, "take an antihistamine only if allergies are causing your stuffy nose, and then take the lowest effective dose." If your congestion is not allergy related, take an oral decongestant, he recommends. Avoid nasal sprays, because your nose can quickly become dependent on them to stay open. You could also try a saline spray. Then you don't have to worry about becomming dependent on it.

ARTIFICIAL SALIVA ADDS MOISTURE

"I use Xero-Lube, a nonprescription aerosol spray, when I wake up at night and feel like my mouth has been cemented shut," says Joyce, a Warren, Texas, woman who has Sjögren's disease. "I'll simply spray the inside of my mouth and my lips. It definitely retains moisture better than water."

Xero-Lube, Salivart and similar products are artificial salivas—preparations designed to mimic natural saliva, both chemically and physically. They contain minerals such as calcium and phosphate ions. Some also contain fluoride.

HUMIDIFIER GOES WITH HER

Only one woman says she complies with Dr. Benninger's number one suggestion for this problem: Use a humidifer. That person is Joyce, also, and she uses a portable cool mist humidifier that she can carry with her from room to room. "It's very dry and dusty where I live, and this definitely does make things more tolerable," she says.

You don't have to live in Texas to experience shrivel-up-and-dry conditions. "A nonhumidified home in the Northeast in the wintertime can be as dry as the Sahara Desert, and that dry air just sucks the moisture out of you," Dr. Benninger says. He recommends keeping a humidifier in your home, particularly in your bedroom at night, and setting it at 35 to 40 percent humidity.

Dry Skin

Techniques to Defeat Dryness

He came, he saw, he scratched. While there's no question Sir Winston Churchill helped rally the English and the Allies from the brink of disaster to crush the Nazi war machine, he seemed to have less success overcoming dry skin.

"This tickle is quite intolerable," Churchill told Lord Moran, who recorded the conversation in his diary. "It kept me awake. Yes, a bloody night. The skin man has given me fourteen ointments or lotions in turn without any theory behind any of them. Just doling out some potion or unguent to keep me quiet. It's a disgrace to the medical faculty."

Although he didn't know it at the time, Churchill's dry winter itch was probably caused by using too strong a soap and not enough moisture, says Jerome Z. Litt, M.D., a Cleveland dermatologist and author of *Your Skin: From Acne to Zits.*

But before you declare war on your own dry skin ("I shall fight it in the bathtub, I will fight it the shower . . . "), consider how our survey takers handle the situation. Here's what they do.

SHE USES EUCERIN

A redhead with pale skin to match, Susanne suffered from extremely dry patches on her arms, legs and face for years. When the condition became particularly bad, she asked her doctor about a solution. He suggested Eucerin, an over-the-counter lotion containing mineral oil and lanolin. It worked. "I noticed a difference right away," says the 47-year-old Yakima, Washington, convenience store owner. "I put it on twice a day, morning and night."

Eucerin works as well as a $50 jar of face cream she bought at a department store cosmetic counter and costs under $10 a bottle, she says.

Eucerin does contain some key ingredients for keeping skin moist, says Dr. Litt. But before you put on Eucerin—or any other moisturizer—you need to prepare your skin. Among the first steps: making certain there's enough moisture in your home by using a humidifier.

"I tell people when their windows fog up over 40 percent humidity—that's just about right, particularly if you live in northern, wintry climes," he says. "No one in the tropics has dry skin because the relative humidity is high."

Next, bathing in lukewarm water 15 to 20 minutes a day will help "plump up" your skin with moisture. A mild liquid soap like Cetaphil lotion or Moisturel cleanser helps clean without drying, he says.

Finally, pat dry only with a soft towel and then apply the moisturizer. This helps seal in the moisture that keeps your skin from drying out, he says. "Glycerine, mineral oil, these are great at keeping in the moisture. Lac-Hydrin Five, another over-the-counter product, also works well," he says.

HE BORROWS A REMEDY FROM THE COWS

A retired corrections officer and farmer, Ernie has a practical approach for treating dry skin on his hands and feet. He says nothing beats Bag Balm—a petroleum-based rub designed to soothe cow udders.

"When the mother cow is nursing, sometimes she'll get bruised, so you'll put that on her to make her feel better," he says. "That's probably how people started using it on their hands. They'd put that on there with their own hands and it would soothe their dry skin."

After rubbing Bag Balm on his dry feet, Ernie says he pulls on some old wool socks to prevent the rub from getting on his bedsheets.

"I've never used Bag Balm myself, but I know a lot of good dermatologists who recommend it, and people love it," says Dr. Litt. (Bag Balm contains lanolin and an antiseptic.)

SHE VOTES FOR VASELINE

About 15 years ago, a wizened old doctor shared some words of wisdom about beating dry skin that Marcia has never forgotten. "He was on the verge of retirement, and he said all you have to do to keep calluses from building up and keep the skin from cracking is rub some Vaseline on your feet," says the Midland, Michigan, day-care center operator. "And if you have any left over, you could rub some on your knees and elbows."

Though the physician passed away a few years ago, Marcia still uses his treatment.

"If I take a bath and get ready for bed, I'll rub on some Vaseline and put on some socks. It was an excellent tip," she says. "I have no problem with cracking."

EDITOR'S NOTE: Vaseline works well at keeping your elbows, knees and feet lubricated—just don't put any on your face, says Dr. Litt. "Vaseline will clog the pores on your face, no question about it," he says.

MAKE HERS HAWAIIAN

A massage therapist, Janie traveled to Hawaii for some training. While touring the big island, she stopped at a store selling locally produced goods. There, among the macadamia nuts, she discovered kukui nut oil, a liquid moisturizer she spreads on her face, shins and hands to keep them from becoming dry.

"It's like vitamin E, but I think it's a little better because it doesn't have that thick feeling and absorbs more quickly than vitamin E," says the 45-year-old Pottstown, Pennsylvania, resident. "It has a very subtle fragrance, very pleasurable, almost uplifting."

After bathing, Janie spreads kukui nut oil on her dry spots. And if she's going outside in cold weather, she spreads an extra coating on her face.

So far, Janie hasn't found kukui nut oil on the mainland but intends to order another batch through the mail.

Although he's never heard of kukui nut oil, Dr. Litt says he would never pooh-pooh such a suggestion. "We're all unique. Everyone responds to different things," says Dr. Litt. "So I tell my patients, if you find something that works for you, then use it."

According to Randolf Wong, M.D., plastic and reconstructive surgeon and director of the burn unit at Straub Clinic and Hospital in Honolulu, kukui nut oil has been a traditional skin-moisturizing method among Hawaiians for hundreds of years. Despite its history, scientists are just beginning to do clinical studies with the oil.

"I am quite excited by the future prospects of kukui nut oil," says Dr. Wong. "We know that it is effective at moisturizing, but we need more scientific data to say why it works so well. I've used it myself for dry skin, and it worked for me. It soaks in quickly, with none of that heavy, greasy feel of a lot of lotions."

If you'd like to try kukui nut oil, you can mail order it. Contact Oils of Aloha, P.O. Box 685, Wailua, HI 96791, for information.

Ear Pain

Approaches to Ease the Pain

Your ear may be tender and itchy. Or it may feel full and near bursting. Whatever the specific symptoms, the one thing all earaches have in common is pain.

Ear pain can come from an infection in the outer canal or in the middle ear, located just behind the eardrum; from blockages caused by swelling or mucus; or from exposure to cold.

Any earache that persists for more than a few hours calls for medical attention, experts say. Even though home remedies may temporarily ease the pain, they won't necessarily cure the problem. They're best used in addition to medical treatments.

Eighty-two survey takers offered a total of nine different home remedies for earaches. Many of their suggestions involve warming up the ear, one way or another.

In fact, gentle heat is very effective at temporarily easing some kinds of ear pain, doctors say. "Warmth tends to increase blood flow to the area, and that relieves pain," explains James Donaldson, M.D., a physician at the Seattle Ear Clinic and professor emeritus at the University of Washington School of Medicine, also in Seattle.

A BLOW-DRYER IS BETTER THAN A BUTT

"My mother-in-law told me she used to blow cigarette smoke into her children's ears to stop earache pain," says Pat, 41, an assistant manager for a blood bank in Cincinnati. "She said it wasn't the smoke, but the warm air that did the trick. She suggested I use a blow-dryer as a source of warm air."

Pat tried the dryer the next time her child had an earache and found that it worked well. "It's important to keep the dryer on a low setting and hold it far enough from the ear to prevent burning," she says. "I didn't have to do it long—just a minute or so relieved pain for a few hours."

EDITOR'S NOTE: To avoid cooking an already painful ear, doctors advise keeping the blow-dryer at least 18 inches away from the ear and moving it slightly back and forth, as you do when you're drying hair. And be sure it's always on the lowest setting.

HOT SALT PACK WORKS FOR HER

"When my kids had earaches, I used my mother's remedy, because I knew it had helped me," says Margaret, a hardware dealer in Granite City, Maryland. "She'd fill a tightly woven handkerchief with about ¼ cup of table salt, wrap a rubber band around it to make a little ball and warm it up in a low-temperature oven. I'd lie down with my ear on the handkerchief, and it seemed to just draw out the pain."

Experts say that the only magic quality to salt, at least in this instance, is that it retains heat well. Two other people recommended this remedy as well, with a very slight variation—using a clean sock to hold the salt.

WARM OIL PROS AND CONS

Thirteen people suggest a popular old-fashioned remedy—putting drops of warmed-up vegetable oil, such as olive oil, into the ear canal.

"I always got earaches when I was a little girl," says Carna, 53, a Zion, Illinois, telephone company engineer. "My foster mother would warm up some cooking oil in a little saucepan on the stove and then, with an eyedropper, put two or three drops in my ear. Then she'd insert a bit of cotton into the ear to keep in the oil overnight."

The oil had an immediate soothing effect, Carna recalls. Usually her earache was gone by morning, when the cotton was removed.

Other survey participants offered variations on the same method. One woman suggests mixing olive oil with tea tree oil (*Melaleuca alternifolia*), available at some health-food stores. "It's nature's antiseptic," she claims. In fact, Australian researchers are investigating tea tree oil's apparent antibacterial properties.

EDITOR'S NOTE: Check with your doctor before trying the warm oil technique. If you have a perforated eardrum, the oil could seep into the delicate middle ear.

And even if your eardrum is intact, Dr. Donaldson has one reservation about this method: "If the oil coats your ear canal, your doctor may need to vacuum or flush it out in order to see your eardrum. That can be an extremely painful process requiring a local anesthetic."

He suggests you stick with a source of heat that doesn't require insertion in the ear. "A heating pad, hot water bottle, hot washcloth—almost anything will work," he says.

In fact, our survey participants offer all those suggestions, along with simply cupping your hands over your ears to retain body heat.

HUG-AN-EAR WORKS FOR BUSY GRANDMA

Nancy, the wife of a retired farmer who lives in Hendrum, Minnesota, offers a variation on the "body heat" remedy. She is now a grandmother, and she took care of her two grandchildren from the time they were born until they started school. "One of the children had terrible colds and ear-aches," Nancy recalls. "Of course, he'd see the doctor, but to relieve the pain, I'd do something my own mother did with me when I was a child. I'd hold him, putting one hand over his ear and pressing the other ear against my chest.

"This was not only comforting to the child, but the heat was very sooth-ing. If I could, I'd have the child lie with me on the bed while I cupped his head against my chest. Sometimes that was the only way either of us got any rest!"

If her own ears hurt, Nancy rests in a reclining chair, rather than lying on the bed. "It helps my sinuses to drain, and keeps my ears open," she says.

In fact, some doctors say the reason so many different home remedies seem to relieve earaches is that administering the remedy requires the per-son to sit up in bed, at least temporarily. "Simply elevating your head at least 20 degrees above a horizontal position makes your eustacian tubes work better and equalizes the pressure," Dr. Donaldson says. The eustachian tubes are tiny passageways that lead from the throat to the middle ears, sup-plying that part of the ear with the air needed to function properly.

FOR "AIRPLANE EARS," DECONGEST

Air travel can cause intense ear pain, especially if congestion or inflam-mation from a cold or an allergy has blocked the eustachian tubes.

But four people told us that using an over-the-counter nasal deconges-tant helps prevent problems with "airplane ears."

"I always had problems with my ears when I flew," reports Teme, an Ar-lington Heights, Illinois, woman. "Now, when I fly, I start taking deconges-tants before I leave. I haven't had a problem in almost three years."

The reason? When a eustachian tube is blocked (as it is when you're congested), the air pressure inside your ear can't equalize with the pressure outside your ear. This can become a problem when an airplane is descend-ing. Even though most commercial airliners are pressurized at 5,000 to 8,000 feet, there is still a fairly rapid pressure change as the plane descends.

As a result of the difference in pressure, the thin tissue of the eardrum is stretched, causing pain. But if you take a decongestant that clears the eustachian tubes, the pressure is equalized and the eardrum tissue relaxes.

EDITOR'S NOTE: Some ear experts recommend a decongestant that contains the ingredient phenylpropanolamine hydrochloride. (Contac Maximum Strength and Triaminic Cold Tablets are two examples.) They advise taking a 50-milligram dose at least one hour before your first descent.

Most doctors, however, recommend a long-lasting nasal spray containing oxymetazoline hydrochloride, such as Afrin, Neo-Synephrine Maximum Strength or Dristan 12-Hour.

"I tell my patients to take one spray of Afrin on each side of the nose about one hour before their first descent and then a second spray in each side ten minutes later,"" says Dr. Donaldson. It's the second spray that relieves the ear pain, he explains. "The first spray opens the nose. The second one shoots way back and shrinks all the mucous membranes." When you spray, you should be sure to inhale deeply, he adds.

BUBBLE GUM FOR MOM, BOTTLE FOR BABY

Chewing, sucking or yawning also help prevent in-flight ear pain, our survey takers report. Experts say that's because each time you swallow or open your mouth to yawn, your eustachian tubes open briefly, which helps keep them clear.

"I chew gum or suck on Life Savers while I fly to keep my ears open," says Carl, a 32-year-old Norfolk, Virgina, private pilot. He adds that he doesn't take decongestants when he's at the controls because they make him drowsy.

Infants too small to handle gum or hard candy can create the same ear-clearing motion by nursing. "To relieve a baby's ear pressure while flying, try giving him a bottle of his favorite milk or juice or plain water," suggests Tina, a Sumter, South Carolina, mother of two. "I used this method when I took two infants on a long flight from Columbia, South Carolina, to Portland, Maine, with stops in just about every city in between. It really helped."

Doctors add another tip: Prop your baby up a bit while he feeds. That helps to direct the milk to the stomach rather than into the eustachian tube.

A FREQUENT FLIER BLOWS AWAY EAR PAIN

"I use a special technique I read about in a magazine called the modified Valsalva maneuver. It keeps my ears open every time," reports a frequent flier from New York City.

Experts say this simple procedure helps keep the eustachian tubes open and equalizes pressure in the middle ear. To do it, hold your nostrils closed by pinching them together right near the bottom. Then blow gently so that your nose balloons out slightly. Begin doing this as soon as you feel pressure build in your ears. You can repeat the procedure each time you feel your ears clogging up.

If you have a cold, though, blow your nose the normal way first to clear it. Once you start the modified Valsalva maneuver, you want to be blowing air, not mucus, toward your ears.

EDITOR'S NOTE: *Experts warn that once ear pain has set in, it becomes harder and harder to open your eustachian tubes by any method. That's because the same vacuum that tugs your eardrums also sucks the eustachian tubes closed, collapsing them. So take measures to keep your ears open the minute the plane begins to descend. If you're not sure when the plane will start its descent, ask a flight attendant.*

COVER UP WHEN IT'S COLD

Earmuffs on a windy day in May? Yes, if you're one of those people whose ears are so sensitive to cold that even a cool spring breeze can start them aching.

"Some people's ears are extremely sensitive to cold," Dr. Donaldson says. "Cold may cause a painful blood vessel spasm in their ears, perhaps as the result of a prior infection." For these people, keeping the ears warm becomes a priority.

But what do you do if you have cold-sensitive ears and you live in northern Idaho, where midwinter temperatures can drop to 30°F below zero? "I wear a felt wool cap with an attached scarf that comes down over my ears," reports Marie, who with her husband tends a large grain farm. "It's much warmer than a knit wool cap. The wind can't blow through it."

IF YOU HAVE A COLD, BLOW GENTLY

For some people, head colds and earaches always seem to go together. That's the way it was for Millicent, a Philadelphia saleswoman, until she figured out how she was contributing to the problem.

"When I'd blow my nose, I would really blow hard," she says. "I thought that was the best way to do it." Then she read in a magazine that such nose-blowing blasts can push germ-laden mucus into the eustachian tubes, setting the stage for a middle-ear infection. Her technique has become more genteel as a result.

"Now, I blow gently, leaving both nostrils open instead of squeezing them shut," she says. "I started doing this three years ago, and I haven't had an ear problem since."

Earwax

Ways to Come Unplugged

Earwax does have merit. It has bacteria-fighting properties that help prevent infection. Plus, it traps dirt and grit before they enter your ear. There's a lot of good in that goo.

Too much of a good thing, however, and you've got a problem—a thick plug of earwax can cause discomfort or hearing loss. Our survey takers offer a host of home remedies for getting unplugged.

THEY OIL IT

Oils of all kinds—sweet, mineral, even olive—won a hardy endorsement for efficient earwax removal during our survey.

Married 48 years, Rusha and her husband have shared nearly their entire life together. So it's no surprise that they share the same remedy for earwax buildup: sweet oil. "Yeah, they say that the longer you're together, the more you're alike," says the 65-year-old Paintsville, Kentucky, resident. "I guess it's true."

After placing a few drops of sweet oil in her ear, Rusha allows it to remain for about a half a day. The sweet oil apparently loosens the wax, which she says she carefully removes with a cotton swab. "You have to tilt your head to one side to make sure the oil gets in," she says. Available at most drugstores, sweet oil also soothes earaches, she says.

Marie, 54, of Paradise, California, says she uses warm olive oil, not only on her pasta, but as an ear wash, too.

Mineral oil meets Joyce's earwax removal needs. The 61-year-old Spokane, Washington, resident says she carefully cleans her ear with a cotton swab dipped in the stuff, and after allowing the oil to remain for several hours, she rinses her ear with warm water and then swabs the area again.

It's no wonder our survey takers are enthusiatic about using oil on their earwax, says Charles P. Kimmelman, M.D., a professor of otolaryngology at

New York Medical College in Valhalla and attending physician at Manhattan Eye, Ear and Throat Hospital in New York City. "This remedy has been around since ancient times. Oils like these actually help soften wax, allowing easier removal," he says. Extremely thick impacted earwax, however, should be removed by a doctor, he says.

EDITOR'S NOTE: Doctors warn against using cotton swabs to clean the ears—they could damage the eardrum. Instead, they recommend using the twisted end of a washcloth.

THEY'RE HIGH ON HYDROGEN PEROXIDE

Hydrogen peroxide has several avid supporters among our survey takers. Among them: Grace, of Tucson, Arizona.

Back in the 1940s, a European doctor who just relocated to the United States gave Grace some simple instructions that she never forgot for removing earwax.

First, he told her to warm some sweet oil and place a few drops in her ear. Follow that with a few drops of three percent hydrogen peroxide. "I can hear the oil working its way through," she says.

In fact, most over-the-counter earwax removal systems contain hydrogen peroxide and some type of oil, says Dr. Kimmelman. "The oil helps soften the earwax, while the effervescence, the bubbles, created by peroxide helps dislodge it and carry it out of the ear. But I tell my patients to use straight peroxide at home. It's less messy."

HE WASHES EARWAX AWAY

Richard, of Ithaca, New York, says he learned from his niece, who is a nurse, that warm water works as well as anything at removing earwax.

Once, when he was suffering from ear ringing and general discomfort, the 62-year-old part-time rehabilitation specialist called his niece for advice. A short time later, she arrived at his home with a water syringe, filled it with warm tap water, and gave his problem ear a gentle squirt. Within minutes, the wax flowed out and his symptoms ceased. "If she hadn't been able to help me, I would have gone to the doctor, but that took care of it," he says.

Since her house call, Richard says he's performed the warm water remedy on himself at least one other time.

EDITOR'S NOTE: Warm water works well for earwax removal, but be careful, says Dr. Kimmelman, and use a syringe made for adults. "An infant syringe or oral ir-

rigator such as a Water Pik will irrigate the ear," he says, "but any time you use force, you run the risk of damage, both from the tip of the instrument or the penetration of the stream. If it's used properly for gentle irrigation, water should dislodge the material and solve the problem."

SHE'S HOT ON HER BLOW-DRYER

When she's not coiffing her curls, one 49-year-old woman turns up the heat on her earwax with her blow-dryer. "I use it on low heat and low speed and direct the air flow into my ears," she explains.

EDITOR'S NOTE: Blow-dryers can be used for earwax and ear infections, but only occasionally, says Dr. Kimmelman. "You probably ought not to continuously apply heat of that type to the ear because you can damage it," he says. "There are so many more effective ways."

Eyestrain

Easy Ways for Soothing Tired Eyes

There's one good thing that can be said for eyestrain. It gives you the perfect excuse to stop working and rest your weary eyes.

Eyestrain isn't considered a medical term, explains Wayne Fung, M.D., ophthalmologist consultant to the Retina Clinic at the California Pacific Medical Center in San Francisco. "People use this word to describe a whole set of symptoms. They may have trouble focusing or concentrating when they are reading. They may have a dull ache in their eyes or feel the need to blink more. Their eyelids may feel heavy, or their eyes may feel like they are being pulled toward the back of the head."

People with eyestrain often feel the need to rub their eyes, or close them, or both, Dr. Fung explains. They may also need to take a break from whatever it is they are doing.

THEY LOOK AFIELD

Take Myra, 45, a psychiatric visiting nurse living in Oklawaha, Florida, for example. Her favorite fix for tired eyes is to stop whatever she's doing—usually sewing or reading—and gaze off into the distance across Lake Fay, which is right off her backyard.

"I never know what I'll see, but I am frequently amazed," she says. "Alligators and all kinds of beautiful birds are common, and I have also seen an otter swimming along on its back. Once I even saw a crane eating a black snake that must have been three feet long. The snake was thrashing around something fierce."

Myra isn't the only one who finds that focusing at a distance relieves her eyestrain. Several other people said they put down their book or needlework or turn away from their video screen to let their eyes rest on some distant, hopefully pleasant, scene.

In fact, putting aside your close work is a good way to relax your eyes, Dr. Fung says. That's because, when you're focusing on something near, the muscles that control the shape of the lens of your eye contract, pulling the lens into a rounded shape, he explains. When you focus at a distance, how-ever, the muscles relax, allowing the lens to flatten.

HE LIGHTS UP HIS LIFE

"I now use a halogen light, and I seem to be able to read for longer pe-riods of time without eyestrain," says William, 74, a retired librarian from New York City with a passion for—what else?—books. "I'll read just about anything except self-help books, which I can't stand."

Compared with incandescent bulbs, which have a warm, yellowish cast, halogen lightbulbs have a cold bluish white light that appears brighter, Dr. Fung explains. That's their only advantage, he says. "Some people don't like the intense whiteness of this light, but people who are developing cataracts or macular degeneration (age-related damage to the retina) need more light to be able to read, do fine work or even just to be able to see. So this light might be a good choice for them."

Reading by candlelight won't make you go blind, but if the light you're using is so dim you need to bring your book up to your nose to discern the type, you strain the muscles that control the position of your eyes. "Focusing this close requires the eyes to converge, or turn in toward the nose," Dr. Fung explains. That makes the eye muscles nearest your nose contract, while those by your temples are forced to elongate. The eventual result is weariness.

THEY PARK THEIR PEEPERS

"I just stop whatever I am reading or working on and rest my eyes for about 30 minutes," writes one woman. "I simply close my eyes, sometimes for just a few seconds every few minutes," says another woman whose work involves a lot of reading. "I spend a lot of time reading from a video screen, so I make a point to get up and walk around for a few minutes every hour," says Frank, 44, a Cleveland shipping clerk. "I find I work faster and make fewer mistakes if I take a breather when I need it."

Resting your eyes is easy and simple, and just about the best thing you can do for eyestrain, Dr. Fung says. Closing your eyelids allows moisture to cleanse and coat the eyeballs and allows the muscles that control focus and movement to relax.

THEY MOISTURIZE THEIR EYES

Some people do more than simply close their eyes. They may lie down and place a warm or cool washcloth over their eyes, cotton balls dipped in ice water, teabags, even cucumber or potato slices.

"I had Bell's palsy many years ago, which paralyzed the left side of my face, so now that eye is dry and doesn't shut tight when I'm sleeping," explains Joy, 71, of Warrior, Alabama. "I use drops in my eyes, and when I've been out in the sun and my eyes feel hot and dry, I'll come inside and lie down with two cold, wet teabags on my eyelids. It does make them feel better."

"Hot or cold is fine, whichever feels best for you," Dr. Fung says. "The moisture helps eyes feel better, and lying down with your eyes covered is relaxing."

The only advantage to using cucumber or potato slices over a cool washcloth, Dr. Fung says, "is that the preparation time involved may induce you to take a longer break from your work."

EYE EXERCISES EASE ACHES

Exercise can shape up just about every part of your body, so why not your eyes? A fair number of people said they do eye exercises to relieve eyestrain.

"When my eyes are tired from reading or driving, I simply roll my eyeballs, very slowly, three times in both directions," says John, 78, a retired insurance salesman from Eau Claire, Wisconsin. "I couldn't tell you for sure what it does, but I think it makes my eyes feel better fast."

Eye exercises work the same way as does rest or gazing out a window, Dr. Fung says. They allow your eye to focus farther away and so let eye muscles relax.

SHE ESCAPES MENTALLY

Eyestrain is often the result of muscle tension in the forehead and cheekbone regions, which can be caused by stress. So it makes sense to relax as fully as possible. If you're having trouble unwinding, you might like to try a relaxing visualization exercise similar to this.

"I'll close my eyes, and to get my mind off a problem, I'll imagine I am somewhere beautiful," says Regina, 47, of St. Augustine, Florida. "For eyestrain, for instance, I might see myself on a beach, watching a distant sailboat. If I am troubled, I might imagine putting my problems in a basket, then putting the basket in a stream and watching it float out of sight. Then, I'll simply watch the empty stream."

Fatigue

Pick-Me-Ups That Boost Energy

Just about all of us are tired occasionally. We come home from work too weary to do more than pry open a can of beans and plop down in front of the television. *C'est la vie.* It passes.

Some of us, on the other hand, are tired most of the time. Such constant tiredness can result from chronic health problems that drain the body's energy reserves.

Whatever the cause, our survey results show that both temporary and chronic fatigue can respond to some lifestyle adjustments—a well-timed nap, for instance, a brisk walk or a careful choice of healthful food. For each individual, finding a balance of activity and rest, work and pleasure, and give-and-take helps to restore both physical energy and a love for life.

Experts do note, however, that it's important to determine the cause of fatigue that lingers for more than two weeks. "Sleeping disorders, depression and all sorts of physical ailments can cause weariness," says Jay A. Goldstein, M.D., director of the Chronic Fatigue Syndrome Institute in Anaheim Hills, California. Many of these conditions can be helped, and with their cure, energy improves.

THEY PARK THEIR DUFFS

You're pooped? So rest. Seems like the logical thing to do, and it is the top suggestion among our survey takers. "Spend the whole day in bed," suggests one person.

"I used to push myself when I was a lot younger," says another. "But now, I find that if I take a few minutes often during the day and enjoy relaxing, swinging on my patio, I feel better."

Yet another brushes aside the idea of a carefree retired life but finds taking the occasional rest a necessity. "My husband is sick, and now I take care of him and everything else as well, so I have more to do than ever," says Doris of East Northport, New York. "There is always work to be done, but I simply can't do as much as I used to. I have to rest now and then, and I simply do."

Don't think that only the geriatric set benefit from an occasional breather. "When my little boy takes his nap, I take one, too, and I need it," says Pamela, 39, a Long Beach, California, mother and part-time graphics art designer.

"Taking a load off" by sitting down, putting your feet up or even lying down is a good way to prevent or relieve the muscle fatigue that can come after long periods of physical activity, Dr. Goldstein explains. It also relieves pressure on joints and the spine that can lead to pain and a sense of physical weariness.

EDITOR'S NOTE: If you are actually sleeping during the afternoon, allow yourself no more than an hour's worth of shut-eye, suggests Wilse Webb, Ph.D., professor in the Department of Psychology at the University of Florida, Gainesville, and one of the country's leading authorities on naps. "More time than that sets you up for problems sleeping at night. If you feel like you need more than an hour's nap, you may not be getting enough sleep at night, or you have a sleeping problem that requires medical attention," Dr. Webb says.

SOME PEOPLE GET MOVING

All things in moderation goes for rest, too. Too much time in bed can backfire badly, resulting in reduced muscle mass and endurance. That's why the flip side of adequate rest is a healthy dose of physical activity, and the people who seem to have the most energy find ways to balance both.

"I find if I go for more than two or three days without much physical activity, I begin to get sluggish and tired and even irritable, and I don't sleep well," says Bill, 43, an insurance adjuster from Fairfax, Virginia.

"I frequently don't have the chance to exercise until 7:00 or 8:00 P.M., and so I often take walks just before I go to bed," says Lynn, 40, a college administrative assistant from Newark, New Jersey. "These walks leave me feeling wonderfully relaxed, so I sleep really well."

Exercise maintains muscle mass, so you can expend energy for daily activities such as cleaning or grocery shopping without feeling exhausted, Dr. Goldstein explains. "It helps to keep your heart strong, your blood pressure normal and your lungs clear," he says. And it circulates blood through your tissues.

Many people say regular exercise gives them a sense of alertness and well-being, which translates into less stress-related fatigue. "Breaking up an afternoon of dreary desk work with a brisk walk really helps me to make the best of the hours from 3:00 to 5:00 P.M.," says Michele, 41, a freelance copy editor from New York City. Since she's on a perpetual diet, she finds a walk followed by a light snack helps her stay within her calorie count. "If I don't walk, I'll find myself reaching for sugary snacks to try to boost my energy level," she says.

In fact, exercise does appear to boost levels of "feel-good" hormones that can also help reduce feelings of fatigue, Dr. Goldstein says.

THEY EAT FOR ENERGY

Don't expect a high-energy performance if you're filling up on low-grade fuel, our survey takers caution. What's considered good fuel? Your basic good diet, from the looks of it. People recommend complex carbohydrates—such as whole grains, fruits and vegetables—and going easy on the fatty meats and sweets.

When it comes to recommending specific nutrients, B-complex vitamins and iron top the list, followed by calcium and magnesium.

"I started taking B-complex vitamins when my kids were teenagers and were driving me crazy," says Rosalee, a housewife from Grass Valley, California. "I didn't start taking them because of fatigue, but because I had read somewhere that they were helpful for stress. Now, I find that if I don't take them for a while, I start to feel tired."

In fact, all the B-complex vitamins are involved in a process called energy metabolism. They help your body convert calories from sugar and carbohydrates into fuel. Without them, energy production lags.

Iron also plays an important role in energy production. It carries the oxygen needed to burn calories throughout the body. Among women who have not yet gone through menopause, iron deficiency is a well-known cause of fatigue. "Iron is also known to be involved in the body's production of neurotransmitters, chemicals that affect alertness, sleep patterns and other brain functions," Dr. Goldstein says. "So iron deficiency can cause symptoms of mental as well as physical fatigue."

"I wasn't just tired. I was out of breath and weak and irritable and thought I was just out of shape," says Sherrie, 28, a public health worker from Norristown, Pennsylvania. "I hadn't been to a doctor in some time, and when I went, one of the first things he checked was my blood iron level. It was quite low, and he prescribed iron supplements." The iron supplements did help relieve her symptoms, she says, but "it wasn't until I had an IUD (intrauterine device inserted in the cervix for birth control) that was causing heavy bleeding removed that my energy level returned to normal."

If you want some assurance that you're getting all your nutrients in adequate amounts, doctors generally recommend taking a multivitamin supplement. If you want to take additional magnesium, iron or B-complex vitamins, discuss these supplements with your doctor.

COFFEE AND SUGAR: SOME SAY NO

What about two quick picker-uppers—caffeine and sugar? Here, responses were mixed. Equal numbers of our survey takers say they use these energy-altering substances to perk up as say they avoid them to maintain their energy levels.

"In my opinion, nothing works better to perk you up than a hot cup of coffee during the wintertime, or a cold Coke during summer," says a Washington, D.C., research librarian, Roberta. One woman even suggests adding a pinch of spicy ginger to a cold cola drink. However, others feel that life without caffeine provides more constant energy levels.

"I used to consume lots of coffee and sugar and felt like I needed it to simply function," says Sharon, a realtor from Detroit. "However, when health problems forced me to change how I eat, I found that, after a time, I had more energy than ever without caffeine or sugar. Now, I don't need my cup of coffee to get started in the morning or to keep me awake in the afternoon."

Although this issue is controversial, some experts agree that some people do better staying away from caffeine and sugar. "Eating sugar provides a temporary rise in blood sugar, which may improve energy levels for a time, but it is often followed by a sharp drop in blood sugar, which leaves some people feeling tired, fuzzy-headed and ready for more sugar," says Robert Thayer, Ph.D., professor in the Department of Psychology at California State University, Long Beach, and a specialist in exercise, mood and cravings.

SOME GRAVITATE TO WATER

Whether it's a soothing hot bath or shower or an invigorating dip in a lake, water seems to have a special power to relax and revive people, according to our survey takers.

Hot weather can be a real energy drainer, and some people have found that water's cooling properties help keep them going. "When I'm working out in my yard and it's very hot, I simply mist my face and arms with the garden hose every once in a while to cool down," says Patricia, 37, a housewife from Emmaus, Pennsylvania. "It revives me well enough to keep going for another half-hour or so."

Sweet Aromas Perk Them Up

"I find a hot bath restores my energy, especially after I've been outside working during the cold winter months," says Ben, a small-engine repairman living in Hill, New Hampshire. His wife sometimes adds herbs such as peppermint to the bathwater. "The scent alone seems to perk me up," he says.

In fact, essential oils from herbs such as peppermint, lavender and rosemary have long been used to revive the faint and restore the weary, says Judith Jackson, a certified aromatherapist and licensed massage therapist from Cos Cob, Connecticut, and author of *Scentual Touch: A Personal Guide to Aromatherapy*.

"Aromatherapists are finding that simply smelling certain fragrances has a stimulating effect, and in the bath, skin exposure to these oils, which have many active ingredients, can also be invigorating," Jackson explains. For a real eye-opening bath, she suggests adding a handful of rosemary leaves and the rind of a lemon to the hot bathwater.

Fever

Putting Out the Flames

F eeling feverish? No sweat. Our survey takers say they've lit up a thermometer or two, only to beat back the blaze with any number of home remedies.

Just what stokes your body's internal fire, anyway? Some experts say your soaring temperature is a by-product of your immune system kicking into overdrive, says William Goldwag, M.D., director of the Center for Preventive/Holistic Medicine in Stanton, California, and a board member of the American Holistic Medical Association. "A lot of symptoms are caused by your body mobilizing its defenses, and fever may be one of them," he says.

When the mercury hits 102°F for kids or 103° for adults, it's probably time to take action. If your fever is accompanied by stiff neck, vomiting or disorientation, you should seek medical help immediately. (It could be a sign of meningitis.) Meanwhile, here's how some handle the heat.

COOLING LIQUIDS LICK THEIR PROBLEM

After aspirin, emergency cooling measures are the most popular suggestions from our survey takers.

If Viola's technique is quick, it's certainly time-tested: She says she learned it from Ella, her 100-year-old grandmother.

Ever since Viola was a child, Ella has treated her fevers and headaches by soaking a piece of a brown paper bag, folded like a washcloth, in white vinegar and applying it to her forehead or wrist. "By the time the bag seems to be heating up, the fever is gone," she says.

As a result, Viola uses the same vinegar and paper bag remedy for her family's fevers. "We never had to use any medication around here for fever, so that should tell you something," she says.

Susan learned from years of experience about rubbing alcohol's effect on a fever. The 44-year-old Haslett, Michigan, homemaker suffered repeatedly from fever as a child. But as soon as her mother splashed some rubbing alcohol on her feet, wrists and palms, relief was usually just 15 minutes away, she says. For tougher cases, Susan's mother would apply the alcohol to her back and legs.

Is it any wonder, then, that alcohol is Susan's favorite fever treatment for her kids? "I have two children, and I used it on both of them," she says. "In no time, it seems like the fever has gone down dramatically."

When Jack was growing up in Salem, Illinois, they were still talking about William Jennings Bryan—a turn-of-the-century presidential candidate and the town's most famous resident. In those bygone days, whether you were a Republican or a Democrat, you couldn't do better for a fever than take an aspirin and a cold bath. "That was about all you could do back then," says Jack. "And from there you just toughed it out."

Today, after raising three boys of his own, Jack still touts the cold bath as a fever remedy. "A child can run a fever at a drop of a hat," says Jack. "But when their temperature starts getting up there, putting them in a cold shower or bath is a good way to get it down in a hurry. I've found a cold washcloth over the forehead also helps," he says. (Doctors recommend against giving aspirin to children with fever because it can cause Reye's syndrome—a potentially fatal illness.)

All these treatments are tough to top because splashing on something cool—water, alcohol, even vinegar—increases evaporation from the skin and as a result, cools the body, says Dr. Goldwag.

"Evaporation cools the blood as it passes close to the surface of the body, particularly in those places where your pulse can be felt easily, like the wrists, armpits, groin and forehead," he says. "You'd have more success cooling your body by putting some sort of liquid on those places than if you'd put some on, say, your abdomen, where there's a lot of fat in between the liquid and the blood flow."

HE LIKES IT HOT

Pearce says he learned how to use heat as a weapon in fighting fever when he was an artillery officer in the Army.

Almost upon landing in cold, wet West Germany, the Arlington, Texas, native felt feverish. And as the days—as well as his company—marched on, he felt even worse. "I just couldn't shake the thing," he says.

When Pearce's company arrived at a mountain position in a town called Wildflecken, he met a West German surgeon and described the problem. The officer told him to go home, take some aspirin, crank up the heat in his stove as high as it would go, get in bed, cover himself with blankets and sweat it out.

Pearce says he followed the man's advice—perhaps too well. "I was sweating so much that, when I got up to go to the bathroom, I nearly froze," he says. But by morning, Pearce says, his fever was gone.

Whenever the 63-year-old Ph.D. candidate suffers from a fever today, he says he augments his heat regimen by also taking a hot bath and drinking a hot cup of chicken soup spiced with hot peppers. "My wife thought it was a little extreme, but it works for me," he says.

Sweating will bring your body's temperature down, but when you have a fever, you probably don't need more physical activity to get the water flowing, says Dr. Goldwag. "I don't know if trying to sweat more is particularly helpful, but, ideally, once you start to sweat, you should come out from under the blankets and actually wipe off the sweat. If you remove the sweat by drying off, you make more room for fluids to come out and evaporate," he says.

EDITOR'S NOTE: Some experts believe that sweating can greatly reduce the length or severity of a viral infection. Just make sure to drink plenty of fluids, so you don't become dehydrated. And don't try working out to bring on the sweat—working out with a fever can damage the heart.

THEY DRINK TEA

A registered nurse for over 30 years, Mary Ann has seen more than her share of fevers—and fever remedies. Yet none has worked as well for her or her children as the simple tea remedy her mother used.

After making a cup of regular tea, adding some sugar to taste and allowing the brew to cool off for a few minutes, the 63-year-old Glenshaw, Pennsylvania, resident adds a single ice cube. She then sips the tea periodically while getting plenty of bed rest. If the fever persists, she'll have a second cup in the afternoon. "I mentioned it to my pediatrician, and he said anything that you use that works is good," she says.

Herbal teas also have their proponents. Roberta, a Garner, Kansas, resident, first read about drinking lemon balm tea for fever in an herb book. She reads a lot of herb books, because she and her husband grow more than 70 varieties of herbs for a living. "My kids don't get sick that much, but I've used lemon balm tea twice to break the fever in them," she says.

After picking some leaves from a lemon balm plant, she dries and steeps them in hot water and then adds honey and lemon—just as she would for regular hot tea. Two or three cups and a few hours later her fever is gone. "And it tastes good, too," she says.

Like chicken soup, tea probably has multiple benefits in fighting fever, says Dr. Goldwag. "Teas are in the same category as chicken soup: Jewish penicillin is what they call it," he says. "The idea is that you are giving fluids, which is beneficial. It also increases the amount of sweating and probably increases the amount of evaporation from your skin. There are all kinds of different benefits claimed for different herbal preparations, and there may very well be something to that; but probably most of the benefit is due to the fluid intake—and maybe that something hot feels good when you're feeling lousy."

They Reach for Onions (and Other Veggies)

The mighty onion once again muscles in on our survey, with two people claiming their fever cure is just a produce stand away.

After frying several chopped onions in a skillet, Pauline puts the onions in a small bag or pillow case, covers her daughter's chest with a towel, lays the bag on the towel, and covers the bag with another towel. A heating pad placed over the top keeps the onions warm. "It's a sticky mess, but you don't mind if it works. It will break a fever faster than anything," says the Michigan resident. "After I used it one time, I had a doctor tell me 'No harm done—it's one of the best real old-fashioned remedies.' "

Between the onions her Irish grandmother put in her socks for her fever and the mustard plaster on her chest for congestion, Carol says she should have grown up to be a salad. "It's a wonder that I lived through my childhood," she laughs.

And yet, Carol swears by the remedy now. When she was a child, her grandmother insisted on putting onion slices in her socks overnight to break her fever. "In the morning, the onions would be black and the fever would be gone," says the Skillman, New Jersey, hospital secretary. "It's wild and it may just be the power of suggestion, but it works." Carol has never tried the remedy on her three boys—perhaps they run too fast.

Also from our "Unusual Vegetable Use" files: Annette, 47, of Virginia, says placing potato slices on a feverish forehead works fine. Two other survey takers claim that when they were kids, tomato slices secured to their feet always helped break a fever.

Can strategically placed onions, tomatoes and potato slices overpower a fever? You just never know, says Dr. Goldwag. "A heating pad and warm onions on your chest might increase sweating, and of course, the bulk of the onions helps maintain warmth," he says. "Stranger things than this have helped, so who am I to say they won't work?"

She Has a Potion from Granny

Elizabeth is so accustomed to taking her fever fixer, she was a little taken aback when we asked her to tell us more about the cod liver oil, lemon juice and honey combination she suggested. "My golly, I thought everyone knew about that," says the 50-year-old Grants Pass, Oregon, resident.

It's her English grandmother's favorite remedy, explains Elizabeth. To make it, she combines two or three tablespoons of lemon juice, ½ teaspoon of cod liver oil and honey to taste. "She used to make up a batch of it and give it to us a teaspoon at a time when a fever or a cold was coming on," says Elizabeth. "But you don't want too much cod liver; you can definitely taste it if you have too much."

This remedy stumped our expert. "I think a lot of people use lemon juice and honey, but I haven't heard of the cod liver oil addition to it," says Dr. Goldwag. "Maybe they add it so it doesn't taste too good—make it taste a little more like medicine."

Flatulence

Easy Steps to Emissions Control

I t's not life-threatening. It's usually not painful. But boy, can it turn your face red.

"It helps if I can laugh about it, but the fact is, it's downright embarrassing at times, and I certainly don't want others making fun of me," says a Massachusetts woman who occasionally has to turn down social invitations because her intestinal gas problem is so bad.

That pretty much sums up the feelings of many of our survey takers who admit to an emissions control problem. The need to be at least semi-civilized has led them to an array of gas-stopping solutions. Here they are.

THEY AVOID GASSY FOODS

Beans and other high-fiber foods such as corn and broccoli deserve their reputation as gas producers, because a fair number of people say they leave these foods off the menu when they can't afford to expel the consequences.

"I always think, 'Where am I going to be, and who am I going to be with, a couple of hours from now?' before I eat anything like corn or lima beans," says Helen, 70, a retired secretary from Chicago.

Beans contain hard-to-digest sugars, and humans do not make the enzyme (alpha-galactosidase) to break them down, explains Roger Gebhard, M.D., a gastroenterologist and professor of medicine at the University of Minnesota School of Medicine in Minneapolis. When these sugars hit the colon, they're fermented by bacteria living there. This process creates gases—hydrogen, carbon dioxide and, in some people, methane and even hydrogen sulfide, with its distinctive "rotten egg" smell.

Several other people said they need to avoid a variety of other fibrous foods, such as onions, peppers, cabbage, apples, prunes and other fruit. "I know I don't eat some foods that are good for me, but my thinking is they aren't worth the trouble," says Susan, 37, a St. Louis, Missouri, manufacturing representative who says she doesn't like to punctuate her sales presentation with unwanted expletives.

The same gas-generating process that gives beans their special talent also occurs when starchy fibers from grains, vegetables or fruits hit the colon, Dr. Gebhard says. "About the only foods researchers have tested that do not cause some flatulence are rice and meat."

Is it worth eschewing an array of delicious, healthful high-fiber foods to relieve a gas problem? Not to the people who have found other ways to deflate this problem.

THEY STOP BEAN BACK TALK

Refried beans, black bean soup, homemade baked beans, devilishly hot chili—people who once avoided these and other gas-producing foods are now finding they can enjoy them without later embarrassment and bloating, thanks to Beano, a product which contains an enzyme that breaks down the indigestible sugars in beans that lead to flatulence. Beano is available in liquid or tablets.

"Beano has helped me a lot," says Charles, a music teacher from Mosinee, Wisconsin. "I like beans and eat them a couple of times a week. My whole family has a problem with gas, but I was always the worst offender, and they were sure to rub it in; so I tried Beano as soon as I heard of it. I use more than the recommended amount, usually about 12 drops per serving, and usually on good old homemade baked beans, chili or lima beans." He admits that Beano isn't cheap. "But one of those little bottles goes a long way for me," he says.

"For many people, this product works pretty well," Dr. Gebhard agrees. "It breaks down most, but not all, of the bean sugars and can significantly reduce gas production."

ACTIVATED CHARCOAL THEIR SURE CURE

Because it absorbs toxins so well, activated charcoal is recommended as an antidote for accidental poisoning. This form of charcoal is purified and steamed—each granule contains many absorbent pores. Besides soaking up poisons, activated charcoal also traps gases, which makes it an ideal choice for people serious about stopping intestinal gas.

"In my experience, it stops gas from any food," says Phyllis, 62, a housewife from Ira, Texas. On the recommendation of a health-food store employee, she started using activated charcoal to relieve gas pain. "My gas came mostly from fruit, and it was the worst when I was lying down." She's been using charcoal for about two years now. "It works very well," she says. "I usually take one or two capsules when I'm eating a food I know will bother me."

In two studies of people eating gas-producing meals, taking activated charcoal along with the meal resulted in less gas.

Yes, but can it relieve gas in dogs, a pressing problem for canine owners nationwide?

"We have given activated charcoal to our dogs when they've had farts so smelly that my husband refers to them as rope burners," says Lee, a dog breeder from Eagle Creek, Oregon. "I don't know why, but dog gas is notoriously smelly. Just a few capsules of activated charcoal does the trick."

EDITOR'S NOTE: "Activated charcoal does absorb gases, but it also absorbs other materials in the intestine, including medications, so it should not be taken at the same time you are taking drugs," Dr. Gebhard cautions. Dr. Gebhard does not know why dog gas smells so bad, either. "Maybe dogs are big hydrogen sulfide producers," he speculates.

DAIRY PRODUCTS WERE HIS BIG PROBLEM

You've heard of cutting the cheese, a euphemism for breaking wind. People who have gas problems with cheese are likely to find other dairy products, such as milk and ice cream, even more gaseous.

"A fair number of foods give me gas, but by far the worst is milk," says Paul, 56, a drill press operator from New Brunswick, New Jersey. He tends to avoid milk, but he has also tried a product, Dairy-Ease, that contains an enzyme, lactase, lacking in many people's intestines, that breaks down milk sugars. (Several other brands of this product are available, including less expensive store brands.) "I thought it worked pretty well," Paul says. "It didn't completely eliminate the gas, but it certainly lessened the amount."

Dairy products can cause several liters' worth of gas—the kind of gas that makes your whole belly swell up, Dr. Gebhard says. "Lactase-containing products break down about half of the milk sugars found in dairy products, so they provide partial relief," he says.

YOGURT CULTURES CUT HER SYMPTOMS

When it comes to gastrointestinal upsets, including gas and diarrhea, yogurt, or products containing the same friendly bacteria found in yogurt, has a fair number of fans.

"If I am having a problem with gas, I usually take two tablespoons of acidophilus (yogurt cultures) at bedtime, and by morning my problem is gone," says Helen, 72, of Olympia, Washington. Others say they eat yogurt at least a few times a week to keep gas problems at bay.

Yogurt cultures help to break down milk sugars and so relieve gas problems associated with dairy products, Dr. Gebhard says. Yogurt may also help to maintain a healthy balance of beneficial bacteria in your intestines. If you want to try yogurt as a gas-reliever, make sure you buy a brand with active cultures—it will say this on the label.

HERBAL TEA TAMES TUMMIES

The very earliest remedies for gas came from the garden, not the corner drugstore. And some people still rely on herbs or spices to dispel a belly full of air.

"I've used peppermint tea for gas, but I find that parsley tea, made with fresh or dried parsley, clears up my occasional gas problem in no time," says Helen, 70, a retired secretary from Chicago. The parsley doesn't cause you to expel the gas, she contends. "It seems to simply make it disappear."

Rather than strain the tea, she often eats the parsley leaves. "Why not?" she says. "They're good for you."

Other people suggest teas made with anise and fennel seeds—both pleasant, licorice-flavored spices. (Some people simply chew a mixture of these seeds.) Peppermint, ginger and chamomile are also popular gas-relieving teas.

"Many herbs, such as anise and fennel, are well-known gas relievers," says William J. Keller, Ph.D., head of the Division of Medicinal Chemistry and Pharmaceutics at Northeast Louisiana University in Monroe. "They contain ingredients that break up and expel intestinal gas." These herbs may also have some sort of action on bacteria in the intestines and may help stop intestinal muscle spasms, Dr. Keller adds.

To make a gas-relieving tea, use one to two teaspoons of anise or fennel seeds per cup of boiling water. Steep ten minutes. If you're using dried herbs, use two teaspoons per cup of boiling water. Steep ten minutes.

EXERCISE EASES OUT EMISSIONS

"It's not like this is anything new," says Melissa, 40, a clothing manufacturer's sales representative from Paterson, New Jersey. "I think most people realize that getting up, moving around, helps them to get out gas." She relies mostly on quick walks. "If I'm working at my desk, I'll simply get up and walk up and down the staircase a few times or around the block," she says.

Since she shares an office area with several people, this tactic also limits others' exposure to noxious odors.

Experts say regular aerobic exercise—walking, biking, swimming and the like—helps to promote normal bowel function, preventing constipation, gas and accompanying problems such as hemorrhoids. Strengthening the abdominal walls with sit-ups may also help bowels function normally to a certain extent. Several types of yoga poses, including torso twists and knee-to-chest poses, can coax a lazy bowel into action and help to move along both gas and feces, says Alice Christensen, founder and executive director of the American Yoga Association in Sarasota, Florida, and author of the association's *Beginner's Manual.* Even vigorous rocking in a rocking chair has been found to relieve painful gas buildup.

Food Sensitivities

Nipping Those Nasty Reactions

Y ou say yum. Your body says yuk. That's not exactly the official medical definition of a food sensitivity, but you get the picture.

When you are sensitive to a particular food, your immune system puts up a minor fuss, producing such symptoms as rashes, nasal stuffiness or a tummy ache. Food sensitivities may be a relatively recent phenomenon, some experts say. That's because eating food grown and manufactured thousands of miles away from your community is only as old as superhighways and chemical preservatives.

As many as 60 million Americans may suffer mild symptoms after eating such things as dairy products, wheat, eggs, corn, chocolate or monosodium glutamate, says Robert Dockhorn, M.D., clinical professor of medicine and pediatrics at the University of Missouri School of Medicine in Kansas City, Missouri, and chairman of the food allergy committee of the American College of Allergy and Immunology.

Although also an immune system response, food allergies can be far more dangerous. In one tragic incident, a boy allergic to peanuts died after eating a sandwich made with a knife that still had a tiny bit of peanut butter on it.

Fortunately, such severe food allergies are rare. However, some of our survey takers do find themselves in the vast group of Americans who are sensitive to certain foods. And they've equipped themselves with strategies for fighting back.

READING LABELS LIMITS HER PROBLEMS

For years, Jean, of Warren, Texas, has tried to keep salt and sugar out of her diet because of the facial swelling they seem to cause. Her vigilance has forced her to develop the investigative skills of a Texas Ranger. "Ever since I found out that I was sensitive to sugar and salt, I've been reading food labels very carefully to make sure I avoid them," she says. "Colorings, preservatives—it's amazing what they put in some of this stuff."

Trading sugar for honey or maple syrup may have been the hardest switch of all. "It seems like the manufacturers sneak sugar into everything," says the 62-year-old.

Although food ingredient labels are more detailed than ever, if you have food sensitivities or allergies, you still need to develop some sleuthing skills, says Dr. Dockhorn.

Starch is one such mystery for food-sensitive people. When food manufacturers use "starch," they don't have to say on the label whether they've used corn, wheat or potato starch. The term vegetable oil on a label seems fairly descriptive—until you discover that the oil may have been made from soybean, corn, peanut or other vegetables. Flavoring agents are also allowed to go undefined, says Dr. Dockhorn. "So if someone has a problem with, say, cinnamon, and the label just says 'flavoring agent,' that doesn't give you a clue what was used." If you have a doubt about what's in a food, avoid it, he says.

In fact, eating foods with a minimum of added ingredients may be the best approach to avoiding food allergies. "Really the only treatment for any kind of these sensitivities is avoidance, because, as far as we know right now, medications only treat the symptoms after the reaction has occurred," he says.

HE LISTENS TO HIS BODY

Though a Wisconsin resident nearly all his life, Charles steers clear of that state's world famous export. For one thing, he's never cared for dairy products. And for another, Charles says cheese may be one of several foods that aggravate his asthma. "I've never been to an allergist or had a food allergy test," says the 72-year-old retired woodworker. "But I can tell the difference if I have something that doesn't agree with me. It really makes breathing difficult."

Charles's self-diagnosis seems sound, says Dr. Dockhorn. "There are several reasons why he may be having problems with cheese," he says. "It could mean that he's allergic to the proteins in the cheese. But also all cheese has some mold in it because of the cheese-making process, and he could be allergic to that."

There are ways to take some of the guesswork out of diagnosing a food allergy or sensitivity, experts say. In addition to having an allergist run a test, you could try what's called an elimination diet. Simply eliminate for one week all the foods from your diet that you suspect are causing your symptoms. If the symptoms disappear, you know you've got the suspect almost corralled. Then every four days, reintroduce one of the suspected foods. If you start suffering from symptoms again, you've caught your culprit.

SHE SAYS NO TO COLA, COFFEE AND TEA

Marie, of Potlatch, Idaho, has discovered over the years that the further she stays away coffee, tea and colas, the better for her stomach. "Mainly, they cause digestive problems, so I just avoid them," she says.

Any one of these beverages can cause unpleasant symptoms, says Dr. Dockhorn. "Lots of people claim that they're sensitive to coffee, and it does tend to cause gastrointestinal problems, nasal stuffiness and, in some, wheezing," he says. "All of these contain a chemical called methylxanthine which can make you feel shaky, nauseated and just plain bad."

THEY KNOW THEIR NIGHTSHADES

Kathie, of McKinleyville, California, is free from food allergies and sensitivities. But her husband isn't quite as fortunate. Unless they're prepared just right, potatoes, tomatoes and peppers make him extremely sick to his stomach, says the 42-year-old nutritionist.

It's not uncommon for someone to be allergic to all of these vegetables, says Dr. Dockhorn. "They are all in what we call the nightshade family of plants, and they do have things in them that can cause allergic reactions like asthma or make asthma worse," he says. "I don't think anyone knows why the nightshades cause so many allergic reactions. But if you are sensitive to one of these, many times you will be sensitive to the others because of the botanical relationship."

But don't just cut out baked potatoes, stewed tomatoes and stuffed peppers and consider yourself cured, says Dr. Dockhorn. People who are sensitive or allergic to potatoes need to look out for potato starch, which is used to expand things like soup broth, he says.

And there just may be something to Kathie's independent discovery about food preparation. "Cooking will alter the chemical composition of the food. And it may change the food enough so you don't have problems," says Dr. Dockhorn.

NO MSG FOR THIS MS.

The waiters at Julia's favorite Chinese restaurant are familiar with her request that comes at the end of every order: "No MSG."

To avoid provoking her food allergies, the 56-year-old Alabama resident strives to avoid all chemical additives, preferring fresh, organic foods and meals "made from scratch most of the time."

Monosodium glutamate definitely has a reputation for causing discomfort, but so far, most experts are only willing to describe it as an intolerance rather than an allergy, says Dr. Dockhorn. Often added as a flavor enhancer in restaurants, MSG has been found to cause flushing, sweating, racing heartbeat, intense headaches and stuffy noses. MSG is also hydrolyzed vegetable protein, found in such foods as soups and chili. (There's another reason to hone those label-reading skills.)

A PILL AND A WALK FIX HER

Amelie has known for some time that she's allergic to milk, chocolate and nuts. "Chocolate is definitely the worst offender for me," says the Aurora, Colorado, resident. "In no time, I'll have swelling in my sinuses. It's real uncomfortable."

Problem is—she loves the stuff. For those rare instances when she allows herself a piece of chocolate cake, Amelie says she's discovered that taking Tylenol Allergy Sinus medication as directed will minimize her symptoms.

Dr. Dockhorn says he recommends antihistamines. In fact, it's the antihistamine in Tylenol that may be helpful. "Histamine is one of the more common chemicals released by the body during a food sensitivity, so we find antihistamines combat rashes, nasal stuffiness and the stomach symptoms quite well."

And when she's out of Tylenol? "I try to force myself to take a brisk walk, something that gets the pulse rate up," she says. "It's difficult when you're feeling incapacitated, but for me, that's the quickest way to recover."

EDITOR'S NOTE: Taking a walk may improve symptoms associated with food sensitivity, but research shows exercise may actually cause problems for someone suffering from a true food allergy, says Dr. Dockhorn.

Foot and Heel Pain

Easy Steps to Happy Feet

There's a lesson everyone can learn from the people who have foot or heel pain: Don't take your feet for granted. If you cram them into too-tight shoes or ask them to carry more weight than they can bear, eventually they'll get your attention—the hard way. They'll ache. And then, it'll be up to you or your doctor to figure out what can be done to restore them to service.

People who expect a lot from their feet have learned what they need to do to keep them in tip-top working order. They offer lots of tender, loving care—hot soaks, massage, relaxing stretches and cushy, roomy shoes, among other things. Here's how they keep ahead of foot pain.

SENSIBLE SHOES SAVE THEIR SOLES

"Comfortable shoes" top our survey takers' list of foot-soothing remedies. High heels and flimsy flats are out; shock-absorbing, high-tech walking or running shoes are in, even with the 60-plus crowd.

"I know a number of nurses, waitresses and school teachers who won't wear anything but running shoes, even if it doesn't go well for their image," says Marion, 70, a former San Francisco city hall clerk now retired to Guion, Arkansas—population 93.

"I started wearing athletic shoes when they first came out 30 years ago, and I was standing on marble floors all day long at work," she says. She still wears such shoes to walk and garden. "I have rheumatoid arthritis and am overweight, so I need shoes that are comfortable."

To keep these trendy shoes from taking a big bite out of her tiny budget, she shops at a discount store. "I buy whatever brand fits me best, and I sometimes buy men's shoes, since my feet tend to be wide," she says. Usually, she can purchase a pair of top-brand sneaks for about $30.

More and more foot doctors are recommending that their patients choose running or walking shoes as their main footgear, says Terry Spilken, D.P.M., a Manhattan podiatrist and adjunct faculty member at the New York College of Podiatric Medicine. "These shoes are designed to protect active feet and are especially good for people who have bunions or other foot or heel pain, or who have to take special care of their feet because of diabetes or arthritis."

If you're concerned that sneakers will clash with your otherwise prim appearance, look for walking shoes, which, these days, come in an array of dress and business styles. Or do as Marion does. Adopt the Arkansas look. Wear blue jeans.

THEY MAKE SURE THE SHOE FITS

"Buy longer or wider shoes," suggests one man. "I've slowly inched my way up from a size 6½ to a 7, and sometimes an 8, depending on the shoe type," reports Katherine, 43, a language teacher from Syracuse, New York, who's had problems finding shoes that accommodate her long second toe.

"Even expensive shoes cause problems if they don't fit right," Dr. Spilken says. To avoid wasting money on a pair of shoes that mangle up your feet, shop late in the afternoon, when your feet are at their largest, wear the same type of socks you intend to wear with the shoes, and take the shoes for a good long test walk, he suggests.

"When the shoe is laced up, your heel shouldn't slip around inside the shoes and you should have enough room in the toes—one-quarter to one-half inch—between the inside of the shoe and the tip of the longest toe," recommends Lloyd Smith, D.P.M., past president of the American Academy of Podiatric Sports Medicine practicing in Newton, Massachusetts. And when you stand up on tiptoe, the shoe should bend easily at the same point where the ball of your foot does.

PADDED INSERTS EASE ACHES

Despite growing acceptance of sneakers as appropriate attire for most occasions, some professional types still feel duty-bound to continue to wear uncomfortable shoes. "I can't wear sneakers, or even nurses' shoes, to work," says Laura, 54, an administrator in the research and development division of a medical and dental equipment company. Instead, she wears good leather dress shoes with a one- or two-inch heel and adds padded inserts to help make these shoes more comfortable.

"I had burning in my feet, which was traced to a problem with inflamed nerves. I felt like I was getting electrical shocks with each step," she says. Full-sole foam inserts helped alleviate some of this pain, as did rest, foot soaks and massage, she says.

It's best to have a doctor determine the cause of symptoms of tingling or burning in your feet, Dr. Smith says. "Padded inserts may help some nerve compression problems, and if the pain is in the ball of the foot, I'd definitely switch from heels to flats," he says.

EDITOR'S NOTE: Foam insoles can cause problems if they make your shoes too tight for comfort. So take your insoles along when you shop for new shoes, and insert them in the shoes you try on, Dr. Smith suggests.

STRETCHES SOOTHE TENDER TOOTSIES

You've probably seen runners lean forward, into a wall, to stretch their calf muscles prior to a race. Well, that same sort of stretch can reduce muscle or tendon pain in the arch or heel of a foot, Dr. Smith says. Such pain is caused by tight tendons, which can become inflamed.

Mastin, of Franklin, North Carolina, used this same sort of stretch to remedy the pain of heel spurs—small growths of excess bone on the bottom of the heel bone, characterized by pain deep in the lower heel.

Instead of leaning into a wall to do the stretch, however, he built a small platform with a 30-degree angle, similar to one in his doctor's office. "I'd stand on the platform, with my heels on the lower end and my back against the wall, several times a day, for a total of about 20 minutes a day," he says. It took only a few weeks for the heel spur pain to be gone for good.

You can also stretch the muscles in your feet by gently pulling your toes forward and backward, and rotating your foot in a circle. That's something Elva, 57, a secretary from Brooklyn, New York, does to keep her feet perky. "I do this when I get home from work and during the day if I get the chance," she says. "I got my foot caught in an old-fashioned subway turnstile years ago, and it tends to ache before the day is over."

"Kicking your shoes off and wiggling and stretching your feet is one of the best and simplest things you can do for them, and it's something people simply forget to do," Dr. Smith says. "It helps to keep your feet strong and flexible."

You won't want to stretch while your pain is at its worst, especially if there's any swelling. "You need to rest your foot then," Dr. Smith warns. But once the initial swelling is over—in two weeks or so—you can slowly and carefully work to lengthen your tight tendons. To do so, place your palms flat on a wall with one leg in front of the other and lean toward the wall, bending at the elbows. Your heel should not leave the floor. You'll feel a nice, deep stretch along the back of your leg and down into your heel. Switch legs and repeat the stretch.

THEY KNEAD AWAY PAIN

The ultimate in foot pain relief? For many people, it's foot massage. By necessity, most people massage their feet themselves, usually after a soak, working in petroleum jelly, hand cream, aspirin-containing ointments or a toe-tingling peppermint salve.

One woman, Audry, 67, of Milwaukee, invigorates her feet by moving them over a rolling pin she keeps under her bathroom sink. "I do this as I set my hair at night," she explains. "My father always kept an extra rolling pin in the bathroom for this purpose, and I find it really does help to keep my feet feeling good and looking good."

You can also use a golf ball or tennis ball to stimulate your soles, Dr. Smith adds.

Another woman, however, is lucky enough to have a husband who enjoys ministering to her feet. "If we're both on the couch at night, I'll put my feet in his lap and wriggle them around until he gets the message," says Melissa, 46, a New York City probation officer. In return, she massages her husband's neck and shoulders.

"Lots of people enjoy having their feet massaged, and it can ease tired, aching feet by improving blood circulation," Dr. Spilken explains. But don't rely on massage to correct bone, muscle or nerve problems, he cautions.

HER FEET SAVOR WARM SOAKS

"I don't know what it does, but it sure feels good, and it helps get me through my work shift," says Pierrette, 49, a Hollywood, Florida, security guard. She's talking about foot soaks, a home remedy that several other people also mentioned. Pierrette immerses her feet in lukewarm water containing Epsom salts each evening for 15 or 20 minutes before she leaves for her all-night job.

"I am on my feet about 12 hours a day and sometimes standing on concrete in the gatehouse for 8 or 9 hours at a time, so my feet burn," she says. Besides soaks, she also brings along a change of fresh cotton socks, and like Marion, she wears running shoes.

"Warm soaks even without Epsom salts are very soothing, but I believe the best treatment for general foot and heel pain is nightly soaks alternating between cold and hot water," says Dr. Spilken. "Soak in cold water for five minutes, then in hot water for five minutes, and repeat. This has a 'massaging' effect that invigorates feet by opening and closing blood vessels."

Does adding Epsom salts to the water, as many people say they do, enhance the benefits of soaking?

"It may," says Arthur Jacknowitz, Pharm.D., professor and chairman of the Department of Clinical Pharmacy at West Virginia University School of Pharmacy in Morgantown. "Epsom salts, or magnesium sulfate, may help to draw fluid out of swollen tissues, which can prevent further tissue damage." He recommends half a cup of Epsom salts per gallon of warm water. For swelling caused by injury, however, stick with cold water initially to reduce swelling.

Cold water should be used with caution by those with poor blood circulation. If you have circulation problems, limit your soaks to about five minutes, says Dr. Spilken.

Foot Odor

Stamp Out Bad Smells

Smelly feet? Not me, you say. Before you move on to the next topic, however, perhaps you should ask your nearest and dearest whether your feet create their own unique atmospheric conditions.

"I can't really smell my feet myself, but when I take my shoes off and my wife wrinkles up her nose and says, 'Yuck' (she's really subtle about it), I know my feet stink," says Jerry, 59, a Rock Hill, South Carolina, music professor who has tried lots of different remedies for his odiferous appendages.

"It's my 12-year-old granddaughter who has the problem," says Alice, 72, of Bedford, Iowa. "But I'm the one who's bothered by the smell, not her. She's used to it."

"If an odor problem develops slowly, it's true that people become desensitized to the bad smell and so often don't even notice it," explains James McGuire, D.P.M., director of physical therapy at the Pennsylvania College of Podiatric Medicine in Philadelphia. "And because it can take a bit of effort to eliminate the problem, many people who are aware that their feet smell usually ignore it until someone else complains."

The 67 people who responded to this question had more than a dozen suggestions, from baking soda soaks to barefoot strolls through dewy grass. Here, then, is what the folks with foot odor—and those who put up with them—recommend to quell the smell.

BAKING SODA SNUFFS SNEAKER SMELLS

They put it in their socks and shoes. They sprinkle it on their feet. They soak in it. They recommend it to friends and family. The product these people use so lavishly is plain, old baking soda—a white powder with well-known odor-absorbing qualities and an ingredient in some over-the-counter body powders.

"I'll put a cup or so into my bathwater, or if I get a chance to soak my feet, I'll put about a quarter of a cup into the warm water, or even make it into a paste and rub my feet with it," says Sarah, 29, of Evanston, Illinois. "I'll also sprinkle it in my shoes. It definitely does cut the odor."

Baking soda powders work, at least temporarily, because they absorb foot perspiration and odors, Dr. McGuire says. He believes they work best, however, when used along with other moisture-reducing measures, such as frequent sock changes.

ASTRINGENT SOAKS STOP THEIR SMELL

Foot soaks help keep feet clean. But soaks can do more than that. With extra added ingredients, a soak can turn into a bacteria-blasting, sweat-stopping extravaganza. Besides baking soda, people say they've successfully used Epsom salts, vinegar, lemon juice, chlorine bleach, black tea and borax to knock out foot odor.

Tops on Dr. McGuire's list, both for effectiveness and safety, however, is a combination of Epsom salts and white vinegar. "I've sent people home with a prescription for this soak," he says. He recommends ¼ cup of white vinegar and two to three tablespoons of Epsom salts per ½ gallon of water. "This soak helps close the pores of the skin and reduce the number of bacteria growing on it."

FRESH SOCKS KEEP HER FEET HAPPY

"At home, I am often barefoot or wear sandals, so my feet don't sweat much," explains Sylvia, 37, a geriatric nurse from Lansing, Michigan. "At work, however, I pretty much need to keep my shoes on, and so my feet do perspire and my socks get wet. So I bring along to work an extra pair of socks to change into at lunchtime. I started doing this, initially, during the wintertime because it made my feet feel more comfortable and kept them warmer. But I soon realized that this also cut back on a lot of odor."

Frequent sock changes are something Dr. McGuire also strongly recommends. "Some patients complain to me that they can't take time to change their socks at work. I tell them everyone gets at least one break to go to the bathroom, and they can change their socks then."

THEY REACH FOR ANTIPERSPIRANT

Feet can get as hot and bothered as underarms, contributing to odor problems, so there's good reasons people turn to antiperspirants to dry up foot odors.

"The doctor I saw for a bad case of athlete's foot suggested I try using an antiperspirant to keep my feet dry," says Michael, 38, a Shreveport,

Louisiana, interior designer. "It did help my athlete's foot, and I discovered that it also eliminated a foot odor problem I'd had for some time."

"I tell people to use a roll-on or pads that contain aluminum chloro-hydrate and to cover the bottom of their feet, including the webbed spaces between their toes. This should be done once a day after washing and drying their feet," Dr. McGuire says. "I don't like sprays, because I don't want people inhaling the stuff."

ZINC STOPS THEIR STINK

Two people in our survey report that zinc supplements stop foot odor. One, our man Jerry from South Carolina, says zinc works better for him than dusting his feet and shoes with baking soda. "My feet sweat a lot, especially when I am physically active," he explains. "My socks get soaked with perspiration." Someone recommended he try zinc supplements. "I did, and I found that within a week or two, my foot odor was significantly reduced." He now takes 15 milligrams of zinc as part of a multivitamin/mineral pill. "If the odor seems to be coming back, though, I'll take a separate zinc supplement of 100 milligrams for a few days," he says.

"Zinc is necessary for healing and for many chemical reactions in the body," Dr. McGuire explains. "Perhaps it somehow makes the skin more resistant to the bacteria that cause odors."

EDITOR'S NOTE: If you decide to try this remedy, it's best to take no more than 15 milligrams of zinc a day without medical supervision. That's because high levels of zinc can interfere with the absorption of copper, another essential trace mineral. If you have a true zinc deficiency, your doctor may initially prescribe amounts as high as 150 milligrams, then cut back as your zinc status returns to normal.

ANTIBACTERIAL SOAPS KEEP HIS FEET SQUEAKY CLEAN

"My doctor prescribed an expensive liquid soap for me to use to wash my feet," says Walter, 78, of Rochester, New York. "After I had used up one bottle, I decided to simply use Dial soap instead, and it worked just as well. Even if I'm taking a shower, I make sure I wash my feet well, using a washcloth and plenty of soap."

"Antibacterial soaps do help," Dr. McGuire agrees. "I tell people to sit down and wash their feet with soap and water and to clean between their toes at least once a day. Simply standing in the shower and letting the water run over your feet isn't washing them."

Gingivitis

Bacteria Busters for the Gums

I t's time to test your knowledge of dental terminology! What preventable periodontal problem causes your gums to bleed after you brush or floss your teeth?

If you said "gingivitis"—dentist-speak for red, swollen, bleeding gums—you're right! Although not a short-term threat to your oral health, gingivitis is the first step on the long road to periodontitis—a condition that eventually leads to tooth loss. And the condition that leads to gingivitis? Bacterial buildup on teeth and gums.

Our survey takers are all too familiar with this condition. After being diagnosed with gingivitis, every single one of them is now brushing and flossing regularly to keep mouth bacteria at bay. "Whether you use a manual or electric toothbrush, you need to thoroughly remove plaque from tooth surfaces and along the gum line at least once a day. This should take about five minutes," says Arthur F. Hefti, D.M.D., acting director of the Periodontal Disease Research Center at the University of Florida's College of Dentistry in Gainesville.

Beyond brushwork, here's what our survey takers recommend to keep their gums in the pink.

MOUTHWASH GETS LOTS OF VOTES

Listerine was one of the top gingivitis remedies named in our survey.

Margie is one such true believer, even if she's relatively new to the faith. "Over the years, I haven't been as careful about my oral health as I should," says the 57-year-old Onalaska, Wisconsin, widow.

Although Margie reports her gingivitis is now in retreat, she really only began paying attention after her dentist broke the bad news. "Now I floss regularly, use that rubber-tipped thing to massage my gums, brush my teeth, and then have some Listerine," she says. "It's a much more concerted effort."

Betty, a 60-year-old staff support person for the Air Force's new stealth bomber wing in Clinton, Missouri, has long considered Listerine her secret weapon in the fight against gingivitis. And so far, she's claiming victory. "I use a capful in the morning after brushing," she says. "I think it kills the bacteria that leads to gingivitis."

Rinsing your mouth with Listerine a half-hour after brushing not only kills bacteria, but it may also prevent any of the microscopic survivors from clinging to your teeth, says Dr. Hefti. "It's a disinfectant, but it also affects the adherence of bacteria onto surfaces—it actually makes it more difficult for the bacteria to grow on your teeth."

Why wait a half-hour before rinsing? Because you don't want to rinse off the fluoride from your toothpaste before it has time to work on protecting your teeth, says Dr. Hefti.

If you'd prefer an alcohol-free mouthwash (Listerine is about 20 percent alcohol) that's also effective against gingivitis, ask your dentist about alternative products, says Dr. Hefti.

THEY ARM THEMSELVES WITH ARM AND HAMMER

So many of our survey takers say they brush with baking soda, you've got to wonder if anyone buys toothpaste anymore.

They don't all brush with their baking soda the same way, however. Stan, 77, hailing from Oregon, combines baking soda and hydrogen peroxide. Peggy, 50, from California, swears by a half salt/half baking soda mixture. Kathleen, 42, also from California, was one of few baking soda purists who scrubs with the powdery stuff solo.

EDITOR'S NOTE: While baking soda can kill bacteria that cause gingivitis, the texture can also be rough on your teeth, says Dr. Hefti. "I would not recommend anyone using baking soda straight out of the box to brush their teeth," he says. "That would be too abrasive. Most toothpastes that contain baking soda, however, are relatively safe to use."

To get the most out of them, let the paste sit in your mouth for a couple of minutes before rinsing. The baking soda needs to sit on your teeth awhile to be most effective.

If you've been brushing with baking soda, ask your dentist if it's caused any abrasion of your tooth enamel. And if you're on a low-salt diet, make sure to rinse your mouth thoroughly after brushing with baking soda.

THESE TWO ARE FOR VITAMIN C

After years of suffering from spongy and receding gums, Lydia, of British Columbia, says fighting off her gingivitis with vitamin C has been a crowning achievement. "At the dentist, it was always the same story: 'Try to work on your gums to strengthen them,'" she says. "I brushed, massaged and flossed, but the problem remained. Then I read that vitamin C helped gums, so I tried taking a daily supplement."

When her next appointment rolled around, Lydia's dentist was surprised—but she wasn't. "What happened?" the dentist asked. "Your gums are firm and not bleeding." Lydia told him about the extra vitamin C she was taking.

Although never diagnosed with gingivitis, Gloria had bleeding gums at the same time she suffered with a toothache that eventually led to a root canal. Gloria doubled both her vitamin C and calcium intake to 1,000 milligrams a day—and hasn't seen any red since. "But I'd read that this might help, so I thought I'd experiment a little, and it did," says the retired Melbourne, Florida, resident.

EDITOR'S NOTE: While there's some research showing vitamin C may actually improve oral health, chewing vitamin C tablets or rubbing powdered C on your teeth can cause erosion, says Dr. Hefti. "Because vitamin C is very acidic, too much vitamin C on the naked tooth surface can actually etch the surface," he says. "If you repeated that daily over a year or longer, you would probably cause erosion—it would wear down the tooth—especially if you used a toothbrush immediately afterward." You can boost your vitamin C intake by eating plenty of fresh vegetables and fruits like broccoli, green peppers, citrus fruits, melons and strawberries. You can also take supplements that you swallow without chewing. Although Vitamin C is considered safe, most doctors recommend you take no more than 1,000 milligrams a day to help prevent side effects such as diarrhea.

MELALEUCA MEETS THEIR NEEDS

Michael had been wearing braces for four years, but it wasn't until last year that his dentist began raving about the condition of his gums and teeth. His wife Kathy suffered from gingivitis, but her latest checkup revealed the problem had subsided.

The source of their dental improvement: a toothpaste made from melaleuca oil (also called tea tree oil), such as Desert Essence, which they purchase in a local health-food store. "I don't know much about it; I just swear by it," says Kathy.

The Annapolis, Maryland, couple began using the toothpaste at a friend's recommendation. "It doesn't have a sweet taste like most toothpastes, more like an antiseptic quality," she says. "But my teeth feel cleaner, and I've noticed that my gums aren't pulling away from my teeth any more."

EDITOR'S NOTE: Tea tree oil may be better for trees than for your teeth, says Dr.

Hefti. "It's certainly not as effective as I would like it to be, mainly because it doesn't stick as long to your teeth as it should—and it may stain," he says.

The leaves and volatile oil of the Melaleuca alternifolia *traditionally have been used as a topical anticeptic for cuts, burns and abrasions.*

SECRET TEA SAVES HER TEETH

It all started with a jug of herbal tea smuggled into Rosetta's hospital room. Laid up after a car accident, the doctors told Rosetta that while she was there they might as well remove some loose teeth.

Rosetta told one of her visitors—a Chinese woman who worked with her at the U.S. Department of Agriculture—about the doctor's plans. Soon after, the woman returned with some home-brewed knotgrass tea. "She said it would strengthen my gums," says the 76-year-old Seattle resident. "So I didn't tell anybody; I just drank this concoction." As a result, Rosetta claims she lost only a few teeth that needed to be pulled anyway. The rest were saved—and she still has them. "My husband said it worked because I thought that it would," she says.

Although Dr. Hefti doesn't know whether Rosetta's secret tea has specifically been cited in research studies, investigators have been taking a closer look at tea and its potential for fighting gingivitis. "Some tea extracts, like Japanese green tea, are actually reasonably effective in fighting plaque and inflammation, apparently because they contain tannic acid," says Dr. Hefti. An herb called bloodroot has been shown to fight the bacteria that cause plaque and to prevent microscopic bugs from clinging to teeth, he says. Bloodroot, also known as sanguinaria, is the active ingredient in Viadent mouthwash and toothpaste.

Gout

Dietary Changes Make a Difference

The classic portrait of a gout sufferer is a rich, portly, middle-aged man sitting in a comfortable chair, one foot resting painfully on a soft cushion, a plate and stein within easy reach.

In fact, most people with gout are overweight, older men. But our survey takers don't fit that bill. They are mostly women past the age of menopause, part of a small percentage of gout sufferers. They say they are not particularly portly. ("Oh, I could stand to lose a few pounds, but who couldn't?" one says.) And they're not what you'd call rich, either. ("One reason I use home remedies is because they're cheaper than most medications," one confesses.) What's more, they are not amused by the presentation of gout as a disease of overindulgence. "I don't fit that image and never did," says Glenna, 74, a certified public accountant from Spokane, Washington.

Of course, gout has other risk factors besides overindulgence: a genetic predisposition, the use of diuretics and lead poisoning can all cause symptoms.

Gout is a form of arthritis and causes the same problems: joint pain and swelling. "Usually, however, the pain is limited to a few distinct joints—the first joint of the big toe, other joints in the foot, the knee, and occasionally the wrist and elbow," explains Jeffrey Lisse, M.D., associate professor of medicine and director of the Division of Rheumatology at the University of Texas Medical Branch in Galveston.

The pain often starts at night and can become so bad that even the weight of bedcovers is intolerable. Gout occurs when crystals of uric acid form in the fluid surrounding a joint. The sharp, painful crystals form when blood levels of uric acid become too high and crystallize in the joints, just as sugar crystals pile up at the bottom of a glass of iced tea when you add too much sugar.

Unlike rheumatoid arthritis, where the connection with diet remains ambiguous, gout has a clear dietary connection. High levels of uric acid are associated with a diet of foods rich in purines—a class of proteins found in organ meats, sardines, anchovies, lentils and yeast (both baker's and brewer's yeast, which is why beer drinkers are prone to gout).

Avoiding purine-rich foods is standard medical advice for gout. Our survey takers agree. They have a few other recommendations, as well.

THEY CUT THE FAT

"It's the same sort of diet you'd follow if you were watching your cholesterol," explains Peggy, 64, a homemaker from Milwaukee. Her lean cuisine eliminates liver pâté, eggs Benedict and roast beef swimming in fatty gravy. It includes lots of vegetables and whole grains.

"This sort of diet offers two benefits," Dr. Lisse says. "It helps you avoid the foods richest in purines and also may help you to lose some weight. Obesity is an additional risk factor for gout."

Naturopathic doctors take the gout diet a step further, adds Joseph Pizzorno, Jr., N.D., a naturopathic physician and founding president of Bastyr University in Seattle. Besides eliminating animal fats and purine-rich foods, they recommend adding fats that have known anti-inflammatory properties—fish oils and certain types of vegetable oils such as flaxseed. They also recommend dark, leafy greens such as kale and spinach, which are rich in folic acid, a B vitamin that some studies suggest helps lower uric acid levels.

SOME ESCHEW THE BREW

"Absolutely no alcohol." Those words from one survey taker echo the experience of many with firsthand experience with gout. Even though they are not particularly big drinkers, some find that even one or two drinks can cause symptoms, especially when the alcohol is combined with a hearty meal.

Because it contains purines, beer is considered the worst possible alcoholic drink for the gout-prone, Dr. Lisse says. "However, any kind of alcohol can cause problems, because it temporarily interferes with the liver's normal metabolic processes," he says. "Your body concentrates on clearing out the alcohol, which means that blood levels of other toxins, such as uric acid, may temporarily rise." Because it draws water out of the body, alcohol can also cause dehydration, another risk factor for gout.

CHERRIES PROVIDE SWEET RELIEF

For years, people have been recommending cherries or cherry juice as a remedy for gout. Our survey takers are no different. They suggest cher-

ries, along with strawberries, blueberries and cranberries—a ve..
salad of pain relief.

Does this stuff work? Those who have tried it say it does.

"My ring finger had been swollen and tender for about two months when I finally saw a doctor," says Phyllis, 68, of Lubbock, Texas. "I thought it was broken, but my doctor said it was some kind of gouty arthritis. He prescribed some medicine, but after I read the list of side effects, I was reluctant to take it."

She was trying to decide what else she might do for her painful joint when she remembered reading that some people eat cherries to relieve gout. "I bought a can of sour cherries, added some sugar to them and started eating one or two dozen a day," she says. "That was no problem, since I like cherries."

In about three days, she says, "I thought I could detect an improvement." And in ten days, she says, "my joint was completely healed." Phyllis continues to include cherries in her daily diet. "I've had an occasional slight spell, and making sure I eat plenty of cherries always clears it up."

Fresh black cherries, when she can get them, work best for Glenna, who, for many years, has used cherries to cure an occasional bout of gout.

"We have a cherry tree in our backyard, so I can pick the fruit off that," she says. She'll also go with the canned variety if necessary. "I eat as many as I can, and if I develop symptoms during the night, I'll raid the jars of fruit on the shelf in the kitchen pantry," she admits. Her midnight forays usually dispel the pain within a day. "I can't be bothered crippling around on a bad foot," she explains.

"I have tried eating cherries and they did work for me," says Janice, 57, of Lexington, Kentucky. "I was diagnosed with gout by my doctor and was put on an anti-inflammatory drug that caused me to retain fluid. I was miserable. I happened to have a book that mentioned the use of sour cherries for gout, and I decided to try it. Instead of my medicine, I ate 20 sour cherries a day for six weeks. My gout cleared up completely during that time, and when I stopped eating the cherries, the gout never did come back. That was about one year ago."

The question, again: Do cherries really cause gout to disappear, or are these women experiencing a natural regression of their disease?

Only one published report from 1950 supports a role for cherries or cherry juice in the treatment of gout. That report, a presentation of three "case studies" by Ludwig W. Blau of the University of Texas, found that consuming one-half pound of fresh or canned Black Bing or Royal Anne cherries per day was very effective in lowering uric acid levels and preventing attacks of gout.

No further research on cherries and gout has been published, however, and most traditional doctors who treat arthritis and gout are very skeptical of cherries' effectiveness, Dr. Lisse says. "In my opinion, it's most likely that the people who started eating cherries or other fruit also stopped eating foods that can bring on symptoms, such as liver or other organ meats," he says.

Dr. Pizzorno suggests some reasons that cherries and some other kinds of fruit may help gout. "Cherries, hawthorn berries, blueberries and other dark red-blue berries are rich sources of anthocyanidins and procyanidins," Dr. Pizzorno says. "These compounds are flavonoid molecules that give these fruits their deep red-blue color and are remarkable in their ability to prevent collagen destruction."

Collagen is a strong, fibrous connective tissue that is part of cartilage, tendons and the fluid-filled capsule surrounding joints. Collagen integrity is known to play an important role in the prevention of joint diseases.

Flavonoids are also known to have anti-inflammatory actions, Dr. Pizzorno says. "These effects make flavonoids extremely useful in the treatment of a wide variety of inflammatory conditions, including gout, rheumatoid arthritis and periodontal disease," he says.

Hair Problems

Tactics for Spiffy-Looking Tresses

Think you're having a bad hair day? You should talk to our survey takers. Judging from the sheer quantity of their complaints, they've had the statistical equivalent of a bad hair decade. But whether the problem was dry hair, frizzy hair, thin hair or oily hair, they say they've clipped their hair problems with a variety of home remedies. Here's what they do.

THEY OIL IT

While dry hair is one of the top hair problems in our survey, it also generates a geyser of remedies, most of them oil-related.

Patricia suffered from dry hair for years—even before she started coloring her hair. That is, until the 58-year-old Lexington, Virginia, resident tapped two products that were as close as her kitchen cabinet: vitamin E and olive oil.

After combining the contents of a 1,000 IU (international units) vitamin E capsule with a tablespoon of olive oil, Virginia massages the mixture into her hair. Next, she ties a plastic bag over her hair, allowing the oil to remain for about an hour. She follows that with a standard wash and style. "Why spend all that money on a hot oil treatment at the beauty shop?" she says. "My hairdresser says my hair is in beautiful condition from this."

Myra from Oklawaha, Florida, says she also uses olive oil once a month to keep her waist-length, strawberry-blonde hair shiny, soft and healthy. The 45-year-old psychiatric nurse says she pours a quarter of a cup of olive oil into a glass, adds a teaspoon of oil of rosemary and heats the mixture.

After shampooing, Myra drenches her hair in the oil and puts on a shower cap. To make sure the oil doesn't soil her bedding, she also covers her head with a wool cap until morning. Shampooing in the morning removes the oil, but not the benefits, she says. "The warmth opens the hair follicles so they can absorb the oil. I don't even need to use conditioners," she says.

233

Oils of all kinds will lubricate your hair, but they can also make styling more difficult, says Carmine Minardi, co-owner of Minardi Salon, one of New York City's most popular hair salons. "You may end up with hair that's in good condition, but when you go to style it or set it, your hair is not going to have the same amount of body," he says. "Oil weighs down the cuticle, the outer protective coating of the hair. It's also tough to get oil out of your hair and scalp."

You can keep your hair from becoming dry by selecting colors and dyes that don't contain ammonia, a leading cause of dryness, he says. And if your hair is still dry, choose one of many hair care products that contain panthenol or taurine amino acids—chemicals that actually help strengthen the inner protein structure of your hair, says Minardi.

SHE FANCIES HERSELF A FRIZZ BUSTER

During the 1980s when her thin, wavy hair was shorter, Amy dutifully plugged in her blow-dryer like everyone else and spent her time at the mirror blasting the strands in place.

But since her hair is longer now, the 28-year-old Berkeley, Illinois, resident has discovered a blow-dryer is among the last hair-care accessories she needs. "I have the kind of hair that really gets frizzy when you use a blow-dryer," she says. "And I've tried so many of the antifrizz gels, but they make my hair oily and weighted down."

Years of experimenting have finally paid off, however: Amy says she's finally developed a technique that keeps her hair looking great. After shampooing, she blots her hair with a towel, making sure not to rub. Next, she combs her hair into place, and allows it to air dry. "The key is to keep any excess air from passing through the hair until the hair is dry at the roots," she says. "I don't finger style or continue to comb the hair at this point either." Amy then styles her hair using gel or mousse.

Not only has Amy discovered a great way to control frizz, but she's also on the cutting edge of a hair-care trend, says Minardi. "There are a lot of people getting into what's called natural drying, meaning no blow-dryers," he says. "If you introduce a blow-dryer to hair that is susceptible to frizz, the heat doesn't damage the hair, but it expands the cuticle; and when the cuticle expands, it appears frizzy. But if you have naturally frizzy hair and put a little gel on your hair or even a little bit of leave-in conditioner and just let the hair dry naturally, the cuticle will lie down. There are lots of other benefits to not using a blow-dryer: you spend less time, it doesn't take as much skill and you use less electricity."

Look for styling gels—also called glissage—and leave-in conditioners that do not contain alcohol, he says.

VITAMINS GIVE HER HAIR VITALITY

After years of fine, thin, lifeless hair, Marilyn read that nutritional supplements might put a little, shall we say, coif in her curls. "It really had no life in it at all," says the 64-year-old Oneida, New York, resident.

Already a supplement user, Marilyn says she added four 800-microgram biotin capsules and three 650-milligram inositol capsules to her daily program and took them faithfully for about a year. (Biotin and inositol are both part of the B vitamin complex.) Needless to say, she liked what she heard recently from her hairdresser. "Your hair is in such good shape," Marilyn recalls the woman saying. She was happy—but she wasn't surprised. "The vitamins made it much thicker and I can't get over how it shines," Marilyn says.

Although he's not familiar with the benefits of biotin and inositol, Minardi says good nutrition in general is vital for beautiful hair. "One of the first things I'll ask clients who have thin, dull or weak hair is whether they're eating right or taking vitamin supplements. I find that a good majority of people who have bad-quality hair don't use any kind of supplements, or they don't eat well," he says.

Experts have discovered that biotin supplements will cause hair growth in lab animals and people who are deficient in biotin. But if you eat enough biotin-containing foods—things like nuts, whole grains and milk—it's unlikely adding more to your diet will stimulate hair growth. For some reason, however, researchers have found that biotin can help wrangle cowlicks into place.

Researchers have also discovered that inositol prevents hair loss in animals. So far, however, there are no studies documenting the same effect in people. The vitamin is found in beans, fruits, grains and nuts.

BAKING SODA BEATS HER HAIR SPRAY BUILDUP

You won't find Rose, of Hurricane, West Virginia, buying bottles of deep-cleaning shampoo for her dark brown, shoulder-length hair. The 31-year-old real estate secretary says she learned from her mother that using baking soda once a week works even better at removing hair spray and gel buildup. "I shampoo once, then on the second shampoo I add a tablespoon of baking soda, mix it in my hand and shampoo," she says. "It makes my hair clean, shiny and soft."

While baking soda may work safely on hair buildup, switching products may eliminate the need, says Minardi. "Low-quality gels and hair sprays are more likely to produce buildup. They use extreme amounts of polymer that adheres to the hair and stiffens and is hard to remove," he says. "Look for sculpting products made with ingredients like mucilage, which is a natural plant extract that gives great hold but is easier to wash out."

Detergent Gets Her Oily Hair Squeaky Clean

Plagued with oily hair for most of her life, Christine, of Jacksonville, Florida, tried virtually every shampoo on the market to slow the flow. "I can't even name all the shampoos I used," says the 30-year-old housewife.

Then, about six months ago, while watching television, she had an idea: If Dawn, a popular dishwashing detergent, removed grease from dishes, wouldn't it have the same effect on her short brown hair? Soon after, she bought a bottle and gave it a try. Her verdict: "It works! I wash my hair two or three times a week now, compared with every day before."

Harsh detergents can damage hair, says Minardi. Don't give up on commercially available shampoos specifically designed for oily hair, he urges. "One company uses an extract of melaleuca—tea tree oil—to create a treatment used once a week that extracts oil from the scalp. This seems to dry up the oil glands slightly, so the daily amount of secretions aren't nearly as high or aren't as obvious."

They Reach for a Brewski

Beer is touted—and toasted—by two survey takers for its hair care qualities. Carol, 59, says she rinses with beer once a week to give her hair body. Another rinses with stale beer every six weeks.

Could soaking your hair in suds somehow enhance your hairstyle? Minardi says yes. "Before we had all these fancy sprays and gels, people sprayed beer on their hair to set it. The alcohol and malt content in beer work as a setting lotion," he says. "And if somebody wants beauty on a budget, and they want a cheap setting lotion, it's not a bad one at all."

After shampooing, conditioning, towel drying and combing, give your hair a spritz from some flat beer in a spray bottle and then you can set or blow dry, he says. "But again here's the caution: You'll smell like a pub," says Minardi.

One Coif . . . with Mayo

Slathered on a BLT or a turkey sandwich seems the right place for a scoop of mayo. But survey takers from across the country say this dressing is good not just for eats.

"I know it sounds weird, but it works," says Mary, 36. Once a week, just like her mother and her mother's mother, she grabs a handful of mayonnaise, rubs it in her hair, wraps a warm towel around her head and allows it soak in. Between 10 and 15 minutes later, the Walbridge, Ohio, resident shampoos the mayo out.

Hold the mustard and your laughter; mayonnaise can help condition hair, says Minardi. "This was very common in the 1960s. You have the protein from the eggs and the acidity from the vinegar that makes it a deep penetrating conditioner," he says.

Before topping your mop with mayo, however, you should probably consider the disadvantages, he says. "The smell may linger, and because it has an oil base, your hair may become flat and hard to style."

MANE 'N' TAIL WORKS FOR HER

Not everything you see on television is completely worthless. Consider what Carolyn, of San Antonio, Texas, caught one night while watching the tube. After seeing a show featuring veterinarians' wives demonstrating animal products that work for people, Carolyn began using Hoof Saver for her nails and her daughter tried a horse wash called Mane 'n' Tail for her hair. "I noticed one day that her hair was looking absolutely gorgeous—soft and curly. I asked her if she got a perm, and she said, 'Guess what, Mom? I used Mane 'n' Tail on my hair.' "

Indeed, neither Carolyn nor her daughter is horsing around: No fewer than eight out of ten bottles of Mane 'n' Tail shampoo and conditioner are now sold for use by people, according to Roger Dunavant, president of Straight Arrow Products, makers of Mane 'n' Tail. "We started out in the horse business, and our human business has taken over our horse business," says Dunavant.

"People started using it because they noticed the sheen, and it helps strengthen thin hair," he says. Is it okay for people to use? You bet, he says, and a 32-ounce bottle, available in most feed stores and some Wal-Mart stores, is $8.95.

Hangover

Dealing with the Morning After

Y ou know where those head-pounding, stomach-churning symptoms came from. Usually, it's a rousing good time the night before—a wedding reception flowing with expensive champagne, a college reunion complete with old drinking buddies, a gee-I-wish-I-hadn't-had-so-many New Year's celebration.

Our survey takers have their share of fun, and they've also had their share of morning-after regrets. Several have remedies they're willing to share for getting rid of unpleasant symptoms.

THEY LOAD UP ON WATER

"I drink eight to ten ounces of water for every beer I have and keep a glass by the bedside to sip during the night," says Vicki, 50, a librarian from Denver. "That completely eliminates my occasional (very occasional) hangover."

Drinking about as much water as you can stand is without a doubt the best cure for a hangover, agrees John Brick, Ph.D., associate professor of biological psychology at the Center of Alcohol Studies at Rutgers University in New Brunswick, New Jersey. "Alcohol causes your body to lose water, so you can easily become dehydrated," he says. That leads to the familiar pounding head, as brain cells shrink and pull at nearby pain receptors, he explains.

Taking in plenty of nonalcoholic fluid while you're drinking, plus more afterwards, helps to reduce these symptoms.

THEY GET "JUICED"

Instead of water, some people prefer an orange juice chaser. "I dilute orange juice with seltzer water; otherwise, it's too acidic for my stomach," says Lauren, 38, a bartender from Queens, New York, who's quick to offer this end-of-the-evening drink to her customers as well.

In addition to its water content, orange juice can help a hangover several ways, Dr. Brick agrees. It contains fructose, a natural sugar that may help the body burn off alcohol faster and that restores blood sugar to normal. (Low blood sugar sometimes contributes to hangover symptoms such as headache, shakiness and fatigue.)

Orange juice also provides a good dose of potassium, a mineral that is lost during urination while drinking. Low potassium levels can contribute to feelings of weakness and shakiness. It also offers vitamin C. One study found that vitamin C helps to clear alcohol from the bloodstream faster.

B VITAMINS CLEAR THEIR HEADS

Speaking of vitamins, several people say they rely on B-complex vitamins to restore them after a hard night of partying. "I take three B-complex vitamin capsules, one before I drink, one while I'm drinking and the third before I go to sleep," says Kellee, 27, a dental hygienist student from Indianapolis. "I've used this many times, and it always prevents a hangover." She learned of the remedy at a health-food store in California.

While there's no proof that B vitamins can do anything to cure or prevent a hangover, it is true that drinking alcohol depletes your body of vitamins, Dr. Brick says. "People who have impairment from too much alcohol may see an improvement in mental fogginess if they take B vitamins," he adds.

A GOOD MEAL SETS THEM STRAIGHT

Several people suggest food as an antidote to a hangover. "Eating something—anything—always makes me feel better. It stops the queasiness and the headache," says Kathy, a nurse from California. Her favorite morning-after meal? A cheese omelet with lots of toast and a big glass of orange juice. Others prefer lighter fare. "Potato soup with parsley is good," says one.

Eating before and while you're drinking, especially protein-rich or high-fat foods such as cheese, is a good idea, Dr. Brick says. It slows the rate at which you absorb alcohol.

THEY REACH FOR ASPIRIN

Aspirin, alone or in combination with lots of water or even with vitamins, knocks out some people's hangovers. "I take two aspirin with a big glass of water before I go to bed, and I usually don't have much of a headache in the morning," says Mike, 40, a government contract worker from East Stroudsburg, Pennsylvania.

EDITOR'S NOTE: Aspirin's fine for a hangover headache, but one study found that taking aspirin before or during drinking increases blood alcohol concentrations and induces a quicker and more severe state of intoxication. So save your analgesic for after the party.

THEY SWEAR BY "HAIR OF THE HOUND"

The best cure for a hangover? A bit more of whatever caused it in the first place, claim several survey takers. "This does not simply postpone the effects. It completely eliminates the hangover and lets you go on with your life," contends Amy, 43, of Macomb, Michigan. "I've tried it several times, and both my father and grandfather have used it."

EDITOR'S NOTE: Dr. Brick agrees, but with a warning. "Alcohol is an analgesic and a central nervous system depressant, so it will alleviate hangover symptoms for some people." However, he warns, "drinking your breakfast is a clear sign of alcohol abuse."

Hay Fever

Resisting a Seasonal Problem

If you have hay fever, you don't need to consult a calendar to keep track of the seasons. You can tell by your runny nose, itchy, watery eyes, and scratchy throat that spring has sprayed tree pollen all over the place or that summer has delivered up a seemingly endless supply of grass pollen or ragweed.

Some of our survey takers are also equipped with their own internal seasonal warning systems. But rather than allowing hay fever to make hay with their sinuses, they've taken a proactive approach to stopping the symptoms caused by pollen and mold allergies. Here's what they do.

THEY GET SWEET RELIEF FROM HONEY

No fewer than a quarter of our survey takers claim that eating locally produced honey gives them sweet relief from hay fever symptoms or has eliminated them altogether.

Laura, 54, is typical. Although she always bought honey from the beekeeper down the block from her Rochester, New York, home, it wasn't until someone told her that locally produced honey could help stop her daughter's hay fever that she considered buying it in bulk.

While discussing her problem at work, some friends said that eating three tablespoons of locally produced honey a day for a year can eliminate hay fever symptoms. And a tablespoon a day after that was supposed to keep them away for good, her friends said. "The girls were having terrible hay fever," says Laura. "So I thought I'd try it."

Laura encouraged her daughters to pour honey on anything needing a touch of sweetener, like cereal or toast. Before long, she noticed the girls were suffering from fewer hay fever–related headaches, stuffy noses and other symptoms.

Five years later, Laura's daughters are still eating locally produced honey to keep their hay fever at bay. "It's a lot better than pumping yourself with medicine all the time," she says.

The use of raw honey for hay fever is widespread, says Bradford S. Weeks, M.D., president of the American Apitherapy Society, a Clinton, Washington–based group studying the medicinal qualities of bee products, including raw honey. "I've treated many people's hay fever with raw honey as a medical doctor," he says. "The rationale is that you get a homeopathic vaccination effect from the pollens which the bee collects from the local flowers and mixes into the honey in little increments. You seem to get kind of a desensitization process. This use for honey is not only widespread, but it's also on the upswing." (Homeopathy is an alternative medical therapy that advocates tiny doses of problematic substances to trigger the body's own healing responses.)

EDITOR'S NOTE: If you decide to give local honey a try, be careful. People with hay fever can also be allergic to the kinds of pollens found in honey. Try eating the honey in tiny amounts months before hay fever season, gradually increasing your intake up to a teaspoon a day. Lessen the amount or quit altogether if you have a reaction to it.

VINEGAR GIVES HER VICTORY

When the summer air begins to hang sticky-thick with pollen over her Cincinnati backyard, Bonnie knows it's time for a tablespoon of her favorite hay fever remedy: apple cider vinegar. "I can't tell you where the idea came from, just that my grandmother made us drink it, and it seems to work," says the 44-year-old savings and loan head cashier. "A lot of us here in Cincinnati will try anything when the ragweed and corn pollen gets bad."

Bonnie says she chokes down the dose in the morning because it seems to reduce or even prevent symptoms like watery eyes, itchy throat and sneezing later in the day. On sky-high pollen count days, she also eats a salad, with lots of, you guessed it, vinegar and oil dressing. "It's not a cure-all, but it helps when the symptoms are moderate."

Perhaps the first known antibiotic, vinegar has been used to treat a wide range of ailments, including chronic middle ear diseases and wounds.

TEA MAKES HER BREATHE EASY

Evelyn has tried and rejected over-the-counter symptom relievers. "They make me feel like I've been drinking," she says. So now when the grass starts going to seed, she simply sips a warm cup of herb tea. Her brew of choice: anything from Celestial Seasonings.

"I'm not sure whether it's the herb in the tea or the steam, but it soothes my throat and unstops my head a little bit," says the 50-year-old Greenville, South Carolina, widow.

While steam from tea could help clear clogged nasal passages, inhaling salt water may work even better, says John A. Anderson, M.D., head of the Division of Allergy and Clinical Immunology at the Henry Ford Hospital in Detroit. "Of course, inhaled steam would help irrigate the nose," he says. "But you can also squirt salt water in your nose and irrigate it that way as well. One brand of sterile salt water you can buy in the store for just this purpose is called Ocean Mist."

If you'd rather make your own salt water, dissolve a teaspoon of table salt in a cup of warm water. Then simply pour some into your palm, hold your hand under your nose and sniff with one nostril while blocking the other, he says.

A WASHCLOTH WIPES OUT HER SYMPTOMS

Grass Valley, California, has the best weather in the world, reports Rosalee. But as the name of the town suggests, Grass Valley has more than its share of you know what.

So every spring when grass pollen and mold starts pounding her sinuses, Rosalee covers her face with a wet washcloth and lies down for a while. "It stops my sneezing attacks and other symptoms that come with it," she says. "By the time the washcloth gets warm, I'm able to get up and get going again."

Rosalee's hay fever treatment may be soothing for several reasons, says Dr. Anderson. "If your eyes are swollen and you put a cool washcloth on them, it's going to feel good because, even if the water itself isn't that cold, evaporation cools the skin," he says. "The eye swelling could be helped by the coolness or the evaporation of the water."

And while you're inside lying down, make sure that your house is sealed off from pollen and your air conditioner is on, says Dr. Anderson. "If you keep your room or the house closed during the pollen season, there will be less pollen in the house than outside. Same goes for the car. If you drive around with the air conditioner on and the windows up, there will be less pollen inside the car than outside. Air conditioning is helpful."

THEY TOUT VITAMIN C

Lori, of Oak Brook, Illinois, remembers giving her boys extra vitamin C when ragweed or mold had them sneezing and wheezing. "We used to keep a bottle of 100-milligram chewables," she says, "but I probably didn't give them more than five in one day."

When Freida, of Mount Carmel, Illinois, read that she could unblock her hay fever–plagued respiratory tract with citrus bioflavonoids (the chemicals thought to give plants their color) and vitamin C, she literally left her over-the-counter antihistamines on the counter. "I took two 1,000-milligram tablets of bioflavonoids after each meal with 1,000 milligrams of vitamin C for two weeks, and it all cleared up."

Because hay fever symptoms are often similar to those of the common cold, vitamin C may actually help, says Dr. Anderson. "Studies have shown that, lo and behold, taking a lot of vitamin C did help a lot of the symptoms of the common cold. So just on that basis, nasal congestion, watery nose and that sort of thing seem to be helped by taking vitamin C. I don't think anyone has studied this in relation to hay fever, but it's possible that it would work," he says.

Bioflavonoids have a checkered past in the United States. Once manufactured and sold by drug companies to help protect blood vessels, bioflavonoids were pulled from the drug market a couple of decades ago by the Food and Drug Administration (FDA) because of insufficient evidence to support health claims for the supplement. More recently, however, research shows that the bioflavonoid quercetin and vitamin C taken together demonstrate antiviral activity. Some experts recommend taking 400 milligrams of the bioflavonoid quercetin twice a day between meals throughout hay fever season for relief. The FDA's ban only prevents doctors from prescribing bioflavonoids; you can still buy them at your local health-food store.

EDITOR'S NOTE: The National Research Council recommends getting 60 milligrams a day of vitamin C. Much higher doses of vitamin C are considered safe, but in sensitive individuals as little as 500 milligrams a day can cause diarrhea and abdominal cramping. If you want to take bioflavonoids and higher doses of vitamin C to combat hay fever symptoms, discuss it with your doctor.

Headaches

Tactics for Banishing Pain

It's fascinating when scientists turn an eye toward the possible reasons an old-fashioned remedy might work. Headache cures provide fertile ground for such research. Headaches are common—a complaint that comes up during more than half of all visits to the doctor's office. And the remedies people use to relieve such pain are truly diverse.

Our survey participants recommend everything from mineral supplements to a headband of potato slices for headache relief. And guess what? All these methods have scientific proof to back them up.

To be sure, not all the people who answered our survey realize there is scientific explanation for their favorite headache cure. And in truth, not all of them care. "I don't need a doctor to tell me what works and what doesn't," exclaims Max, a wastewater treatment supplier from Corvallis, Oregon. At least one woman, however, is grateful that she has been vindicated. "I am happy to hear that the remedy that helped me so much many years ago seems to stand up under scientific scrutiny," says Margaret, 74, of La Puente, California.

Headaches have a multitude of causes. The most common type—the tension headache—may develop from painful muscle spasms in the neck, jaw and head. It may also come from chemical changes in the brain or may be related to stress and tension. Migraine headaches may originate as an electrical change in brain cells, followed by a disturbed blood flow to the head—blood vessels that first constrict, then dilate to throb painfully. Migraines may also be associated with an inflammation of the arteries of the meninges (the covering of the brain). A number of triggers can set off a migraine, including hormonal changes in women, bright lights, a change in sleep pattern, and food or chemical sensitivites.

Experts agree that many kinds of headaches respond to simple measures. They do, however, issue a warning: See a doctor if it's your first bad headache or your worst headache ever, or if your headaches become frequent or sudden and severe, or if they are accompanied by fever, confusion or stiff neck. "These are all signs of potentially serious problems," says Alan Rapoport, M.D., codirector of the New England Center for Headache in Stamford, Connecticut, and assistant clinical professor of neurology at Yale University Medical School in New Haven.

For the occasional, unavoidable headache, here are a number of tips from those on the leading edge of experimental medicine—just regular folks trying out things at home.

OTCs Ease Their Pain

They're quick, they're cheap, and they work, which is probably why over-the-counter drugs are very popular for headache relief. More than one-third of the people answering this question said aspirin, ibuprofen or acetaminophen provides all the relief they need.

"I simply take two aspirin or one ibuprofen and, if I can, lie down for a few minutes. That always helps," says Maria, 46, a health care systems analyst from Princeton, New Jersey.

Over-the-counter pain-relieving drugs work by numbing the nerve endings in the skin, tissues and blood vessels that lead to the brain. Some are also combined with caffeine, which has an added effect on blood vessels.

Several people also say that using a decongestant helps a headache, whether it's sinus-related or not.

"Many decongestants contain phenylpropanolamine, a drug that constricts blood vessels and so may relieve a headache," Dr. Rapoport says.

EDITOR'S NOTE: All headache drugs, including the nonprescription kind, have a mean side to them if misused, Dr. Rapoport points out. "If you use them more than twice a week, you risk developing a condition called analgesic rebound," he says. "Your body becomes dependent on the pain reliever, and your headaches become more severe, longer-lasting, and harder to treat. When you stop taking it, your headache comes back, worse than ever." An analgesic rebound headache can last as long as two weeks before it tapers off. "That's why finding other means of headache relief besides taking frequent pain-relieving medication is important to people who get frequent headaches."

Ice Eases Their Throbbing Heads

Some 30 percent of our survey takers say that applying ice to the head, usually the back of the neck or forehead, is a fast, reliable way to abort a headache. A smaller number—about 20 percent—prefer heat, and some use a combination of both.

"I get icy cold hands when I'm about to start a migraine, as well as during one," says Cemela, 46, a health researcher from Allentown, Pennsylvania. "Sometimes plunging my hands into a basin of hot water helps to short-circuit the headache. But the best is a hot bath, where I lie with the back of my head and neck immersed as well as my hands and feet. And because the veins in my temples and around my ears become exquisitely tender, I use a frozen gel pack on the front of my head."

Ice helps both tension and migraine headaches by constricting blood vessels, especially if you use it on yourself at the very first signs of a headache, says Seymour Diamond, M.D., executive director of the National Headache Foundation and founder of the Diamond Headache Clinic in Chicago, the world's largest and oldest private headache clinic.

Some people like the feel of a flexible ice pack or a cold gel pack that can mold to the shape of the neck, so the cold can be concentrated at the base of the skull. (If you're sensitive to cold, you might want to wrap the ice pack in a small towel to buffer the effect.)

Heat can also have a soothing effect, Dr. Diamond says. Placing a heating pad on tight neck muscles for 20 or 30 minutes might relax them and ease a tension headache, he says. Some people enjoy the sensation of a hot shower pounding down on their skull, Dr. Rapoport adds.

SOME SLEEP IT OFF

Fighting off fatigue can be a head-pounding experience, and 15 survey participants take an aching head as a sign that it's time to take a nap. Those with a preference say they choose a dark, cool, quiet room. But they'll take what they can get! "Sometimes, sleep is the only thing that works for my headache, and so I'll stop and nap in my car if necessary," says Louise, 38, a medical equipment salesperson from Elizabeth, New Jersey.

"I don't get many headaches, but when I do, I often have other symptoms, too, such as an upset stomach," explains Mary, a management analyst for the U.S. Department of Defense who lives in Holland, Pennsylvania. "If I have the opportunity, I take a couple of aspirin and take a little nap, usually only 10 or 15 minutes. It always helps me feel better."

"Sleep often helps tension or migraine headaches, but it can make cluster headaches worse. Cluster headaches are characterized by an excruciating, sharp, boring pain in or around the eye and only last for about 1 to 1½ hours," Dr. Rapoport says.

EDITOR'S NOTE: *Too much sleep, though, can also cause headaches. People who sleep longer than usual on weekends, for instance, may wake up with a headache by Sunday morning. "Any change in sleep pattern upsets your body's natural rhythm, leading to fluctuations in your brain's chemistry, which may increase susceptibility to headaches," Dr. Rapoport explains.*

THEY WALK AWAY FROM PAIN

Stress and headaches seem to go together, and some of the people who get tension headaches say that getting out for a walk to blow off some steam works as well as aspirin to relieve a headache.

"It's almost like I am getting something out of my system," explains Max. "I'll get up and walk and try to breathe deeply, which is pretty easy around here, where the air is fresh and clean. Pretty soon, my anxiety and my headache are gone."

"Exercise can sometimes nip a tension headache in the bud," Dr. Diamond agrees. And while exercise might make an established migraine headache worse, people who begin to exercise regularly generally find they have fewer sieges, he says.

THEY KNEAD AWAY TENSION

Hands-on healing in the form of massage is particularly popular with our survey takers.

"My husband does something for me he learned from his chiropractor," says Verna, a homemaker from Nicholasville, Kentucky. "He rubs my shoulders and the back of my neck and head. When he finds a particularly sore spot, he rubs his thumbs in circles on it for a minute or so. Sometimes it hurts initially, but then I begin to relax, and it feels really good. I sit and relax for a few minutes after this, and my headache usually feels better."

Massage helps relax spasms of the scalp and neck that accompany many headaches, experts say. You can also lightly massage your temples.

SHE BRUSHES HER PAIN AWAY

Is it a mother's loving touch that eases the pain? Or a nervous system reaction that improves the circulation of blood through your head? Whichever it is, hair brushing seems to ease some people's headaches.

"I brush my hair gently. I used to do that for my daughter, too, and my mother did it for me when I had a headache," says Elva, 57, a doctor's assistant from Brooklyn, New York. "I brush all over, but especially, I brush upward from the back of the head, and away from the face at the temples. I don't know why, but it is very soothing."

Friction rubs, including hair brushing, are a common form of therapy. Medical experts speculate that brushing stimulates blood flow to the area of the body that is being brushed.

MAGNESIUM STOPS HER MENSTRUAL HEADACHES

"I don't take aspirin for any headache," reports Connie, a homemaker from Romulus, Michigan. Instead, she believes the calcium and magnesium supplements she takes every day (650 milligrams of calcium; 400 milligrams of magnesium), along with other supplements such as vitamin C, help keep her from developing the menstrual-related headaches that she and other women in her family are prone to get.

"Occasionally one will start, usually if I go for a few days without taking my vitamins, so then I will temporarily increase the amount I take by up to one-third, which comes to about 800 milligrams of calcium and 550 milligrams of magnesium," she says. "I've been doing this for about 15 years with success, and other women who have tried it also say it works."

Connie's relief is more likely to be coming from the magnesium in her supplement than from the calcium, says Alexander Mauskop, M.D., director of the New York Headache Center in New York City. "Research shows that people with low blood levels of magnesium are more likely to have one of many different kinds of headaches, including migraines and menstrual headaches," he says. There are a number of case reports of magnesium helping headaches, he says.

EDITOR'S NOTE: *The recommended Daily Value for magnesium is 400 milligrams. Ingesting up to 700 milligrams is considered safe. Amounts in excess of that could prove toxic, especially to people with weak kidneys. It's best to take supplementation only with your doctor's approval.*

POTATO SLICES THEIR PAIN

Several people tell us they tie a towel or bandana tight around their head at the temples for headache relief. Three say they take this remedy one step further: They tuck potato slices in the band.

As strange as it sounds, this apparently is a custom in several countries, explains Margaret. "A friend made up this remedy for me one day long ago when I was terribly sick with a headache, and it worked wonders," she says. "She soaked the slices in vinegar, tied the bandana on, then tucked the slices into the bandana at my temples and forehead. I left it on for a few hours. When I took it off, the potatoes were hot and dry, and my headache was gone."

In fact, a combination of cold—which would come from the moist potato slices—and pressure may well do the trick. According to medical experts, applying cold and gentle pressure to different parts of the head, including the nape of the neck and temples, can be helpful for a headache.

Heartburn

Dousing the Flames

F eel like acid strong enough to dissolve nails is burning a hole through your chest? Maybe it is!

Stomach acid is strong stuff, about as strong as battery acid. Normally, the mucus-secreting tissues protecting your stomach lining allow stomach acid to digest food without digesting you, too. But sometimes stomach acid leaks upward, through the circular muscle valve that separates your esophagus from your stomach, and irritates your lower esophagus. That's heartburn, and it often feels like a smoldering ember right under the breastbone.

Television commercials correctly point out that overeating is a common cause of heartburn. But it's not the only cause. Problems with delayed stomach emptying or disordered peristalsis—muscle problems that interfere with the wavelike contractions that move food through your digestive tract—can precipitate heartburn. So can malfunctions of that little muscular valve that separates your lower esophagus from your stomach.

If you have heartburn daily or even several times a week, see a doctor. "Frequent symptoms could be an indication of an inflamed esophagus or a beginning ulcer," says Ronald L. Hoffman, M.D., director of the Hoffman Center in New York City and author of *Seven Weeks to a Settled Stomach.*

Moderation in just about everything seems to be a key component of heartburn control. When our survey participants overdo it, their stomachs let them know it. "I just don't eat or drink the way I used to, and I feel a lot better for it," says Denis, 34, a power plant worker from Loudon, New Hampshire, who uses gingerroot tea to ease his occasional heartburn. Other people say that losing weight, eating smaller meals or not eating right before bedtime have improved their problem. Here are the details.

STOMACH-SOOTHING DRUGS THEIR TOP CHOICE

Tums, Mylanta, Rolaids, Maalox, Pepto-Bismol, Gaviscon . . . sounds like a shopping list for someone with a B-A-D case of heartburn. But those are only some of the many over-the-counter antacids our survey participants depend on to ease their acid stomach. "I chew a couple of Tums and the heartburn is gone, so why bother with anything else?" says Frank, 61, a retired aircraft mechanic from San Diego.

Antacids do help some people, Dr. Hoffman agrees. He prefers that his patients take an antacid that contains calcium carbonate and no aluminum compounds. Aluminum compounds have been linked with Alzheimer's disease and can also be absorbed by the body, preventing adequate mineralization in bone, he explains.

Some antacids contain an additional helpful ingredient—alginic acid— a gel derived from seaweed which floats on top of the acidic stomach contents and acts as a barrier between the acid and the esophagus. One survey participant, Lothar, a machinist from Deerfield, Michigan, uses kelp tablets for this same reason. "I think they're good for a number of stomach problems, but they're especially helpful for acid stomach," he says. He takes five tablets at the first sign of a problem.

Spicy Ginger Tea Helps Him

"I use a remedy I learned from my karate teacher and which I think works better than any over-the-counter antacid," says Denis, our New England power plant operator. Denis has problems with heartburn when he is pumping iron or shoveling in pizza.

"I take a two- or three-inch piece of fresh gingerroot, slice it very thin and simmer it in a quart of water," he explains. "Then, I sip it as lukewarm tea, two or three times a day, for three or four days, or until my stomach feels better. One quart of tea and my stomach feels better for months."

"Ginger has a long history of use as a stomach soother," explains Daniel B. Mowrey, Ph.D., a psychologist and director of the American Phytotherapy Research Laboratory in Lehi, Utah. "We're not sure how it works in this regard, but it seems to absorb the acid and have a secondary effect of calming the nerves."

Baking Soda Cuts Their Acid

About 20 percent of our survey takers recommend downing a glass of water containing a teaspoon or so of baking soda. "I don't have heartburn very often, but when I do, I simply drink some baking soda in water," says Edna, 55, a day-care worker from East Rockaway, New York. "It's handy, and it works real fast. Why go out and buy something when you have something that works right at hand?"

Editor's Note: It's true that baking soda is alkaline and has the capacity to neutralize stomach acid, but Dr. Hoffman discourages its use. Baking soda is extremely high in sodium. Anyone on a sodium-restricted diet should not use this remedy at all.

"Baking soda is loaded with salt (½ teaspoon contains almost 500 milligrams of sodium); in a few rare cases, people's stomachs have exploded from the combination of a large meal followed by a glass of baking soda and water," he says.

At least one case of baking-soda explosion has been reported in the medical literature. The case involved a man who consumed mass quantities of Mexican food, went home, got indigestion, drank a baking soda and water mix, and developed stomach pain so severe he required emergency medical care. Doctors discovered his stomach had been torn open from the extreme pressure of the food and the release of bubbly carbon dioxide from the baking soda.

THEY TREAT ACID WITH ACID

It seems strange that people would claim an acid—apple cider vinegar—helps reduce a stomach acid problem, but that's exactly what seven people told us. "One tablespoon of apple cider vinegar in some water and heartburn is gone in seconds," writes one.

"It's true that too much acidity is the problem in some cases of heartburn, but an equal number of cases are caused by inadequate acidity," Dr. Hoffman says. Trademarks of low stomach acidity: sour stomach and a feeling of fullness. "People say they feel like food is stuck in their craw," Dr. Hoffman puts it.

What happens is this: Food is improperly digested and remains in the stomach. The esophageal sphincter (that circular muscle we mentioned earlier) then relaxes and allows the food to reflux, or back up in the esophagus.

"I see this in a number of my patients," Dr. Hoffman says. "They've taken all kinds of antacids, with no relief. We perform a certain test which tells us that they have low stomach acid rather than high, and we feel justified in using a trial of additional stomach acid. We use hydrochloric acid tablets, but an old-fashioned way to do the same thing is vinegar."

CHARCOAL TO THE RESCUE

Our survey participants must be onto something. They recommend activated charcoal for a number of digestive problems—gas, indigestion, irritable bowel and heartburn.

"I don't get heartburn too often, because I'm careful about my diet, but when I do eat something like tomatoes and end up with heartburn, one capsule of activated charcoal takes care of the problem," says Helen, 76, of Saddle Brook, New Jersey.

Activated charcoal—charcoal that's been steam-processed to make it extremely porous—is considered a universal antidote. It's used in emergency rooms around the country to treat people who have been poisoned. In fact, Helen used it once to treat her husband, who accidently swallowed a vial of prescription pills, thinking they were vitamins. "I gave him the charcoal, then called the doctor," she says. "The doctor said I had done the right thing and to simply watch my husband for a few hours to make sure he was alright. Well, he was just fine."

EDITOR'S NOTE: Activated charcoal absorbs just about anything and will interfere with your body's ability to absorb medicines you need. So don't take it along with medicines. Activated charcoal may also interfere with nutrient absorption, so you won't want to take it with every meal, Dr. Hoffman says.

AFTER-DINNER WALK USURPS HER BURP

Taking a postprandial stroll—rather than a nap—is one way several people say they avoid heartburn, especially after they know they've overdone it.

"I usually feel uncomfortable after I've eaten a big meal; I feel stuffed, whether I have heartburn or not. And so I have made it a habit for years to get out for at least a short walk after eating," says Linda, 41, of Northampton, Massachusetts. "In fact, this has turned into a tradition of sorts with my family at holiday meals such as Thanksgiving and Christmas. Anyone who wants to can go out with me for a stroll through the countryside after dinner, and anyone who's not washing dishes usually does come along."

Walking's a great digestive aid, Dr. Hoffman agrees. But you'll want to avoid vigorous exercise, such as running, which can cause heartburn after a big meal.

BIGGER BELT EASES HIS SQUEEZE

Think of your stomach as a tube of toothpaste. If you squeeze the tube in the middle, paste goes in two directions—out the top and to the bottom of the tube. So you can imagine how a tight waistband around your middle could make trouble for your stomach by squeezing food upward. Doctors have been saying for years that as simple a measure as using suspenders instead of a belt, or wearing clothes with a generous waistband, can alleviate a heartburn problem. And the people who have tried it say it works!

"I was surprised how much it helped my heartburn," says Ray, 52, a drill press operator from Lawrence, Massachusetts, whose doctor suggested larger trousers. "I even look better now, since I am not trying to squeeze into too-tight pants. They weren't real tight when I was standing, but when I'd sit down, I could feel the squeeze around my waist. I just didn't do anything about it, because I kept hoping I would lose weight. I even feel like I can breathe easier and move easier now. This sure beats taking antacids."

Heart Palpitations

Fix-Its for the Flutter

Suppose your heart sometimes goes pitter-kerplunk instead of pitter-pat. Does your love life need a tune-up—or your heart?

Sorry, Valentine: In this case, a letter to Ann Landers won't cut it. Unless you've been dumped recently (and really hard), only your doctor can truly tell whether you've developed heart palpitations—a sometimes serious symptom characterized by a skipping, racing or hard-beating heart.

"There's no way you can be sure what's going on in this situation if you haven't seen a doctor," says Lou-Anne Beauregard, M.D., director of the Heart Station and Pacemaker Follow-up Center at Cooper Hospital/University Medical Center and assistant professor of medicine at the University of Medicine and Dentistry of New Jersey/Robert Wood Johnson Medical School, both in Camden. "Even people with healthy hearts skip beats, but if you notice it happening, you should probably get it checked out."

Once your doctor says your ticker is as sound as a Swiss watch—or diagnoses a problem and prescribes treatment—consider what our chest-thumping band of survey takers learned about their conditions.

MEDICATION MAKES HER UNEASY

Eleanor's allergy medication knocked out her congestion like a round-house right. But a short time after she began taking the prescription tablets, the 73-year-old Palm Coast, Florida, resident noticed a new symptom: heart palpitations. "It was a really strange feeling," she says. "A few times I almost blacked out."

Concerned, the retired drug company secretary read the warning that came in the drug package. To her surprise, heart palpitations were listed as a possible side effect. To test her theory that the medication might be causing her problem, Eleanor skipped the tablets for a few days. Sure enough, her palpitations stopped. She hasn't taken that allergy medicine since. "I'd rather suffer than have a heart attack," she says.

Over-the-counter and prescription medications are two of the leading causes of irregular heartbeats, says Dr. Beauregard. Over-the-counter cold and allergy capsules, for example, often contain decongestants that not only shrink mucous membranes to help you breathe easier, but constrict blood vessels and make the heart beat faster and harder, which can lead to heart palpitations. "A lot of the cold and allergy medications contain common ingredients that sort of turbocharge the heart," she says. "If you have heart or thyroid disease or high blood pressure, you should be very careful using these medications."

The best way to avoid a potential problem: Check the package label or dose instructions. "Often, the warning will be right on the package, and if you see a warning like that, it should tip you off that it has some effects on the heart," she says. If you do choose to use an over-the-counter cold or allergy medication, also keep an eye on the amount you're taking: "It's somewhat dose-related. You might be able to take Actifed or Sudafed at 30 milligrams and be fine but at 60 milligrams have palpitations," says Dr. Beauregard.

Editor's Note: Do not stop taking a prescription medication on your own. Discuss any side effects with your doctor. It's often possible for your doctor to switch your medications or alter the dosage.

MAGNESIUM SETTLES HIS HEART DOWN

In spite of the medicine he was taking, George's rapid heartbeat grew so frequent he was sometimes having two episodes a day.

His life changed when he read the condition might be caused by low magnesium levels and bought a multivitamin supplement with magnesium. "The results after taking the supplement were dramatic. In the 2½ months following, I had only three light attacks," says the Hartsville, South Carolina, resident.

Magnesium supplements for those with a deficiency may be a magnificent way to reduce heart palpitations because this mineral seems to stabilize the heart's electrical system, says Dr. Beauregard. "Magnesium is enjoying a resurgence in popularity in the cardiac-care community," she says. "It's been used to treat some very dangerous rhythm problems that result from the heart's electrical system firing at will."

So how do you know if you have a magnesium deficiency? If you take diuretics (water pills) for high blood pressure, you could be a candidate, says Dr. Beauregard. "Ordinarily, a normal diet would contain enough magnesium, but there are certain situations where you might not be getting enough, or you may be washing it out of your system with the water pills." And because magnesium is stored in the bones, you're also at risk for a deficiency if you have osteoporosis, she says. But before you rush out and buy

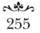

some magnesium supplements (some on the market contain both calcium and magnesium), check with your doctor, she says. "If you have kidney problems, magnesium accumulates and can become toxic in your blood," she says.

CAFFEINE IS MEAN TO THEIR HEARTBEAT

Several of our survey takers seem to have registered seismic activity from their heart while sipping java, eating chocolate or, for that matter, ingesting anything with caffeine. Says one 56-year-old: "Less coffee or none at all works best for me."

Can forsaking coffee or chocolate put your heart palpitations in check? "Certainly if people experience palpitations, they should avoid caffeine and probably watch out for chocolate, which contains a chemical similar in effect to caffeine," says Dr. Beauregard.

Too much alcohol can also cause heart palpitations, she says. In fact, researchers have documented irregular heartbeats in frat brothers two days after they drank excess alcohol at a fraternity party.

ICE WATER WORKS WONDERS FOR HIM

Sam, 61, of Marietta, Pennsylvania, is a cut-up. He's even got a recording of Rich Little doing Jack Benny on his answering machine. But doctors take his remedy for heart palpitations seriously: a glass of cold water.

Doctors aren't sure why, but they suspect swallowing food or fluid actually can press the esophagus against the left atrium of the heart in just the right way, ending palpitations, says Dr. Beauregard. Another possibility: The heat or cold somehow affects the heart in a similar way, she says. "We know it works; we just don't know why," she says.

AVOIDING FOOD DYE DOES IT FOR HIM

For nine years, Mary's son was troubled by rapid heartbeat. And even though he was given a drug for his symptoms, three of these episodes sent him to the emergency room. But it wasn't until the Oshkosh, Wisconsin, resident did some label reading that she found the answer to her son's problem.

"I noticed that his attacks always came after he'd eaten a packaged product like pudding, cake mix, snack foods and some drinks," she recalls. "I read the labels and saw that all these items contained a food dye, FD&C Yellow No. 5 (tartrazine). Since eliminating this dye from his diet, he hasn't had any more attacks, and with our doctor's help, we gradually tapered off his medication. I'm sure if he stays away from Yellow No. 5, he'll never have another spell."

Although heart palpitations caused by food coloring are probably rare, they shouldn't be overlooked as a possibility, says Dr. Beauregard. "I haven't seen a tremendous body of literature about it, but people are sensitive to certain things, and a reaction to a component like food coloring could be possible," she says.

HAWTHORN BERRIES ARE HER CHOICE

For years, Aletha suffered from frightening heart palpitations that temporarily boosted her blood pressure. "They would come on suddenly," she says. "I had no way of knowing when they would strike."

So when a friend recommended that she try an over-the-counter remedy featuring hawthorn berries, cayenne pepper and lecithin, the 72-year-old Modesto, California, resident was more than willing.

Just over 20 minutes after the first pill, she says she felt relief. Now when her familiar heart problem starts, she reaches for a hawthorn herbal capsule. "I just relax and let it work," she says.

While hawthorn berries aren't known to have any antipalpitation action, they do contain chemicals (vasodilators) that can increase blood flow, which could assist in treating heart palpitations, says Dr. Beauregard. "I suspect this person was feeling better either from the vasodilator components of these capsules or the placebo effect," she says.

Hemorrhoids

Soothing Treatments for Where You Sit

Here's a hemorrhoid joke you've probably never heard: A comic who callously wrote hemorrhoid jokes for years rushes to the doctor one day, frantic about a strange new pain that's making his behind ache and itch.

After listening politely for a while, the doctor can't resist: "Don't be too concerned," he says, "many people get it in the end."

Our suffering jokester has lots of company. There are several reasons why hemorrhoids are so common. Repeated straining during bowel movements or childbirth, wiping too hard or even passing a sharp object in your stool are some of the most likely causes.

But there's no shortage of remedies to soothe a savage case of hemorrhoids—our survey takers have shown us that. And while these techniques may not leave you laughing, our survey participants say they've kept them out of stitches (rectal surgery, that is).

THEY HAIL WITCH HAZEL

Few remedies for any ailment in our survey cast a spell over our survey takers like witch hazel. Nearly half say this plant extract works like magic to relieve hemorrhoid pain and swelling.

Jean has witch hazel on ice just in case her hemorrhoids act up. But the 65-year-old Catskill, New York, resident doesn't just place a bottle in the fridge. Jean says she soaks cotton pads or balls in witch hazel for those moments when she'd rather stand than sit. "I leave one on for five or ten minutes and it really soothes," she says.

Another witch hazel aficionado, Marge, 74, of California, says a sanitary pad dunked in witch hazel and warm water and applied to hemorrhoids "reduces swelling and relieves pain."

Witch hazel works so well against hemorrhoids that it's a common ingredient in some over-the-counter treatments like Tucks pads, says Lester

258

Rosen, M.D., associate clinical professor at Hahnemann University School of Medicine in Philadelphia and a board member of the American Society of Colon and Rectal Surgeons. But be careful: "Sometimes, witch hazel can aggravate an itching problem," he says. "Some people find it relieving and cooling; some people find it makes itching worse."

THEY PUT THEIR PAIN ON ICE

Ice—both crushed and cubed—rates a block-solid second place among our survey takers' home remedies.

Sharon, a 40-year-old Jackson, Kentucky, hospital lab manager says a nurse suggested ice to her after she bore her first child. When she needs relief, she fills an ice bag with ice—"crushed if I can get it"—adds a little water, and then sits on the bag. Gently. "By the time the ice has melted, I'm feeling better," she says.

Pamela, a 44-year-old rental agent in Mansfield, Massachusetts, says she also started using ice for hemorrhoids after having a child.

A nurse at the hospital told her to chill Tucks pads before applying for best results. But when Pamela discovered a short time later that the coldness seemed to provide more benefit, she traded in her pads for an ice pack. For even greater relief, Pamela lies on her couch or bed and elevates her feet. "It really seems to bring down the inflammation," she says.

EDITOR'S NOTE: Ice may be nice for some, but prolonged use could cause other problems, says Dr. Rosen. "It's not generally recommended to put ice on hemorrhoids. They're very sensitive, and ice may worsen clotting by slowing blood flow."

WATER POURS ON THE RELIEF FOR THEM

A warm water soak gets raves from long-time hemorrhoid sufferers like Sharon for relieving pain.

Not only does the condition run in her family, but for many years, the Taylorsville, Indiana, resident didn't eat enough fiber. And to top it off, she had children.

But she wasn't destined to suffer forever: She's discovered the soothing potential of a long, hot soak. "If you have hemorrhoids, you're going to find out what causes them and what cures them," says the homemaker and home-based business owner.

Sharon says she fills up a bath with warm water and adds a few squirts of antibacterial soap. "When I have an acute attack, it's the best thing I can do for temporary relief," she says. "The warm water and the antibacterial soap speed up the healing process, and it feels so much better."

Antibacterial soap may not be necessary, but a soothing soak is one of

Dr. Rosen's favorite remedies. "A hemorrhoid occurs when blood in a vein gets stopped up," he says. "And when your rectum is tight, it prevents the blood from flowing out, putting more pressure on your hemorrhoid." A warm soak tends to relax the anal sphincter muscle, and as a result, makes you more comfortable, he says.

NOXZEMA MEETS HER NEEDS

Tina's been a Noxzema fan for years, spreading the creamy white concoction on virtually every sunburn she's ever had. So it wasn't much of a jump from there to treat burning where the sun doesn't shine, she says. "Good old Noxzema is really the best thing I've found for them," she says.

Brandishing a tissue, the 60-year-old Franklin Park, Illinois, office clerk says she scoops some Noxzema out of the jar and then onto her hemorrhoids. She leaves the tissue in place "to keep from getting Noxzema all over my undies," she says. "It's really soothing and takes away the itch." Tina says she tries to leave the Noxzema on overnight.

EDITOR'S NOTE: Itchy, burning hemorrhoids may best be treated with zinc oxide rather than topicals like Noxzema, says Dr. Rosen. "Zinc oxide is usually good for people who are itchy, because it coats the area and, in a way, decreases the ability of people to scratch, allowing healing to take place." Desitin, an over-the-counter product sold to treat diaper rash, contains zinc oxide and is great for hemorrhoids, he says.

VITAMIN E HELPS EASE THEIR PAIN

Jim's itchy hemorrhoids were so tender that even wiping with regular toilet paper could make the blood flow. And over-the-counter preparations? "I tried them, but they seemed to make me more irritated and itchy," he says.

In desperation one day, the 52-year-old Rochester, New York, resident spread some liquid vitamin E over his toilet paper before wiping. To his amazement, the blood flow was cut to a trickle. "I'd say the oil has cut bleeding by 90 percent," he says.

Karen, 42, of Oregon, combines equal parts of liquid vitamin E, aloe vera and lecithin in a cup and applies the mixture two or three times a day to treat her hemorrhoids.

Wiping with Tucks pads or baby wipes should cause even less irritation than using liquid vitamin E, says Dr. Rosen. But in other cases, the solution may be as simple as wiping less vigorously and with softer toilet paper, he says. "There are many on the market now that really are gentle," he says.

HE FOCUSES ON HYGIENE

Rollo, from Port Orchard, Washington, says he was bothered with bleeding hemorrhoids until he read a story that changed his bowel hygiene habits. "I keep a small pan of water by the toilet. After the bowel movement, I wipe only once with a piece of toilet paper, then put the pan over the toilet. I squat over it and wash good with my fingers and then, using a paper towel, pat it dry . . . it has worked for me for years. But woe is me when I travel and have to be in motels, restaurants, et cetera, and have to use only toilet paper," he says.

As simple as it sounds, proper hygiene can help prevent aggravating hemorrhoids, says Dr. Rosen. "It's important that you're reasonably clean," he says. "That's why we sometimes suggest using baby wipes or Tucks wipes rather than wiping really hard and persistently."

THEY FIGHT WITH FIBER

Fred has never had hemorrhoids. But then again he probably never will. The 65-year-old Richmond, Virginia, resident drinks no less than 64 ounces of water and eats more than 25 grams of fiber a day.

He wasn't always this concerned about his diet: A former restaurant owner, Fred downed an average of four steaks a week! Today, he typically starts the day by eating a shredded wheat and all-bran cereal combination with skim milk, gobbles half a fiber bar by midmorning and includes a carrot at lunch. His dinner appetizer: raw cauliflower and shrimp cocktail sauce. "I just started reading about it, and before long, I knew I had to make some changes," he says.

And rather than chugging the water in one sitting, Fred says he slowly sips from a plastic bottle he props on his desk.

Sharon, from Illinois, is also high on fiber as a hemorrhoid preventive, eating five servings a day. "I love fresh garden vegetables," she says. "So that's where mine come from."

Getting adequate fiber and water may be the best preventive against hemorrhoids, says Dr. Rosen. "Fiber is good because it stimulates the bowel to form a rather solid bowel movement, and when you go to the bathroom, you feel a complete emptying," he says. "People strain and give themselves hemorrhoids because they have difficulty initiating a bowel movement."

But fiber isn't the only problem, says Dr. Rosen. "Too much junk food, coffee and dairy products like cheese, chocolate and ice cream make the stool mushy, almost like baby stool. Babies have mushy stool because they drink milk and formula and not much else," he says. "When you have mushy stool, you have trouble going to the bathroom. You are forced to bear down or go a little more frequently, and those are things that lead to hemorrhoid formation."

Over-the-counter fiber preparations like Metamucil, Konsyl or Citrucel taken after breakfast are all convenient ways to increase fiber intake, he says. And when you're eating lots of fiber, drinking six to eight glasses of water a day becomes even more important, because it helps prevent your stools from becoming too hard, says Dr. Rosen. And it keeps hemorrhoids at bay.

Hiccups

Tips for Stopping the Spasm

I f you complain about having hiccups, you're more likely to get a laugh than some sympathy.

But if you're trying to lick those hiccups, you're in for some TLC. It seems everyone has a favorite hiccup remedy, ranging from the basic, like breathing into a brown paper bag, to the bizarre: An Israeli doctor recently reported that he successfully treated hiccups with anal manipulation.

Though not nearly as controversial—or potentially uncomfortable— our survey takers also produced a prodigious supply of hiccup remedies. Here's what they say.

SUGAR HALTS THEIR HICCUPS

A simple spoonful of sugar delivers sweet relief to more than a sprinkling of our survey's hiccup sufferers.

For decades, Gwen's used a teaspoon of sugar to treat hiccups in herself, her children and her grandchildren. But her latest success came at work just recently. While walking past an adjoining office, the 53-year-old Fayetteville, North Carolina, secretary heard hiccuping coming from inside. Stopping, she poked her head in the door. "Is that you?" she said to a woman sitting there. The woman blushed: "It's me and I've got the hiccups."

Gwen described her remedy to the woman and helped her track down a pack of sugar. Seconds after swallowing the sweet spoonful, the woman's hiccups were gone. "I've never known it to fail," says Gwen. In fact, she even gave her infants a teaspoon of sugar water any time they suffered from hiccups.

Marjorie, of Yardley, Pennsylvania, has friends who have gone as far as standing on their heads and drinking water simultaneously to get rid of hiccups. But the 50-year-old apartment manager says any time her children suffered from hiccups, she would give them a teaspoonful of sugar, and that was the end of the problem. "It would stop immediately," she says.

Sugar hasn't become the sweetheart of hiccup remedies for nothing. The texture of sugar may provide just enough sensation to stop a spasm in your diaphragm, the true source of hiccups, says Lloyd M. Loft, M.D., professor of otolaryngology at New York Medical College and attending surgeon at the Manhattan Eye, Ear and Throat Hospital in New York City.

"Things like eating or drinking, even emotion, can sometimes irritate nerve receptors that control the diaphragm, causing spasms," says Dr. Loft. "Once the spasm in the diaphragm starts, this creates what's known as a reflex arc—a nerve message that travels back and forth from the organ to the brain like a circle. You need something to break the arc. I think sugar is effective because the same nerves that generate the spasm are used in swallowing—and the texture and taste of sugar provide a sensation that stimulates those nerves."

BROWN BAGGING WORKS FOR THEM

A hefty percentage of our survey takers say breathing into a brown bag is an effective hiccup remedy.

Take Bernice. Her son never had hiccups, but the way the 80-year-old Milwaukee resident remembers it, every time she turned around her cousin Darwin had lapsed into another round. More than once, Darwin's mother came over to Bernice's house in a huff, wondering what to do to end his hiccups. And more than once, Bernice suggested that Darwin breathe into a brown paper bag. "We'd have him breathe into the bag until he stopped hiccuping and that was it," she says.

Brown bags may actually help beat hiccups for several reasons, says Dr. Loft. There's some evidence that mentally focusing on a task, like breathing into a bag, may also break the reflex arc. But carbon dioxide, expelled from your lungs after every breath, may play an even greater role, he says. "Some experts occasionally suggest inhaling a preformed mixture of 5 percent carbon dioxide for hiccups," says Dr. Loft. "When you breathe into a bag, you expel carbon dioxide; so when you breathe it back in, you're raising the carbon dioxide in your blood."

THEY SOUR THEIR HICCUPS

Don't call these folks sourpusses, but they use lemon or pickle juice to lose their hiccups.

Rhonna knows her remedy's a dilly, but the 34-year-old Topeka, Kansas, dental assistant says she gets rid of hiccups by drinking a tablespoon of pickle juice. "My husband will back me up on this," she says. "It ends them immediately."

A friend's mother shared the secret with her years ago, and she's been using it ever since, says Rhonna. And because they almost always have a jar of pickles in the refrigerator, it's a convenient remedy.

Dede tried holding her breath. But it wasn't until a family friend suggested sucking on a lemon wedge that she finally found a cure that worked, she says. "It works immediately every time for me," says the 49-year-old Camarillo, California, resident. Dede says she simply cuts off a lemon wedge and sucks on it. "And because we live in California, we've always got lemons around."

Cam's lemon remedy came in handy when a family member developed hiccups at a restaurant. "Someone had a lemon slice in their drink and I said chew on that. They did and their hiccups went away," says the 64-year-old Sante Fe, Texas, resident.

Like sugar, the strong taste of lemon or pickle juice could shock your diaphragm's nerves out of spasm, says Dr. Loft. "These are very potent flavors to have in your mouth," he says. "They really stimulate the taste receptors, even cause you to swallow or gag a little bit. This strong stimulation of the nerves is just what you need." An ice water gargle is also an effective way to shock your diaphragm into behaving, says Dr. Loft.

Brain Teasers Top Their List

Stephanie has a theory about hiccups: The retired 71-year-old Llano, Texas, resident says if she catches them early, she's able to prevent an attack. If not, she's likely to spend the next five minutes making that awkward, yet familiar, gasping sound. "It seems like once these things get established, they become an automatic reflex that is hard to get rid of," she says.

So as soon as she hears the first hic, she repeats to herself, "This is going to go away. I'm not going to have any more hiccups." And according to her, she doesn't. "Most people would probably say pooh to that, but it works," she says.

Robert, 61, of Kentucky, also finds concentrating on something to be effective. Another survey taker is more specific: He says trying to recall the names of ten bald men works well.

Phyllis, of Greybull, Wyoming, says she practiced the game show equivalent of this technique on an unsuspecting hiccupper at a local laundromat. While the woman was folding clothes, Phyllis says she asked, "When was the last time you saw a white horse?" At first, the woman seemed to ignore her. A short time later, however, she answered the question. And after she did, Phyllis says the woman's hiccups were gone.

Although just concentrating may help end hiccups, Dr. Loft says concentrating on performing a task seems to generate the best results. "I'll give you an example: Some people talk about drinking from the wrong side of a cup. Did you ever try this? This is tough! You have to think about how you would do it," he explains. "Medically, I can't think of why that would work other than it takes a lot of concentration. And there's some evidence that intensely focusing on something else is an effective remedy."

THE EARS HAVE IT HERE

Cheryl's hiccup cure may require the dexterity of a circus juggler, but that hasn't stopped the 41-year-old Brighton, Michigan, mother and former nurse from using it on her children. "It was my mother's surefire technique," she says.

Just like her mother many years ago, Cheryl instructs her son to gently insert a single finger in each ear. Next, Cheryl gently pinches his nostrils shut with one hand while offering him a glass of water with the other. "The idea is to have him take as many little swallows as he can," she says. "Somehow this must block the eustacian tubes in the ear and put pressure on the diaphragm to relax."

A slight variation on this multiple-orifice approach comes from Tom in Mishawaka, Indiana. "What I do is fill a glass with water and put a straw inside. Then I take my two index fingers and put them firmly in my ears," he explains. "After exhaling, I suck the water through the straw without taking any breaths of air. When I'm finished, I wait half a minute and take my fingers out of my ears very slowly. It works."

According to the medical journal *Lancet*, sticking your fingers in your ears temporarily short circuits the nerve that controls hiccuping.

A TICKLE WORKS FOR THEM

Shelly and family used to try to scare one another any time one of the clan contracted hiccups. The Addam's Family they weren't. "It's hard to scare someone when they're expecting it," says the 38-year-old Norcross, Georgia, homemaker.

Their new technique: tickling. "Tickling the one with hiccups so they laugh hysterically has worked 100 percent of the time in my family," she says. "You have to make sure that the person is laughing, though."

Could a little coochy-coo cure hiccups? In fact, tickling or scaring someone affects them in much the same way, says Dr. Loft. "Reflexes are controlled by the nervous system," he says. "When you frighten someone, when you tickle them, it changes the outflow of nerve patterns to the brain, so once again, in a basic way, you fool the nervous system into breaking the reflex."

While less enjoyable, gagging can also help end hiccups. "Gagging is a powerful, protective reflex stimulating lots of nerves, and that may break the reflex arc," he says. Painless ways to make yourself gag: putting your finger in your throat, touching the back of your mouth with a tongue depressor, or even tugging lightly on your tongue, he says.

High Blood Pressure

Pointers for Dropping Those Numbers

Most of the 50 million Americans with high blood pressure have what doctors call primary, or essential, hypertension. That means there is no underlying disease—no kidney or hormone condition, for instance—creating the problem.

Medical experts say the exact cause for this kind of high blood pressure is unknown. Many doctors who treat high blood pressure, however, argue that many of the contributing causes are well known: Obesity, a high-fat or high-salt diet, smoking, alcohol abuse, too much everyday stress and not enough physical activity all combine to send blood pressure creeping upward over the years.

In fact, instead of turning directly to medications, these days some doctors advise their patients with high blood pressure to take at least six months to attempt to lose weight, quit smoking and drinking and begin exercising, says Robert DiBianco, M.D., director of cardiology research at Washington Adventist Hospital in Takoma Park, Maryland. "If their blood pressure is still too high at the end of that time, they'll begin using drugs to treat it," he says.

Many of the 83 people who talked to us about our question on high blood pressure use a number of tactics to keep their condition in line. Most are under a doctor's care, and some use drugs. But they also rely on dietary changes such as eating more garlic and onions, lowering salt intake and increasing their intake of potassium, calcium and magnesium.

Some of the survey takers are primarily vegetarian. One man even contends that simply drinking more water has dropped his blood pressure. And these people use exercise both to trim their weight and relieve the stress they believe contributes to their problem.

Because they used a combination of these remedies, it's often difficult for them to say exactly what's helping and what's not. While that might make it hard for them to compare, for instance, the effectiveness of the calcium supplement they take each day with the beta-blocker their doctor prescribes for them, it's probably the best approach they can take, Dr. Di-Bianco says. "It's not very scientific, true. But a combination of treatments works best for most people," he says.

Here, then, is what our survey participants say helps keep their blood pressure normal.

THEY GO FOR GARLIC

Almost half of those who recommend a home remedy for blood pressure come up with the same thing: garlic. Most use fresh or cooked, some use powdered garlic capsules or tablets (so-called deodorized garlic) and a few prefer garlic oil. No one we contacted, however, said they rely solely on garlic to control their blood pressure.

"I microwave two or three cloves in water until they are soft, let them cool, then just dip out the cloves and eat them," explains John, 78, a retired insurance salesman from Eau Claire, Wisconsin. "That kills the strong odor and softens the garlic. It gives it a pleasant, nutty taste without overcooking it," he says.

John's had high blood pressure since he had a kidney infection some 15 years ago and has been eating garlic every day for about three years. "I also eat a low-salt, low-fat diet with very little meat and have been taking blood pressure medication," he says. Using these methods, his blood pressure remains normal.

Garlic remains a controversial treatment for high blood pressure, says Yu-Yan Yeh, Ph.D., associate professor of nutrition at Pennsylvania State University in University Park. "In animal studies, the benefits do seem to be clear," he says.

In a study done with laboratory animals, for instance, a diet containing the equivalent of five to six cloves of garlic a day led to a 40 percent drop in blood pressure.

"Most studies with humans show about a 10 to 15 percent reduction in blood pressure," says Dr. Yeh. "These studies have been done mostly on people with high cholesterol, in an attempt to lower cholesterol. The reduction in blood pressure was a secondary effect."

Should you add garlic to your diet? "I personally believe there is merit in the preventive use of garlic," Dr. Yeh says. "However, I would use it in addition to other, proven dietary changes, such as a low-salt, low-fat diet."

THEY SHOOK THE SALT HABIT

About 25 percent of the people who answered say a low-salt diet has helped them control their blood pressure. "I think I've been pretty successful at reducing salt in my diet by eliminating high-salt foods or choosing reduced-salt versions," says Leona, 63, a housewife from Des Moines, Iowa. Both she and her husband have borderline high blood pressure.

Lunch meats, hot dogs, canned soups, most processed foods and snacks such as crackers, popcorn and nuts are just some of the items she's learned require label-reading. "I try not to buy anything that has more than 500 milligrams of sodium per serving," she says. Her one weakness: cheese. "I love it, and although I can tolerate the low-fat versions, the low-fat, low-sodium kind is tasteless as far as I'm concerned. So I don't buy more than a quarter pound at a time, because I know I'll eat it up fast."

Not all people with high blood pressure find that cutting out salt helps, but enough—about 25 percent—can see a reduction of three or four points in both the high and low readings if they cut their sodium intake in half, experts say. People who are salt-sensitive are most likely to benefit, but there are no tests readily available (at least, not yet) to weed out salt-sensitive individuals.

EXERCISE ADDS TO HER RESOLVE

About 10 percent say they use exercise, mostly walking, to help control their blood pressure. "My doctor says the exercise I do has a lot to do with my blood pressure staying down," says Betty, 56, a retired schoolteacher from Greenville, North Carolina, with a family history of high blood pressure. "I walk for 30 minutes, four or five times a week, around my neighborhood. I wanted to lose weight, too, and I think the walking helped me to lose about ten pounds." She also takes medication for her problem.

Studies suggest that people who exercise cut their risk of developing high blood pressure by 35 to 50 percent compared with sedentary people, regardless of their body weight. "Many doctors believe exercise is worthwhile simply because it is an aid to weight control, and being overweight is a major risk factor for high blood pressure," Dr. DiBianco says.

SHE GETS A DAILY DOSE OF DOG

Studies show that, at least for people who like animals, petting a dog or cat or even just gazing at an aquarium of fish lowers blood pressure, at least temporarily.

Well, Rose Marie, 59, a cleaning lady from Winton, Minnesota, fully appreciates the demands that her little dog, Ralf, puts on her. Like any self-respecting canine, Ralf likes to get scratched behind the ears ("I find it very soothing to do, too," Rose Marie says). And he insists on a daily walk. "I get home around 3:00 P.M., and we walk about two miles, every day except Sunday, before it gets dark," Rose Marie explains. "Both my mother and father had high blood pressure, and mine was about 220/110 at its highest. Now it's about 130/80, or lower." She attributes this to her blood pressure medication, 1,000 milligrams daily of supplemental calcium, a low-salt diet and a daily dose of dog.

THEY TAKE A FISH TO LUNCH

Several people say that fish is on their menu two or three times a week. "I've read so many times about how fish is good for your heart," says John, 67, of Newark, Delaware. "I don't know what it's doing for my blood pressure, but it's sure nice to be able to eat something I really enjoy and that's good for me, too." His top choices are grilled salmon or tuna. "And try fresh mackerel in mustard sauce, if you can get it," he recommends. "Certainly, fish can be part of a heart-healthy, low-fat diet," Dr. DiBianco says.

POTASSIUM AND OTHER MINERALS AID SOME

Just as too much salt can raise blood pressure in some people, too little of certain minerals seems to be associated with an increase in blood pressure.

Potassium is one of those minerals, and six people we surveyed say they go out of their way to make sure they get enough of it. "My doctor told me to eat a handful of dried apricots each day for potassium," says Rose Marie of Winton. That's a good choice. Half a dozen whole dried apricots offer about 600 milligrams of potassium (and about 100 calories). Potatoes with skins, pinto or lima beans, raisins, orange juice and bananas are also loaded with potassium.

Several people also say they take calcium and magnesium supplements. Increased intakes of both these minerals have also been associated with lower blood pressure. But researchers say they need to understand more about how these minerals may affect blood pressure before they recommend increased amounts.

"For now, I'd simply recommend you make sure you get the recommended Daily Value of these two minerals," Dr. DiBianco says. That's 800 milligrams of calcium, and 350 milligrams of magnesium. Potassium has no DV, but doctors studying potassium and blood pressure say you should aim for 3,000 to 4,000 milligrams a day. Most people get only about 2,500 milligrams a day.

EDITOR'S NOTE: Over-the-counter potassium supplements are restricted by law to contain less than 100 milligrams of potassium per tablet—the amount found in about one inch of banana. So your best potassium sources are fresh fruits and vegetables and their juices. Higher-dose potassium supplements are available only by prescription, with good reason. The compound these supplements most often contain, potassium chloride, can cause intestinal ulcers.

HE TAKES WATER

"I know it sounds too good to be true, but I believe it has really helped me," says Ed, 65, a retired steak house owner from Richmond, Virginia. He's referring to his new habit of drinking at least 64 ounces (eight 8-ounce cups) of water daily. "My blood pressure dropped about ten points within three weeks of starting to do this," he says. Ed also takes about 600 milligrams of supplemental potassium a day.

His method is based on the book *Your Body's Many Cries for Water*, by F. Batmanghelidj, M.D., founder of the Foundation for the Simple in Medicine, in Falls Church, Virginia. Dr. Batmanghelidj believes that high blood pressure and many other illnesses result from chronic dehydration, which he says, interferes with the natural two-way flow of fluids in and out of cells and causes constant constriction of the blood vessels, leading to higher blood pressure. Dr. Batmanghelidj recommends drinking two eight-ounce glasses of water before every meal.

"Drinking more water is generally not harmful unless you have some sort of kidney disorder that interferes with fluid excretion," Dr. DiBianco says. "In fact, water has beneficial effects for all the organs in your body. However, studies do not indicate that people develop hypertension because they are dehydrated. I wouldn't count on water to lower anyone's blood pressure."

SOME SEEK CALM

They meditate, breathe deeply, listen to soft music or simply try to stay calm in the face of day-to-day minor disasters. "I really think it does help to have some quiet time each day," says Martha, 54, a church secretary from Chicago who was recently diagnosed with mild high blood pressure. "It helps keep you calm when the going gets rough."

Does relaxing really help reduce blood pressure? Researchers know that certain kinds of activities, such as resting with your eyes closed or breathing slowly and deeply, can drop blood pressure temporarily. Whether or not such techniques can contribute to a significant long-term reduction in blood pressure is unknown, says Peter Kaufmann, Ph.D., chief of the Behavioral Medicine Branch of the National Heart, Lung and Blood Institute in Bethesda, Maryland.

"Studies have had mixed results, and results have not been strong enough for review committees to make recommendations to the public," he says.

None of these activities is harmful, however. If you feel that staring at fish in your aquarium or anything else that helps you relax is having a positive effect on your blood pressure, go for it.

High Cholesterol

Bringing Those Levels Down

Ten years ago, if your doctor warned you that your cholesterol was too high, you might have nodded your head solemnly, then later pondered his statement while eating a good cheeseburger.

What a difference a decade makes. Of course, heart disease is still the nation's leading cause of death, made possible, in large measure, by gooey Mr. Cholesterol sticking to your arterial walls. But our survey shows that more than a third of the participants know that there are simple and effective ways to reduce this dangerous buildup.

Pointing to their plunging cholesterol levels (and shrinking waistlines) with pride, they say getting cholesterol levels to drop below 200 is as easy as cutting the fat out of your diet, getting regular exercise and, in some cases, taking vitamin and mineral supplements. And that's also the prescription shared by some of the country's leading health experts.

LIVING THE LOW-FAT LIFE

Our survey takers tend to know that a low-fat diet is crucial—but they each have their own tips for eliminating fat.

Judy, for example, has a weakness for bacon, lettuce, and tomato sandwiches—and the more creamy mayo the better. "What can I say, I'm a sandwich person," says the 52-year-old Goodland, Kansas, resident.

And yet, once Judy restricted her beloved BLTs to once a month and adopted other fat-reducing measures, in a year her cholesterol dropped nearly 100 points and she lost 20 pounds.

Also, instead of loading up on fatty lunch meats like bologna, Judy now favors low-fat fare like broccoli, green salads, turkey and fish.

Helen, on the other hand, still hasn't mastered a low-cholesterol Christmas: Peanut butter balls and chocolate marshmallow fudge are as certain to appear on her holiday menu as gifts under the tree. Come New

Year's, however, the North Tazewell, Virginia, resident shifts into high cholesterol–fighting gear. "We just tried a low-fat banana nut cake a few days ago, and it was pretty darn good," says the 62-year-old grandmother.

Helen has also traded her two percent milk for skim, eggs for low-fat egg substitutes, lunch meat for turkey slices, and regulation mayo for fat-free condiments like mustard. Fried chicken, another longtime favorite at her home, has become a rarity. "Now I grill or bake chicken," she says. She's also added more fruit like grapefruits, oranges and bananas, and vegetables like broccoli, cabbage and green beans to her plate.

The fruits of her labor? In just a few months, Helen's cholesterol reading went from 240 to 203.

Margie tells a similar story. There's no other way to describe the old Margie: She was a beef and potatoes person. But it was the beef rather than the potatoes that pushed her cholesterol level over 300. (Well, maybe all that butter on the potatoes had something to do with it.)

For a time, Margie's doctor urged her to simply switch to chicken and vegetables to get her cholesterol down. But when the 71-year-old cafeteria worker didn't respond quickly enough to those changes, he advocated adding fish, oat bran and niacin to her diet. Within a year, her cholesterol level dropped to 185.

"He was really surprised by the drop, but I guess I really did change my eating habits quite a bit," she says. "I used to eat fried potatoes and scrambled eggs with cheese. Now I eat a lot of fruit salad and vegetable salad. And low-cal potato salad with nonfat mayonnaise. I used to do a lot of frying, and now I bake things like chicken or fish with all kinds of seasonings."

Margie learned firsthand that some people aren't as efficient at metabolizing dietary fat and, as a result, need to take more dramatic steps to prevent the progression of heart disease.

"The good news is that, if someone is willing to make big changes in his diet, cholesterol levels may come down by 40 percent on average," says Dean Ornish, M.D., director of the Preventive Medicine Research Institute in Sausalito, California, and author of *Dr. Dean Ornish's Program for Reversing Heart Disease* and *Eat More, Weigh Less*. "But it requires much more change than conventional recommendations. Unfortunately, many people think that a 30 percent–fat diet is a low-fat diet. But eating like that won't really do much. Ideally, a 10 percent–fat diet is what our research shows to have the most dramatic impact. That means most people, optimally, should have no more than 20 grams of fat a day." (The 10 percent he's referring to is 10 percent of total calories from fat, by the way. He doesn't mean that for every nine bites of potato you can add a pat of butter.)

"If your blood cholesterol is elevated and you don't have heart disease, you can begin by making moderate changes," says Dr. Ornish. "If that's enough to bring the cholesterol level down substantially, then that may be all you need to do. If not, it doesn't mean that you've failed at dieting, it means that you need to make bigger changes—and a simple cholesterol test would tell you that."

LEARNING TO SPARE THE FAT

Roberta never had what you'd call high cholesterol—at its peak a few years ago, the 50-year-old Midland, Michigan, native chalked up a reading of 193. And after taking a healthy cooking class and an herb supplement and starting a new exercise program, her cholesterol level has hit an impressive new low: 139. She's also lost 15 pounds in four months. But the irony is that Roberta wasn't even trying to bring her cholesterol down. "I just wanted to be healthier and help my husband lose some weight after he quit smoking," she says.

Among cooking tips, Roberta says she discovered that ground turkey meat can have almost as much fat as ground beef if the turkey's skin is ground up with the meat—a common practice. She also learned that non-fat yogurt can be used as a tasty, but skinny, substitute for fat-laden salad dressings and potato toppings. Other beneficial swaps she's instituted in the family meal plan: nonfat cottage cheese for ricotta cheese in lasagna and olive oil instead of margarine or butter.

"I get some flack from my family for using so little fat, but someday they will thank their mother for their health," she says.

And her husband? "He's lost about 20 pounds, too, although he still has a little left to go."

Roberta's cooking classes have paid off handsomely, but she may do even better if she reconsiders oil's role in her food preparation, says Dr. Ornish. "Oils are 100 percent fat and all oils—even olive oil—have some saturated fat. If people did nothing more than eliminate all oils from their diet, including cooking oil, their weight and blood cholesterol levels would come down, sometimes substantially. The best kind of oil is no oil because oil is the single most concentrated form of fat. One tablespoon of oil is 14 grams of fat. If people have to use oil, they can spray a little Pam on their cooking utensils, but you don't really even need to use oil when you cook; you can sauté using water, even juice," says Dr. Ornish.

WALKING AND RUNNING CHOLESTEROL DOWN

There was nearly unanimous agreement among survey participants that exercise plays a powerful role in reducing cholesterol.

Marcie's three dogs—Corky, Daisy and Keesha—are so rambunctious that walking them together is like adoption day at the pound.

"Honestly, they're like a bunch of teenagers when they get together," she says. "You just can't control them." So the 43-year-old Allegan, Michigan, housewife walks each dog separately for at least one mile each day.

She doesn't stop at walking her dogs, however. Three times a week, Marcie begins the day carefully stretching for 40 minutes and then performing 20 minutes of aerobics at home to contemporary Christian music. Then, twice a week she follows along with Jane Fonda for a 60-minute step aerobic workout.

As a result of exercise combined with a low-fat diet, within a year Marcie's cholesterol has dropped from 248 to 216.

As you're probably aware, cholesterol is divided into good and bad varieties. The good cholesterol—called HDL (think H for helpful)—actually helps clean your arteries. LDL (like L for loser) clogs your arteries. Studies show that regular aerobic exercise, like walking or dancing, actually helps increase your HDL, while sending the evil LDL packing. To obtain those benefits, however, most experts suggest getting 30 minutes of moderately vigorous exercise like walking, jogging, biking or aerobics three to four times a week.

DROVES PREFER GARLIC CLOVES

Garlic is cited as a pungent key player in many a cholesterol-reduction strategy.

Consider Henry. The 68-year-old Strongsville, Ohio, resident says he gobbles no fewer than three to four cloves a day to help reduce his cholesterol.

This is the new Henry we're talking about. Years ago, back when he was working as a driver for a bakery in Cleveland, Henry was more likely to stuff a deep-fried dessert in his mouth—specifically, a beloved apple-filled pastry that was coated in sugar. Eating one or two of those high-fat treats a day while on the job helped him pack on 50 extra pounds and pushed his cholesterol sky-high. "I can't remember how high it was, but the doctor said he wanted me to check into the hospital. I said you can check me in but I'm not going. I just don't believe in those places."

Henry did take the matter to heart, however, and began walking (sometimes as much as three miles a day), jogging and watching the fat in his diet. Among other things, his beloved pastries went by the wayside.

Meanwhile, Henry also started eating raw, finely chopped garlic, washing it down with little more than a glass of water, and taking a liquid lecithin supplement that he bought at a local health-food store.

His cholesterol level is now at 207, and Henry is 50 pounds lighter. And when he takes his daily walk, people tell him so, says Henry. "Just the other day, one of the gals in the development where we live said, 'Hey, you used to have a pot belly.' I said, 'Yeah, but not anymore.' "

Garlic can add firepower to your blood-fat reduction strategy. Just don't use it as your only weapon, says Dr. Ornish. "The problem with things like garlic and oat bran is that people often view them as a magic bullet that will enable them to eat a lot of fat and cholesterol without making meaningful changes in their diet. And that's when it becomes a problem," says Dr. Ornish. "One patient once told me he had a cheeseburger, but he had it on an oat bran bun."

Much of the research seems to show that raw chopped or crushed garlic—just like Henry eats—has the most benefit. During crushing or chopping, the raw garlic releases a chemical called ajoene that apparently inhibits blood clots. According to Varro E. Tyler, Ph.D., professor of pharmacognosy at the School of Pharmacy and Pharmacal Sciences at Purdue University in West Lafayette, Indiana, and author of *The Honest Herbal*, ajoene from fresh garlic "is at least as potent as aspirin" in thinning the blood.

There is also some suggestion but no hard evidence yet that lecithin may help reduce cholesterol.

THEY TURN ON THE JUICE

With her cholesterol topping the charts at a life-threatening 330, Myrna had little choice but to take drastic action. Checking into a San Diego–based natural health center, the 63-year-old Brooklyn, New York, reading specialist was treated to nothing but fresh fruit and vegetable juices, salads and exercise.

Two weeks passed. Time enough for her to think about her health. Time enough to give her a new lease on life: Myrna's cholesterol dropped to 203. "I absolutely believe that the more raw fruits and vegetables I eat, and the more fat I cut out of my diet, the lower my cholesterol will be," she says.

Among juices they now prepare at home for themselves, Myrna and her husband prefer watermelon, carrot with beet and parsley, grape and apple, and strawberry. She and her husband also drink something called wheat grass juice.

Although her cholesterol edges up during the winter when she sometimes succumbs to the temptation of high-fat holiday foods, Myrna says it hasn't been over 250 for years.

Gleena's interest in juicing to keep her cholesterol in check came with her second marriage. Except for an occasional chicken and turkey, her wiry Seventh Day Adventist husband shunned most meats and other high-fat foods in favor of fruits and vegetables.

After her husband died, the 75-year-old Spokane, Washington, great-grandmother spent a week eating whatever she wanted for dinner, including prime rib, Chinese food and chicken. Even before she put down the last drumstick, however, Gleena says she was feeling groggy and lethargic. "Really, like dead weight, without any energy," she says.

Gleena still eats chicken occasionally, but now she lives almost exclusively on raw fruits and vegetables and the juices she makes from them. Her cholesterol level: 180.

There is plenty of research to explain why this works. A fiber called pectin, which is found in fruits, vegetables and seeds, binds up cholesterol, actually preventing its absorption in the blood, experts say.

THEY VOTE FOR OATS

Nearly 70 percent of our survey participants thought sowing their diet with oats was good for keeping cholesterol down.

While growing up, Karen watched her father grow his career in the oil business, provide for his family and, unfortunately, develop high cholesterol. The problem came to light when he flunked a stress test while applying for life insurance. Further tests revealed a 90 percent blockage of at least one coronary artery and a cholesterol level of 275, says the Columbus, Ohio, resident.

Since the blockage was surgically cleared, Karen says her dad has been eating like a new man, including reading food labels to determine their fat content. "Not something he was ever known to do," she says.

And his new favorite food: oat bran muffins. "He swears by those things. He's got to have at least one a day," she says. For exercise, he plays golf every day.

Since then, Karen says her dad has lost 20 pounds, and his cholesterol comes in at about 220.

With a family history of borderline high cholesterol, Ruth has always kept tabs on her diet. No kielbasa for this 61-year-old Urbana, Illinois, resident. She's good about exercising, too: It's rare when Ruth doesn't do either ten miles on her indoor bike, walk a few miles with her husband or perform some low-impact aerobics in front of the television at home.

So when her cholesterol still wouldn't budge below 240, Ruth decided to try oat bran—or "my daily ration of horse food," as she calls it.

Mr. Ed never had it this good. Ruth says she creates her own muesli by mixing together about ⅓ cup of oat bran that she purchases in bulk at a health-food store, ⅔ cup of Fiber One cereal, some raisins or dried fruit and walnuts or hazelnuts. And rather than using milk, she pours on apple or orange juice.

"It wasn't much of a dip," says Ruth, "but it's come down a little, and that says to me that the oat bran has helped."

Oat bran contains soluble fiber that has been shown effective at reducing cholesterol. In one study, ten people ate 41 grams of oat bran (about three muffins) each day for about six months. The result: Their cholesterol levels dropped 26 percent each.

Oat bran alone will never tame a wild cholesterol level, says Dr. Ornish, but used properly, it can help.

Iron Man Uses Vitamin E

Vitamin E may be making headlines for its cholesterol-busting ability, but that's nothing compared with John's seemingly miraculous comeback—due in part to vitamin E.

Seemingly in top condition, John dropped over dead while cutting grass in 1985. Revived by paramedics, surgeons later found that nearly all his major arteries were clogged with plaque—even though he's always exercised and eaten a fairly low-fat diet.

Six months after quadruple bypass surgery, John was taking prescription cholesterol medication and jogging again. His cholesterol level dropped from 310 to 185. Worried about side effects from the drug, however, John switched to 500 IU (international units) of vitamin E a day at the suggestion of Veronica, his wife. Briefly, his cholesterol level went to 210 but has held steady at 185 for a year. A few months ago, John, 60, completed a triathalon—a grueling competition that features cycling, swimming and running.

"People don't believe what happened to him until he takes off his shirt and he shows them the scar," says Veronica, a Carpinteria, California, resident.

Bonnie, of Boulder, Colorado, is also a devoted vitamin E supportee. She's been taking 150 IU of vitamin E a day for the past decade. With a history of heart problems in her family—her brothers and sisters have all suffered from conditions like high blood pressure, high cholesterol, even angina—Bonnie wasn't taking any chances. Between eating low fat and taking vitamin E, her cholesterol stays around 200. Her husband, Joe, started taking the vitamin a few years after Bonnie. His cholesterol level: 200. "It's kind of hard to argue with success," says the 67-year-old. "The stuff works."

Vitamin E, an antioxidant which helps slow the aging of cells, has, in fact, been found to help provide relief for such cardiovascular problems as intermittent claudication and angina, as well as helping to improve your cholesterol levels. One study showed that 500 IU of vitamin E each day can raise HDL, your good cholesterol, as much as 14 percent.

EDITOR'S NOTE: Among other foods, vitamin E is found in nuts and whole-grain cereals, but it is difficult to get the potential healing amount through diet alone. If you want to go on a supplement program, discuss it with your doctor.

NIACIN MEETS HIS NEEDS

It was a midlife crisis that sent Brian to his doctor to get his cholesterol checked. But it was a little help from his wife, Brenda, a new low-fat diet and niacin supplements that helped get his cholesterol level in check.

When he first began taking 1,500-milligram doses of niacin at his wife's suggestion two years ago, Brian was annoyed by a commonly reported side effect of the supplement: flushing. But when he switched to a time-released formula and began taking it at night, the side effects subsided.

His cholesterol level has dropped from 250 to just under 200, says his wife, adding, "even his suits are a little big for him now."

At least two major studies have confirmed niacin's cholesterol-reducing properties. One researcher reported good results using as little as 1,200 milligrams of nicotinic acid (a type of niacin) a day.

EDITOR'S NOTE: Some experts suggest only using niacin as a last resort. In his book Natural Health, Natural Medicine, *Andrew Weil, M.D., associate director of the Division of Social Perspectives in Medicine at the University of Arizona College of Medicine/Arizona Health Sciences Center in Tucson, warns: "You should have liver function tests before starting niacin therapy and discontinue use if nausea or other gastrointestinal symptoms take place. And don't take high doses of niacin if you have coronary heart disease, diabetes, gout, liver disease, gallbladder disease, ulcers or are pregnant."*

You should not try to self-treat high cholesterol with niacin. Niacin can cause unpleasant symptoms, including flushing, so it's a good idea to take therapeutic doses only under the supervision of your doctor.

THEY SWEAR BY PSYLLIUM

Fiber-rich food additives like psyllium get an enthusiastic thumbs up from a number of cholesterol fighters.

Originally, Evelyn started taking psyllium for her spastic colon—the fiber kept her regular and seemed to prevent bloating and pain. But the 51-year-old Greenville, South Carolina, resident is also convinced that her daily glass of Metamucil, which contains psyllium, has helped keep her cholesterol level at an impressive 160.

"It used to be like drinking a glass of oatmeal," says Helen. "It tastes a lot better now. But even if they never changed the taste, I'd still be drinking it because I know it's helped."

Helen's hunch just may be right. Psyllium contains soluble fiber that has been shown to lower cholesterol. Other sources of soluble fiber include beans, dried peas, fruit and oats.

Hyperventilation

Bagging Improper Breathing

You can't find a lower-tech device. Yet no home remedy in our survey—not one—is more widely hailed as a successful treatment for hyperventilation than the paper bag. Nearly all of those who have remedies for this condition—which features rapid breathing, chest tightness and heart palpitations—say they use a paper bag to sack their symptoms.

THEY'RE ALWAYS READY

Lots of folks have heard of using a paper bag for hyperventilation. But how many people carry one in their purse or pocket in case a relative, friend or stranger has an attack? Probably more than you think.

Helen, a Hendrum, Minnesota, farmer's wife, carried one for years after her son and niece each suffered severe cases of hyperventilation.

Overcome by grief at his grandfather's funeral, her son Bobby hyperventilated until he nearly passed out. Unfortunately, no one had a paper bag handy that day, says Helen.

A few years later, Helen's niece Maureen suffered an attack while playing high school basketball. Maureen's mother, acting on Helen's advice, was ready for the emergency. She whipped out a paper bag. A few minutes after slowly breathing into the bag, Maureen's symptoms disappeared.

Bedridden with a bad case of the flu, Adrienne felt awful. Imagine her concern when a wave of nausea turned into hyperventilation. "I was breathing so rapidly and shallowly that I was taking in way too much oxygen," says the Fleetwood, Pennsylvania, media buyer. "I even started losing voluntary control of my fingers and joints—I thought something really terrible was happening."

Adrienne cried out to her husband, who quickly phoned their doctor. His diagnosis: hyperventilation. The recommended treatment: breathing into a paper bag.

283

After just a few seconds of puffing into a paper bag held over her nose and mouth, her symptoms subsided. "I was still nauseous, but I wasn't hyperventilating anymore," she says.

Linda has never hyperventilated, but she knew what to do when a friend had an episode at the end of a church service one warm Sunday.

The congregation was singing the closing hymn when the 49-year-old Granite City, Illinois, resident noticed Lucille, a recent widow, breathing rapidly. "You could tell she was having a really tough time," Linda recalls.

Linda quickly got her brother's attention—he's an emergency medical technician—and the two walked Lucille to a pew in the back of the church. A small crowd began to gather, but Linda gently urged them to give Lucille room to breathe and sent the most animated among them to the church basement for a cold washcloth. While she and her brother quietly comforted her, Linda also pulled a brown paper bag from Lucille's purse—one that she carried for such occasions—and told her to breathe with the bag covering her nose and mouth. Within a few minutes, Lucille was fine.

Paper bags work so well for treating hyperventilation that even hospitals use them, says Betty Booker, a registered respiratory therapist and pulmonary rehabilitation coordinator at University Hospital in Denver.

What makes them work? For one thing, when you breathe into a paper bag, you're expelling carbon dioxide. Then, when you breathe in the carbon dioxide, you reduce the amount of oxygen you're breathing in, which has a normalizing effect on your respiratory system, says Booker.

Also, to accomplish the task of breathing into a paper bag properly—creating a seal around your mouth and nose and breathing for about a minute—you have to focus on what you're doing. And that temporarily takes your mind off what may be causing you to hyperventilate, she says. Playing mental games with yourself and using self-talk—suggestions from two other survey takers—serve a similar purpose, she says.

STRETCHES WORKED IN THIS SCENARIO

A professional sprout grower until she was 76, Alice was working in her greenhouse one day when a friend came in hyperventilating. The North Hollywood, California, resident stopped what she was doing and told her friend to stretch her arms as high as possible and breathe deeply. Within a few minutes, the symptoms subsided. "I've known about it longer than I can remember," says the 85-year-old.

Stretching is a fine technique for halting hyperventilation, says Booker.

"Often, hyperventilation starts when you're not breathing deeply enough. You're taking shallow breaths rapidly," she says. "Stopping to stretch would cause you to take some deep breaths and, again, focus on something else. But you would exhale that air slowly, allowing the lungs to empty."

If you really want to make sure you're breathing as deeply as possible, place your hand on your abdomen. Each time you inhale, try to push your hand away with your abdomen.

Hypoglycemia

Tips to Even Out Highs and Lows

Hypoglycemia—low blood sugar—is something of a medical mystery. A fair number of people are convinced they have this problem. And they have at least some of the symptoms that go along with it—flushing, heart palpitations, tingling, sweating, hunger, light-headedness, weakness, anxiety, difficulty concentrating and sleepiness.

You could have these symptoms and not be a true hypoglycemic. That is why most doctors believe that a large proportion of people do not have this condition, says Stanley Mirsky, M.D., associate clinical professor of metabolic diseases at Mount Sinai School of Medicine in New York City and author of *Controlling Diabetes the Easy Way*.

Often, people with these symptoms are actually suffering from stress, says Dr. Mirsky.

Still, a number of our survey participants say low blood sugar is a problem for them. Many also say their symptoms disappear when they stick with standard suggestions for controlling low blood sugar—such as avoiding sugar, caffeine and alcohol and having a snack or two during the day.

Needless to say, people whose low blood sugar is caused by a health problem need to be under a doctor's care, says Dr. Mirsky.

Then, if it's a decent bet that low blood sugar is causing your symptoms, try these diet and lifestyle changes offered by our survey participants. Most say a combination of several of these suggestions works best for them.

MINI-MEALS SOOTHE THEIR SYMPTOMS

More than half our survey participants recommend nibbling throughout the day to keep hypoglycemia at bay.

"I've found that eating about six times a day, making sure I eat before I get really hungry, does a lot to relieve my symptoms," says Cheryl, 47, a secretary from Santa Monica, California, who's had problems with low blood sugar as long as she can remember. "I carry food with me so I am assured of always having something good to eat." Her favorites: baby food jars of oatmeal and unsweetened applesauce.

"I get spaced-out—unable to concentrate—unless I have something to eat every two or three hours," says Lucille, 39, an elementary school teacher from Des Moines, Iowa. Others say they get shaky, sweaty or "weak in the knees" if they don't fuel up often.

Most experts agree that frequent, small meals can counteract the most common form of low blood sugar, called reactive hypoglycemia. Dr. Mirsky recommends eating breakfast, lunch and dinner as well as small snacks at 10:30 A.M. and 3:30 P.M.

SUGAR'S OUT FOR THEM

It's true that ingesting sugar will temporarily perk up flagging blood sugar levels. But a fair number of our survey takers say that filling up on sugary foods only fuels their problem. So they steer clear of soft drinks, sugared teas and coffee, candy, cakes, pies and other desserts.

"My symptoms don't manifest if I stay away from sugar," says Lori, 47, a piano teacher from Oak Brook, Illinois, who calls herself a "recovering sugar addict."

"I try to keep sweets out of the house, and I make a point not to eat sweets, especially early in the day, when I really feel the effects," she says. "I may be able to handle a dessert after dinner."

People who believe their symptoms are associated with sugary foods or drinks should replace those foods with a balanced diet of vegetables, fruits and whole grains, while trying to keep protein and fat to a minimum. They should also eat smaller portions of food, but more frequently, says registered dietician Audrey Lally, a diabetes educator with the Mayo Clinic in Scottsdale, Arizona. "These foods provide nutrients they need, along with fiber, which helps to stabilize blood sugar by prolonging absorption time of sugar in the intestines," she explains.

HE SAYS NO TO ALCOHOL

"When I first started having symptoms 20 years ago, I thought I had mononucleosis; I was that weak and tired," says Ron, 43, a city employee from Thousand Oaks, California. Although his doctor never did diagnose a problem, Ron says he started reading and decided his symptoms were from a poor diet and too much alcohol.

"I started eating better, eating several small meals a day, getting more protein and complex carbohydrates and taking vitamins," he says. But it wasn't until he stopped his nightly visits to the local tavern that his symptoms disappeared for good. "I can pretty much eat what I want now, although I still need to avoid overeating sweets," he says.

Too much alcohol can cause hypoglycemia, Dr. Mirsky agrees. "Alcohol interferes with the conversion of sugar from protein and inhibits the release of sugar from the liver's stores," he explains. That means your body can't rely on sugar stores to boost blood sugar when you haven't eaten for a while.

THEY CHROME-PLATE THEIR DIETS

Three people tell us chromium supplements help relieve their hypoglycemia symptoms. Several more say that brewer's yeast—which contains glucose tolerance factor, a form of chromium—alleviates their symptoms.

One chromium user, Daryl, 38, of Alto, Michigan, is an emergency room physician. "I had profound postprandial (after meals) hypoglycemia, and it was something I'd always had," he says. "Apparently my body was reacting to a meal by producing too much insulin, and if I wasn't careful to eat every two or three hours, I would have lethargy, sweating and headaches.

"My wife read about chromium in a magazine. We did a little more research, and I decided to try it. It did even my blood sugar out and made it possible for me to eat less often without getting symptoms. Within a couple of days I had more energy, and over time I got much better."

Daryl continues to take 600 micrograms of chromium picolinate a day and says his symptoms tend to return if he fails to take it for a few days.

Chromium, an essential trace mineral and the same shiny stuff that's used to put a gleam on car bumpers, has been found in several studies to improve symptoms of hypoglycemia.

"It seems to work by improving insulin efficiency, or the ability of insulin to escort glucose into cells, where it is burned for fuel," explains Richard Anderson, Ph.D., a biochemist at the Beltsville Human Nutrition Research Center in Beltsville, Maryland. "It seems to normalize insulin levels and insulin function, which in turn normalizes glucose levels." (Insulin is a hormone that your body produces to help you handle glucose—the simple sugar that your body uses for fuel.)

In one of Dr. Anderson's studies, eight women with symptoms of hypoglycemia who took 200 micrograms of chromium for three months showed a significant improvement in their symptoms.

EDITOR'S NOTE: While there are no known toxic effects from chromium, any trace mineral can be toxic in large amounts.

Most experts recommend you take no more than 200 micrograms a day. A normal individual will respond nicely to 200 micrograms, but people with diabetes, hypoglycemia or certain other disorders may need more to see beneficial effects, says Dr. Anderson. He believes up to 600 micrograms of chromium daily is safe under medical supervision.

Needless to say, if you have diabetes or severe hypoglycemia and want to try chromium supplements, do so only with close medical supervision.

Good food sources of chromium include whole grains, black pepper, thyme, meat and cheese.

THEY JUNK THE JAVA

"Coffee and doughnuts always did me in," says Lorraine, 44, a Souderton, Pennsylvania, waitress who once worked the extra-early-bird shift at an all-night diner. "By ten o'clock in the morning, I'd be a zombie—tired and unable to concentrate."

Passing up the doughnuts for whole-wheat toast or yogurt and granola for breakfast relieved most of her symptoms. Still, she found that long workdays that included countless cups of coffee—cream, no sugar—would bring on symptoms.

Indeed, coffee may be a previously unsuspected accomplice to jelly doughnuts when it comes to symptoms of hypoglycemia, says Robert Sherwin, M.D., director of the Diabetes Endocrinology Research Center at Yale University School of Medicine in New Haven, Connecticut.

Dr. Sherwin and colleagues found that healthy, normal-weight volunteers who drank the caffeine equivalent of three cups of drip-brewed coffee developed some symptoms of hypoglycemia—trembling, sweating and heart palpitations—at a blood sugar level that was within a low but normal range.

"Caffeine does two things," Dr. Sherwin explains. "It constricts arteries and so decreases the flow of blood to the brain. At the same time, it increases the use of sugar by brain cells. So caffeine may, theoretically, induce a relative shortage of sugar in brain cells, which would explain why some people have symptoms of low blood sugar when their blood levels are within a low-normal range."

MUSCLE BUILDING TAMES HER BLOOD SUGAR

"I used to literally feel like I was on a roller coaster," says our Santa Monica secretary, Cheryl. In addition to frequent snacks, she has found regular exercise, including pumping iron with the boys from the mail room, relieves her symptoms. "I'd get easily irritated when I hadn't eaten for a while," she says. "For me, exercise is like a giant tranquilizer."

Since exercise burns sugar, she finds it helpful to keep some fruit juice or food on hand. "If I exercise even 20 minutes longer than my usual hour, I start to develop symptoms of shakiness and weakness," she explains. "If so, I usually drink four ounces of fruit juice and then try to follow that soon with something more substantial."

EDITOR'S NOTE: It's true that exercise builds up muscle mass and whittles away fat. It also helps your body use and store sugar more efficiently, says James Barnard, Ph.D., professor of physiological sciences at the University of California at Los Angeles. However, he warns: "Exercise is not the answer to hypoglycemia. A person whose hypoglycemia is being caused by an oversecretion of insulin may find his condition becomes worse, not better, if he suddenly starts exercising. Anyone with true hypoglycemia should start an exercise program only with medical supervision."

Impotence

Suggestions for Ending the Slump

Few health problems trouble a man like those that make him question his very maleness. And impotence—the inability to achieve or maintain an erection—is one of them.

As medical experts and our survey takers know, there are a variety of remedies that can transform even a not-so-temporary slump into newfound sexual success. "There are so many things that can be done. Impotence is almost always curable," says Sheldon Burman, M.D., FACS, founder and director of the Male Sexual Dysfunction Institute in Chicago.

Here's what our survey takers recommend.

USE IT OR LOSE IT

Rollo's strategy for overcoming impotence is as straightforward as a kiss on the lips. "Use it or lose it," says the 80-year-old Port Orchard, Washington, resident. His preventive regimen: sex with his wife at least once or twice a week. A doctor shared the secret with him years ago while he was being treated for prostate problems.

"You see, that muscle is the same as any other muscle," says Rollo. "If you don't use the muscle, it will get weak and soft. If it gets weak and soft, then you are surely going to have trouble."

Both Rollo's remedy and physiology are rock solid, says Dr. Burman. "Erections bring large amounts of oxygenated blood into the penis," he explains. "As you get older, these do not occur as often and, consequently, there is oxygen deprivation. As a result, all that smooth muscle becomes progressively replaced with scar tissue. Those penises that are involved in sexual intercourse will probably retain their tone over a longer period of time."

If you're already having trouble maintaining an erection, Dr. Burman says you may improve your performance by placing a rubber band around the base of your penis just before intercourse. The rubber band helps close off veins that are supposed to clamp shut after you become sexually excited and your penis is engorged with blood. Just don't put the rubber band on too tightly or forget to remove it after sex, he says. (The rubber band should be snug, but not tight.)

CALCIUM CORRECTS HIS PROBLEM

Richard says he started taking calcium supplements to help heal his back. Before long, however, he noticed the capsules strengthened something else.

"A few years ago, I started to have intermittent trouble achieving an erection," says the retired Miami Beach resident. "I started taking 4,000 milligrams of calcium each day because of a weak back that several doctors had not been able to help. My back is getting better, but I also noticed that I stopped having problems with erections."

EDITOR'S NOTE: "Every medical student knows that calcium is needed to cause muscular contraction and that it plays some role in potency. But there's just no evidence to support that lack of potency is due in any way to calcium deprivation nor that potency can be restored by calcium administration," says Dr. Burman.

Most experts say calcium supplementation of up to 2,500 milligrams daily is safe, however. Doses above this are not recommended. You can also get calcium from milk, yogurt and green leafy vegetables.

FOOD AND DRINK GIVE A LIFT

Several foods (and at least one beverage) show up in our survey takers' recommendations for putting an end to impotence. Chris, 56, of Connecticut, says wine and eggs are helpful, while Austin, from (where else?) Texas, eats plenty of asparagus and dates.

In fact, several factors, including food, can determine whether you're likely to suffer from impotence, says Dr. Burman. "Those factors that induce or hasten the occurrence of vascular disease, like high blood pressure, type A personality, obesity, lack of exercise, high cholesterol, cigarette smoking and family history—all those known cardiac risk factors—are the same risk factors that produce early impotence. The penis is a vascular structure, erection is a vascular phenomenon and those things that retard the occurrence of cardiovascular disease will also retard the occurrence of impotence." (The word "vascular" refers to anything having to do with blood vessels.)

As a result, Dr. Burman says, a committment to good health can help prevent impotence. That means doing things like eating a low-fat diet, getting regular exercise and quitting smoking, he says.

A glass or two of a drink containing alcohol can calm the performance anxiety that leads to impotence among some, says Dr. Burman. But encouraging words and kind acts from a supportive partner have as much or more effect. "A man's state of mind and a woman's contribution to that state of mind can make a big difference," he says.

Incontinence

Ways to Stop the Flow

It's a common enough problem, but it's so hard to talk about it. Helen, a 74-year-old New Jersey woman with urinary incontinence, pretty much sums it up when it comes to this troubling problem. "It is embarrassing, and I'm glad, at least, that people aren't so reluctant to mention it to their doctors these days. I got help, and I bet a lot of other people can, too."

Although there are things you can do at home for urinary incontinence, it's important to see a health professional about it, too. That's because only they can determine exactly what's causing the leakage and suggest the best course of action. It may be due to muscle weakness, a side effect of drugs, a bladder infection or a more serious condition. If you're a man with this problem, it's important to have a doctor check for prostate problems. For women, it could signal an estrogen deficiency.

"Most people who have incontinence can be helped, and that includes the elderly. Urinary incontinence is not an inevitable consequence of aging," says Catherine DuBeau, M.D., an instructor in medicine at Harvard Medical School and a member of the Gerontology Division and the Continence Center at Brigham and Women's Hospital, both in Boston.

Most of our 23 survey participants who answered this question have mild stress incontinence. That means they leak when they laugh, lift something heavy or sneeze. A few also said they have urge incontinence—they leak urine when they cannot get to a toilet soon enough after perceiving the urge to urinate. All of them suggest a number of flow-stemming tactics. Here's what they say has worked for them.

THEY PUT THE SQUEEZE ON

Those who do Kegel exercises to stem the flow report anywhere from minimal to "very helpful" relief from the problem.

Kegels target the slinglike group of muscles that stretch from the pubic bone in front to the tailbone in the rear. These muscles surround the anus and urethra (the tube that drains the bladder). Squeezing them can cut off the flow—like a clamp on a hose.

"Kegel exercises saved me from having to have surgery for incontinence," says Eileen, 68, a hospital laboratory worker from Croton-on-Hudson, New York. "My bladder was protruding into my vagina, causing some urinary leakage, and my gynecologist told me how to do this exercise to strengthen the pelvic muscles."

The first step in learning these exercises was stopping the flow of urine when she was on the toilet, she says. That taught her how to work the proper muscles. "Now, I do them anywhere and everywhere," she says. "It does take some concentration, but it's worth it. It beats having surgery."

In studies, about 70 percent of people who received instruction and who regularly did Kegel exercises reported improved control over stress or urge incontinence. You can practice isolating the appropriate pelvic muscles on your own by turning the flow off and on when you urinate. You can check if you're exercising the right muscles by placing your hands on your thighs and buttocks. If they're contracting, you're using too many muscles.

COLD TURKEY ON COFFEE HELPED HER

"I was drinking a lot of coffee and tea and was having occasional diarrhea and leakage of small amounts of urine when I would cough or lift," says Susan, 43, a college secretary from Lafayette, Indiana. "I wanted to cut back on the amount I drank, but I wasn't very motivated to do so until I read in a magazine that coffee can irritate your bladder and cause leakage. I decided to stop drinking coffee—and my leakage stopped almost immediately," she says. "I can still drink a few cups of tea a day with no problems."

Coffee contains substances that can be irritating to the urinary tract, agrees Andrew Weil, M.D., associate director of the Division of Social Perspectives in Medicine at the University of Arizona College of Medicine/Arizona Health Sciences Center in Tucson and author of *Natural Health, Natural Medicine.* "If you have reason to avoid coffee, stay away from decaffeinated coffee as well," he advises.

EDITOR'S NOTE: Other foods besides coffee have been associated with leakage, says incontinence expert Katherine Jeter, Ed.D., executive director of Help for Incontinent People (HIP), an advocacy group based in Union, South Carolina. Among the foods HIP members associate with leakage: milk, sugar, corn syrup, honey, alcoholic beverages, carbonated beverages, tea, chocolate, citrus juices and citrus fruits, tomatoes and highly spiced foods. "This doesn't mean you need to eliminate all these foods from your diet," Dr. Jeter says. "Remove only one at a time for a week or so to see if it helps."

BLADDER TRAINING HELPS HER

"My problem wasn't real serious, but I did need to get up several times during the night to urinate," says Mary Alice, 75, of Pinellas Park, Florida. Her doctor suggested bladder training—scheduling times to go to the bathroom. She started by going every two hours, gradually working her way up to every four. "That, along with limiting fluids after dinner, did help my nighttime problem, but ultimately, I needed to take drugs to stay dry during the night," she says.

Most people train their bladders by going every hour or so for a few days, Dr. DuBeau says. Then, if they remain dry, they go on a two-hour schedule. "If you feel an urge to go in between times, stop and make your bladder relax, then walk slowly to the toilet," she suggests. "The goal is to go every three or four hours during waking hours." People on this daytime program are less likely to get the sudden urge to go at night because the bladder is trained for a regular schedule.

FLUID RESTRICTIONS HELP SOME

Several people said that they restrict the amount of fluid they drink, especially before bed or prior to leaving home.

EDITOR'S NOTE: Although this may be helpful, the possibility that you will get so little fluid you become dehydrated is very real for older people who restrict their fluid intake, Dr. DuBeau warns. "People should check with their doctor before they restrict fluids," she says. "Keeping track of the amount you urinate for a few days will help your doctor determine if your incontinence is a result of drinking too much."

SHE STANDS LIKE A MAN

"I stand to urinate at least once a day," says Joyce, 62, a busy crocheter from Spokane, Washington. "A woman doctor suggested this when my mother was having problems with incontinence. I decided to try it myself for the little leakage I sometimes have. I found that if I urinate standing up before I go to bed, I don't have such a full bladder that I have to rush to the bathroom first thing in the morning. It seems to help me empty my bladder better."

No, she doesn't have to worry about missing her target. "I use a glass that holds two or three cups, then simply empty it in the toilet and rinse the cup out," she says.

"Standing to urinate may be helpful in some women whose bladder has prolapsed or dropped a bit," Dr. DuBeau explains. However, this technique isn't for everyone. "For many women, standing may make the bladder drop more, making it harder to empty completely while urinating, Dr. DuBeau says.

OLD-TIME HERB OFFERS HER RELIEF

"My urinary leakage was due to bladder infections, which I used to get fairly regularly, until I figured out ways to avoid them," explains Claudia, 47, a Hopewell, New Jersey, arts administrator and freelance musician. She no longer has the problem. Here's how she got rid of it. At the first signs of an infection (frequent need to urinate and burning), she'd use an herb recommended to her by a health-food store employee—uva ursi, also known as bearberry. "It worked, as long as I used it right away," she says. "I would not try it for a full-blown infection." She used capsules, following package directions.

The dried leaves of uva ursi have been used for hundreds of years as a folk remedy. They contain the chemical arbutin, which breaks down in the body to hydroquinone, a substance that serves as a urinary antiseptic.

EDITOR'S NOTE: Uva ursi should not be used by children or pregnant women, herbal experts warn. Nor should it be used for prolonged periods of time in high doses. If you want to use this herb for urinary incontinence, you should talk to your doctor first.

Indigestion

Stomach-Soothing Tips

Indigestion is a kind of grab-bag term for just about any upper abdominal symptom—belching, rumbling, fullness, pain, burning and sour stomach. Sometimes these symptoms can be linked with a specific disorder, such as a stomach ulcer or gallbladder disease.

Often, however, no specific cause can be discovered. And so, it's up to the individual to manage the symptoms with changes in eating, drinking and smoking habits, with weight loss, and, where appropriate, with drugs, says Ronald Hoffman, M.D., director of the Hoffman Center for Holistic Medicine in New York City and author of *Seven Weeks to a Settled Stomach*.

Many of our survey takers who have frequent bouts of indigestion say they have stomach symptoms for reasons that seem to stump their doctors. And their simple remedies—apple cider vinegar, Coca-Cola, honey, peppermint tea, gingerroot, cardamom seeds or simply eliminating a particular food—often leave their doctors puzzling for an explanation of why they work.

"My doctor wanted me to take an ulcer drug, even though I didn't have an ulcer, for my stomach pain," says Martha, 71, of Baltimore. "I did take it for a while, but then I decided to try some dietary changes instead—eating smaller meals and avoiding fatty foods, for instance. I also started to take a short walk after meals. These things worked well enough that I haven't needed drugs. I asked my doctor why he didn't recommend these things first, instead of drugs, and he didn't have an answer."

Here, then, is what people say helps them overcome this common problem.

A SOUR SIP SOOTHES HIS STOMACH

As we're discovering, many people swear apple cider vinegar is a sure cure for a wide variety of ailments. That includes indigestion. Several say they drink apple cider vinegar mixed with water (and sometimes, a spoonful of honey) for quick relief from stomach pain.

"Sometimes I wake up with a sour stomach," says Rollo, a robust 80-year-old who frequents the buffet at a restaurant in his town of Port Orchard, Washington. "Maybe I ate too much, drank too much or ate something that disagrees with me. Whatever, I take one teaspoon of apple cider vinegar in a glass of water and walk around the room for five minutes, and during that time, my stomach settles down just fine." This remedy has worked for him, he says, "100 percent of the time. I think it replaces the hydrochloric acid that my stomach doesn't produce as much of since I am older."

Current medical thinking holds that the condition of low stomach acid, common in older people, does not cause symptoms and does not require treatment, experts say.

"That is the conventional viewpoint, but it happens to be wrong," Dr. Hoffman says. "Some people really do benefit from extra acidification, which is one reason that apple cider vinegar may provide relief."

People whose stomach problems don't respond to acid-blocking drugs may find their symptoms relieved by prescription capsules containing hydrochloric acid, he says. Bacterial overgrowth, which can cause inflammation and ulcers, is less likely to occur in a stomach that is properly acidified, he adds.

HER CURE IS SWEET

"I used to have stomach cramps so bad, for three or four hours at a stretch, that I would end up in the emergency room, where they would give me painkillers," says Alisa, 33, a forestry student at the University of Georgia.

Who would have dreamed that a remedy as simple as a tablespoon or two of honey would abort her symptoms before they became gut-wrenching? "Someone suggested I try it, and I thought, 'What do I have to lose?' " she explains. "I do this now whenever I feel symptoms coming on, and within a half-hour, my stomach is back to normal."

The healing benefits of this sweet, thick liquid go back to the days of hieroglyphics—somewhere between 2600 and 2200 B.C. The ancient Egyptians used honey to help heal wounds and soothe stomach ailments. "Honey is being found to have some interesting antibacterial properties, but I'm not sure how it would work in this case," Dr. Hoffman says.

PAPAYA IS HER PANACEA

"I use a product called Super Papaya Enzyme Plus, made by American Health, and it is fantastic," says Linda Mae, 44, an accounting student from Waco, Ohio. "I used it for the first time when I had stomach pain so bad that

I thought I was going to die. I had eaten some cabbage that just didn't agree with me. Now, I use it whenever I eat gassy, hard-to-digest foods. It prevents all the gas, stomach upset and nausea and freshens your breath as well."

Papaya has a long-time reputation as a digestive aid. An enzyme in papaya, papain, is said to resemble two well-known digestive enzymes in the stomach—pepsin and trypsin. Papain is used as a meat tenderizer and, in fact, does help to break down protein. But because there is no good scientific proof that it actually helps to aid digestion, the U.S. Food and Drug Administration no longer allows papaya products to make that claim. The products continue to be available in health-food stores, however, and people continue to buy them as digestive aids. (You just won't see anything about digestion on the label.)

THEY TAKE CHARCOAL

"My major problems are sweets or gassy vegetables, which give me all sorts of stomach and intestinal pains," says Phyllis, 62, of Ira, Texas. To avoid discomfort, she takes a capsule of activated charcoal along with the offending food. "It works every time for me, for any food," she says.

Activated charcoal is an all-purpose antidote, used in hospital emergency rooms for most types of poisoning. So it's no wonder several of our survey participants say they use it with great success to alleviate an array of stomach ills.

SHE PREFERS A FIZZY FIX

"I don't have much trouble with my stomach, but when I do, I use an old-fashioned remedy that always seems to work," says Bobbie, 50, a New York City real estate broker. She mixes a teaspoon or so of baking soda in a glass of water and drinks it down. "It does make you burp, and the burp seems to relieve bloating," she explains.

EDITOR'S NOTE: Baking soda—sodium bicarbonate—does a fine job of relieving stomach gas and neutralizing stomach acid, experts say. In fact, it's the main active ingredient in a number of over-the-counter antacids. However, baking soda is high in sodium, and for that reason, some doctors suggest you reserve it for only occasional use. "I'd much rather have someone use a low-sodium antacid," Dr. Hoffman says.

CREAM OF TARTAR TAMES HER TUMMY

"My grandmother used to give me cream of tartar in water years ago if I had an upset stomach," says Jeanne, 68, of Vacaville, California. "I haven't had to use this much in the last few years, but I do very clearly remember two things about it—it didn't taste bad, so I didn't mind drinking it. And it worked. Within 15 minutes my upset stomach would always be gone."

Unless you're a serious baker—cakes, pies, breads and the like—you may not have heard of cream of tartar, an ingredient in baking powder. Like baking soda, this white powder is an old-time remedy for aching bellies. And, like baking soda, it produces a healthy burp, relieving gas and the feeling of fullness. An ingredient in some gastrointestinal drugs, cream of tartar is a residue found in the sediments left when grapes ferment to produce wine.

SHE CHEWS CARDAMOM SEEDS

"I chew cardamom seeds for a tummy ache," reports Bernice, of Corvallis, Oregon. "Within ten minutes, the pain is gone."

Many fragrant spices—fennel, coriander, cardamom, ginger and others—have a long history of use as digestive aids. These spices contain oils or other ingredients that may relieve nausea, soothe intestinal spasms, and promote gas expulsion, even as they sweeten the breath. Cardamom, a key ingredient in curry powder, tastes like gentle ginger, with a pinch of pine.

KELP TABLETS EASE HIS UPSET

"If I'm having problems with my stomach, especially acid indigestion, I take five kelp tablets," says Lothar, a self-employed mechanic from Deerfield, Michigan. The tablets ease the pain, usually within a half-hour or so, he says, adding, "I simply swallow them whole, with water."

This solution doesn't seem so far-out once you realize that kelp and many other seaweeds contain substances that help form gels to bind up stomach acid and so soothe the stomach, explains Arthur Jacknowitz, Pharm.D., professor and chairman of the Department of Clinical Pharmacy at West Virginia University School of Pharmacy in Morgantown.

EDITOR'S NOTE: "Since seaweed is high in sodium, Dr. Jacknowitz cautions that it should be avoided by those individuals who must limit their salt intake."

ARITHMETIC DIET HELPS SOME

Some subtract, some add, and a fair number do fancy equations with foods that aid or alleviate their stomach pains. They subtract milk and coffee and may add fiber or yogurt. James, an Alexander City, Alabama, resident says he has taken to eating two or three radishes with every meal to combat stomach problems he's had with spicy or hot foods. "I don't know why it works, and neither does my doctor or any dietitian I've talked to," he says.

Doctors' comments on this? Use common sense, says William Ruderman, M.D., chairman of the Department of Gastroenterology at the Cleveland Clinic Florida in Fort Lauderdale. "Most people tolerate a broad spectrum of foods without difficulty. But if you are having trouble with certain foods, then you'll want to avoid them, just as you'll want to continue to eat the foods that make your stomach feel better," Dr. Ruderman says.

EDITOR'S NOTE: It's important to have a well-balanced, healthful diet, so don't go overboard. If you are eliminating so many foods that you can no longer eat healthful, balanced meals, it's time to see a doctor about your problem.

Ingrown Hairs

Nailing Those Nasty Nubs

If you're suffering from severe ingrown facial hair—a common problem for African-American men—chances are your doctor will tell you to grow a beard. "If you have many of these on your face or neck, that's really the best thing you can do," says Libby Edwards, M.D., associate clinical professor at Bowman Gray School of Medicine and chief of dermatology at Carolinas Medical Center in Charlotte, North Carolina. "Many ingrown hairs are very difficult to treat. But if you leave them alone long enough, they will pop right out on their own."

If the thought of looking like Grizzly Adams is absolutely, well, unbearable, fear not: Our survey takers who have suffered from ingrown hairs share their tips for treating this annoying problem—something that can happen anywhere your body sprouts hair.

HE PULLED THE PLUG

Milton the surgeon was forced to practice his craft on his own face every few weeks to extricate ingrown hairs—until he gave up his electric shaver. "Even though it was quick and efficient, it seems like it was forcing some of the hair under the skin," says his wife, Celia.

But since he replaced his electric razor with a Gillette Sensor, reports the Albuquerque, New Mexico, housewife, Milton hasn't had any ingrown hairs.

If switching from an electric shaver to a razor doesn't improve the situation for you, you may want to consider a special kit designed for those who suffer from ingrown hairs on their face, says Dr. Edwards. "The kits may include a small hook that's used to carefully pull hairs out, lotions to soften whiskers and razors shaped in a way that is supposed to maximize cutting and keep hair from ingrowing as much," she says. You may be able to find a kit at your local drugstore. If not, ask your barber if he can order you a kit through his supplier.

SPONGE SPEEDS THEIR HEALING

Suzanne treats her ingrown hairs like a mobster handles his adversaries: She rubs them out.

But instead of wielding a machine gun, the Charlotte, North Carolina, native arms herself with a loofah and some herbal castile soap, both purchased at a local health-food store.

"When I get them, they show up on my thighs," she says. "The brisk rubbing action takes off a layer of dead skin cells, rubbing the ingrown hairs out. And the castile soap is better than other deodorant soaps, because it has natural oils that are healing—they remoisturize the skin as they clean."

Evelyn says she's found a soak in a warm bath filled with Aveeno Shower and Bath to be the best prep for a loofah self-treatment. The 66-year-old New York resident says she completes the procedure by applying a lotion that contains aloe vera.

Loofah treatments will likely provide positive results, says Dr. Edwards, but it's best to to take a warm bath first. And be prepared for potential skin irritation. "Scrubbing with a loofah sponge makes a lot of sense," she says. "Remember, though, that abrasive things like that can be irritating to some people's skin." But once the hairs have reemerged, consider allowing them to grow. "When you trim hair, you give it a sharp point; and if it's curly hair, it will tend to curl right back in and pierce the skin again."

You can slow the rate of ingrown hair growth in problem areas with waxing or electrolysis, she says. "When you have your hair waxed, wax or a waxlike substance is painted on the skin, hardens and then gets pulled off, pulling the hair off with it," she says. Because the hair is literally pulled out at the root rather than simply cut off, it takes much longer for the hair to grow back, she says. Electrolysis destroys the hair root with an electric current, she says.

BACON FAT HELPS HIM

Bacon as a home remedy for ingrown hairs is a technique passed down from Janet's mother-in-law, a former farmer. Any time her husband, Leo, suffers from one of those nasty nubs, the retired Cleveland resident helps him trim a sliver of raw bacon fat from the slab in the fridge. Applied with an adhesive bandage directly to the spot and left on overnight, the bacon fat seems to soften the surrounding skin and loosen the hair, making it easier to remove with a pair of tweezers, she says. "It seems to make the skin and hair a lot more pliable," she says. "Those farm people have lots of great ideas like that."

While there may be no harm in treating ingrown hair with pig fat, you can spare Porky and his pals by simply using Vaseline, says Dr. Edwards. "I expect that a little dab of Vaseline would do the same thing as bacon. And it's likely that even the bandage by itself would work. It's a matter of getting the skin and hair moist so that it's softer, and that may certainly make it come out easier."

He Pinpoints His Problem

Gently probing with a sterilized needle is Paul's approach to removing an ingrown hair. "I have to be careful not to push the needle too deeply into the skin," says the Basking Ridge, New Jersey, resident. "But if I get underneath it just right, I can gently lift the hair out and then trim it with a razor."

Paul's approach seems sound—just as long as he doesn't probe too deeply with that needle, says Dr. Edwards. "You should just barely pierce the skin, or hook the edge of the hair and pull it out," she says. "If you feel the need to go digging around, you probably should at least learn how to do it from a doctor, because you could end up with scarring and changes in skin color that will not make you happy." Dab with an antiseptic like witch hazel if you want to, but Dr. Edwards says water works fine.

You can sterilize a needle by holding the tip over a flame, wiping it with alcohol or submerging it in boiling water, she says. And, of course, never use a needle someone else has used to pierce their skin—sharing a needle is one of the fastest ways to contract a communicable disease like AIDS, she says.

Insomnia

Snooze Inducers for the Sleepless

All of us need our Zzzs, but for one reason or another, some of us find sleep eludes us. A number of our survey participants say they've struggled with occasional sleeplessness, usually due to stress. And they've found many different ways to get to sleep faster and to stay asleep through the night.

One they all seem to agree on: Worrying about falling asleep or trying to force yourself to do so is a sure way to prolong tossing-and-turning. So some of them naturally do exactly what sleep experts recommend: They distract themselves until sleep comes naturally.

Experts say you should see a doctor if you have trouble sleeping more than a few days a month or if your sleeping problem is associated with breathing problems such as heavy snoring or with depression or other mental problems.

"I strongly suggest people not rely on sleep aids, natural or otherwise, to cover up a sleeping problem," says Joseph Pizzorno, Jr., N.D., a naturopathic physician and founding president of Bastyr University in Seattle. "People should be addressing the real causes of their insomnia, such as stress or too much caffeine."

Reducing stress and staying away from after-dinner coffee, tea or chocolate are among the many slumber-inducing tactics our restless sleepers suggest. Here's what they say.

MONOTONY BEGETS SLUMBER

If you've ever fallen asleep during a church sermon or while studying for an exam, you know that boredom can lull your brain into unconsciousness. Several people take advantage of that tendency to drift off. They read familiar verses from the Bible, watch television or turn on the radio. One mentally packs a trailer to fall asleep. Another says she starts with *A* and works her way to *Z*, "thanking God for all he has done for me." And one woman, Myrna, 65, a reading teacher from Brooklyn, New York, recites childhood poems.

"I have been saying poems to put myself to sleep for a long time," she says. "I find them soothing and reminiscent of different days and times. I have a very active mind, and reciting poems takes my mind off my problems and relieves the stress I might have had if I continued to think about what I really had on my mind. My poems took me through some very long nights during a recent bout with breast cancer." Among her favorites: "The Rime of the Ancient Mariner," "The Rubiyat of Omar Khayyam" and "Gunga Din."

Such distracting, relaxing activities allow the brain to naturally facilitate sleep, explains psychiatrist Henry Lahmeyer, M.D., professor of psychiatry and behavioral sciences at Northwestern University Medical School in Chicago. "They beat trying to make yourself go to sleep, which takes active thinking and which fights your natural tendency to go to sleep," he says.

NUZZLING LEAVES HIM NODDING

Speaking of distractions—hopefully not too monotonous—Robert, of Indiantown, Florida, is the only survey taker to admit that a bit of snuggling sends him straight to dreamland. "The trick is not to get too relaxed too soon," he cautions. "If you roll over and go to sleep right away, your wife will get mad at you. Of course, I have never had that complaint."

Some researchers have found that hormonal mechanisms triggered during sexual activity help enhance sleep.

CREATURE COMFORT LULLS HER

In wilder times, having a dog by your side during the night was something of a security blanket. You could sleep soundly, knowing your trusty companion, with its keen ears and sense of smell, could detect trouble on the way and sound the alarm.

These days, a pet (or two) in the bed functions more as, well, companionship for a couple of our survey takers who say they like creature comforts.

"I sleep with my white little dog, a Bichon Frise, and an alley cat, usually one on each side, although sometimes the cat will try to sleep on my chest," says Linda, 46, a professional artist from Southold, New York. "If I'm tossing and turning because of a problem, I usually end up petting them, and that makes me drowsy and keeps them quiet, too."

Several studies show that, in people with close attachment to animals, pets induce calmness and reduce blood pressure, says Linda Hines, director of the Delta Society, an organization that promotes the role of animals in therapy. "By focusing attention outside ourselves and our problems, animals can relieve the stress that is interfering with sleep," she says.

SHE BURNS THE MIDNIGHT OIL

Counting sheep? Perhaps you should take a tip from a true night owl, Sharon, a small-business owner from Taylorville, Illinois. She turns her sleepless nights into truly productive time.

"I never was a real good sleeper, so I take all sorts of things with me to bed," she says. At any one time, you might find buried in her bedcovers a tape recorder, books, pencil (ouch!) and paper to write letters and an electronic keyboard. "I also direct a choir, and if I have extra time during the night, I'll play and review music for the choir," she says. "About the only thing I won't do at night is yard work, although I have been known to get out of bed and repot house plants."

All this nocturnal activity does eventually catch up with her. "Sooner or later, my body becomes tired enough to sleep," she says.

But isn't her tail dragging when daybreak comes along? She says no. "I've found I can get by on a lot less sleep than you'd think. I haven't actually counted the number of hours I sleep each night, but I must be getting enough, because I am functional and productive."

Not everyone can burn the midnight oil as lavishly as Sharon does, Dr. Lahmeyer explains. "Some people do fine on as few as 4 hours; others need up to 12 hours," he says. Extreme night owls, he says, often sleep in the morning if their job allows it. Signs that you're not getting enough sleep: daytime drowsiness, trouble concentrating or learning and memory problems.

HOT BATH LEADS TO LANGUOR

An evening bath is a stress-draining experience for several of our survey participants.

"I have a whirlpool bath, which really relaxes me right before bed," says Laura from Pittsford, New York, an administrator for a company that designs medical equipment. Sometimes, she'll read in the tub. "And the best thing, then, is to be able to get into a bed with clean sheets," she says.

"Taking a warm bath an hour or two before bedtime increases the deep stage of sleep," explains Dr. Lahmeyer. He speculates that the warming effect of the bath triggers sleep-inducing biochemicals in the brain. "But timing is very important," he says. "Taking a bath right before bedtime is too stimulating and will keep you awake rather than help you sleep."

FRIDGE FORAYS HELP SOME HIBERNATE

Think cookies and milk at bedtime is just for kids? You're missing out on a potent sleeping aid. Besides this traditional fare, our survey participants rely on cereal and milk or simply warm milk to help them sleep.

"I find a cup of warm milk especially helpful when I am dieting and would otherwise go to bed wide-awake, hungry and thinking about food," says Marie, 43, a nursing instructor from Staten Island, New York, who needs to get up early to beat the traffic to work.

Milk helps you sleep because it contains tryptophan, an amino acid (protein) used in the body to manufacture serotonin, a calming brain bio-chemical, Dr. Lahmeyer explains.

EDITOR'S NOTE: Tryptophan used to be sold as a dietary supplement that was used by some as a sleeping aid. It was removed from the market in late 1989 when a contaminated batch was apparently linked to approximately 40 deaths, with an additional 5,000 to 10,000 illnesses, says Lori A. Love, M.D., Ph.D., director of the Clinical Research and Review staff in the U.S. Food and Drug Administration's Office of Special Nutritionals.

It's perfectly safe to consume food sources of tryptophan, of course. And adding a bit of sugar to milk helps tryptophan cross into the brain, Dr. Lahmeyer adds. "Actually, any snack containing protein and sugar will help you sleep," he says.

MINERALS HAVE THEM NODDING OFF

Several people say that a combination of calcium and magnesium helps them relax and sleep.

"After many years of sleep problems, I discovered, quite by accident, that calcium supplements cured my sleeplessness," says Eve, 71, a retired personnel manager and a volunteer literacy tutor from Gold River, California. It has been a blessing to me. It's better than sleeping pills."

And one woman says that grape juice does the trick for her. "I used Welch's—the purple kind—which is full of potassium, to help me sleep while I was in the hospital years ago," says Alice, 71, a real estate agent from Oakland, California. "A nurse's aide tried it herself and said it made her sleep like a baby."

There is no scientific research to support the use of calcium or potassium as sleep aids, but there's a bit of evidence supporting the use of magnesium as a muscle relaxer, Dr. Pizzorno says. "Intravenously, magnesium does promote muscle relaxation, and I would speculate that oral doses work the same way," he says. He recommends taking 400 milligrams of magnesium, along with 50 milligrams of vitamin B_6, a vitamin that interacts with magnesium, two hours before bedtime.

HERBS SEND THEM TO DREAMLAND

"The side effects I experienced from taking prescription sleeping pills scared me so much I stopped taking them," says Carolyn, 51, who runs a scholarship search business in Medford, Oregon. Instead, she decided to try an herbal product, Silent Night, which contains valerian, hops and skullcap.

"I don't need to take it often," she says, "but when stress leaves me struggling to sleep and I want something that works quickly, I'll take a capsule, and I'll be drowsy within ten minutes. If I wake up during the night, I'll also take one if necessary. I've never had any kind of side effects or morning drowsiness doing this."

A number of our survey participants say they choose herbs to help them sleep. Some take teas containing herbal mixtures, such as Sleepytime or Good Night. Others take capsules of an herbal mixture or a particular herb.

Herbs have long been tucked into pillows, brewed into potions or ground into sleep-inducing capsules. They remain popular as gentle promoters of sleep because they can work and because, properly used, they can produce less lingering drowsiness and fewer side effects than do prescription and over-the-counter sleeping pills, explains Daniel B. Mowrey, Ph.D., psychologist and director of the American Phytotherapy Research Laboratory in Lehi, Utah.

Passionflower, valerian and hops have the strongest tranquilizing effects, Dr. Mowrey says. "All three work on the central nervous system in one way or another to induce a relaxing effect," he says. "When people use these herbs, they aren't bothered with the anxiety, tension and problems that would normally keep them awake."

Some of the other herbs mentioned—catnip, chamomile, and sage—are much weaker sleep promoters, Dr. Mowrey says.

"I will recommend herbs to help people sleep, but only to help them break the cycle of sleeplessness and until lifestyle and nutritional changes have taken effect," Dr. Pizzorno says. "Herbs, like drugs, should not be used regularly to induce sleep." Capsules of powdered herbs are typically stronger than teas made from the same herbs, he adds.

THEY PLAY HARD TO SLEEP WELL

"I always sleep well after a hard day of work or walking," says Lorraine, 44, a Souderton, Pennsylvania, waitress. A number of other people couldn't agree more. They rely on regular exercise to help them get a solid night's shut-eye.

"I don't really notice how much it helps me unless I haven't had the chance to exercise for a few days," says Peter, 42, an energy systems engineer from Pittsburgh. "Then, even if it's bedtime, I'll have trouble falling asleep or drift in and out of sleep. I feel restless until I get a good workout."

One woman says she'll often go out for a leisurely walk just before bedtime to help her sleep better. "I'll do it if I've had a particularly stressful day and no other opportunity to exercise," says Lori, 37, a college administrator from Ithaca, New York.

"Exercise helps to reduce stress and induce sleep by depleting biochemicals such as norepinephrine and epinephrine, which activate the body," Dr. Lahmeyer says. Some research indicates that exercising in the late afternoon or early evening has the best effect on sleep.

GENTLE STRETCHES INDUCE SLEEP

Three people say they do stretches—in bed, or even hanging over the bed—to summon the sleep fairies.

"I'll sit in bed with my legs straight out, pull my upper body down, point my toes, and hold that pose for a few seconds," says Bonnie, 43, head cashier for a Cincinnati savings and loan association. Then, she'll stretch her arms and legs out as far as they'll go. "I try to take deep, slow breaths while I'm stretching, to deliberately slow myself down, and that really does seem to help," she adds.

Stretching and relaxed breathing can help induce sleep, agrees Alice Christensen, founder and executive director of the American Yoga Association, Sarasota, Florida, and author of the association's *Beginner's Manual*. "Stretching promotes good circulation, which makes you more restful," she explains. "But rather than rely on your own contrived stretches, which may not be the best or safest, why not learn a few yoga techniques, including progressive relaxation, in which you gently relax all muscles one by one, to help you sleep better?"

Irritable Bowel Syndrome

Solutions for an Aggravating Condition

I t's something of a medical mystery. Doctors have no idea what causes irritable bowel syndrome (IBS). In fact, some readily admit that IBS is one of those important-sounding names that doctors use when they're not exactly sure just what the heck is wrong with your body—or, in this case, your digestive system.

As it turns out, several of our survey takers refuse to let this condition make them miserable—and set out on their own quest to find out what is ailing them. Their stories may surprise you. If you're suffering from some of the most prominent symptoms of IBS—alternating diarrhea and constipation, severe pain, bloating and mucus in your stool—these stories may also give you hope that a cure is possible in some cases. That, at least, is the intention of Chris, of Pekin, Illinois, in sharing her story. Her daughter Lori suffered from IBS for four years until they finally banished it from their lives. "If this helps one person, all the pain that Lori and the family went through would be worth it," she says.

TAKING ACIDOPHILUS HELPS HER

Lori's irritable bowel was so unpredictable that she had to be tutored at home for the last two months of her senior year in high school. The problems didn't stop when she got her cap and gown, either. They followed her to college—even though she was taking three different prescription medications. "It was an ordeal just to lead a normal life," says her mother.

Unhappy with the drugs' results, Lori turned to acidophilus tablets, an over-the-counter supplement suggested by her mom and an employee at a local health-food store. At first, Lori had to take as many as eight acidophilus tablets a day to obtain relief, but before long, her condition im-

312

proved, and she was able to reduce the dose as long as she consistently took two or three a day.

Research shows introducing acidophilus into your system, like Lori did, can actually help tip the battle between good and bad bacteria fighting for control of your gut. "There's a very careful balance between the good guys and the bad guys in the colon," says Jorge Herrera, M.D., spokesperson for the American Gastroenterological Society and associate professor of medicine at the University of South Alabama College of Medicine in Mobile. "The good guys are constantly producing substances that kill off the bad guys. But when you upset that balance, you've got problems."

One thing that's very likely to tip that delicate balance: taking antibiotics. These powerful drugs wipe out good and bad bacteria indiscriminately—a massacre that sometimes allows the bad bacteria to repopulate unchecked. Live acidophilus, like the kind found in some yogurts, supplies the good bacteria that can control the growth of bad bacteria, he explains.

SHE CANNED THE COLAS

It wasn't until relatively recently, however, that Lori found herself completely free from IBS. And that, according to her mother, came when she gave up caffeine-containing beverages like colas, tea and coffee. "We're convinced giving up caffeine really made the difference," she says. A recent road trip confirms her theory. While touring with a friend, Lori accidentally drank a soda containing caffeine. The symptoms returned briefly, her mother says, and then went away. "I'm really pleased that we found out about this big offender," she says.

Cracking this case is quite a coup, says Dr. Herrera. "All of the things she did here make sense," he says. "Caffeine, without any question, is a bowel stimulant. If you have irritable bowel syndrome and drink more than three cups of coffee or cans of soda a day, chances are you'll get diarrhea."

And caffeine isn't the only offender in soda: All those innocent-looking bubbles can put an IBS sufferer's tummy into turmoil, says Dr. Herrera. "People with IBS are extremely sensitive to gas. Anything that distends your intestines, like carbonated beverages, will cause a lot of pain," he says. Some sodas and gum also contain sorbitol or sucrose—indigestible sugars that can have the same effect as a laxative in an IBS sufferer, he says.

"A few pieces of gum won't bother you," he says. "But there are people out there who will buy those packs that have 45 sticks and eat two of those packs a day. That's like taking two Ex-Lax a day."

ALOE CALMS HER COLON

Joann credits aloe vera gel with helping ease her IBS, brought on, she believes, by the stress of an 11-year-old daughter stricken with pelvic cancer. "Any time I hear some bad news, I literally can feel my colon go into spasm," says the single mom. "Doctors' medications help a little. But this most wonderful plant treats my symptoms immediately."

A Boca Raton, Florida, resident, Joann says she drinks ½ cup of gel purchased at a local health-food store immediately after her symptoms start. "The cramps subside very quickly, almost like a miracle," she says.

Although he's had patients who reported success fighting IBS after drinking aloe vera gel, Dr. Herrera says he's not sure why it may work. But be careful, he warns. Some aloe vera gel users have suffered from upper intestinal burning or indigestion after taking a drink.

CHARCOAL DAMPENS HER DIGESTIVE FIRE

For two years, Phyllis suffered from severe pain, diarrhea and gas nearly any time she ate fruit, beans or baked goods. But the 62-year-old Ira, Texas, resident didn't wait for a diagnosis of IBS to begin her search for a cure. Finally, she read about charcoal capsules, and within 20 minutes of swallowing the first capsule, she felt relief.

"This stuff takes all the toxicity, all the irritants, out of my system," she says.

Convinced that charcoal capsules helped cure her digestive problem, Phyllis shared her secret with a friend. Her friend confirmed the theory when she said her great-grandfather, a cowboy, added charcoal from his campfires to his coffee to soothe his stomach out on the range.

Phyllis has rustled up a quality pain reliever in charcoal tablets, but she should also keep gas-producing foods off the old chuck wagon. "People with IBS are sensitive to any amount of gas," says Dr. Herrera. "And even normal amounts of gas will cause them to have cramps and bloating because gas tends to get trapped in pockets of the intestine, which causes distension, which, in turn, causes pain."

Foods to avoid include: beans, cabbage and other green leafy vegetables, dairy products and processed foods containing milk. If you can't avoid them, try over-the-counter antigas products like Beano or simethicone that destroy gas in the upper intestine, says Dr. Herrera.

The active ingredients in charcoal tablets, like the ones Phyllis is taking, prowl the lower bowel for gas, soaking it up on contact, he says. Be aware, however, that taking charcoal tablets can turn your stool black, he says. It's nothing to worry about, but it can certainly give you a start if you're already worried about the health of your colon.

EDITOR'S NOTE: While activated charcoal does absorb some gas, it also absorbs medications. Don't take it if you're taking other drugs.

FIBER MAKES THEM FEEL BETTER

Imagine planning your morning around five to eight trips to the bathroom. That was Gwen's fate—until she discovered Metamucil. "It got so bad, I could not drive the ten miles to work without having to stop at a fast food place," says the Fayetteville, North Carolina, resident. "I was generally miserable and had to get up at least two hours before leaving home so I could get my bathroom routine over with."

Today she mixes a heaping tablespoon of Metamucil in a glass of water before she goes to bed. "With the Metamucil, I'm down to two to three morning trips," she says. "What's more, there is none of the crampy feeling I used to experience. My condition is 75 percent improved."

Metamucil also made a profound difference for Susan. But not before the 44-year-old Haslett, Michigan, homemaker spent $2,100 in an attempt to pinpoint the cause of her stomach problems. Even removing dairy products from her diet didn't help. "I couldn't function," she says. "I had severe pain, constipation, vomiting, cramping, gas—you name it. I must have gone through 10 or 11 different tests."

Her doctor was right on target when he told her about Metamucil, however. Two weeks after she began stirring a tablespoon into a glass of orange juice each day and drinking it, her symptoms stopped. Now the only time she has trouble is if she ignores her doctor's advice and eats peanuts or popcorn. "It's done wonders for me," she says. "But if I eat those, I've got real problems."

You won't see it in any insurance policy (yet), but Shelly, of Norcross, Georgia, says she and her husband each down a few tablespoons of fibrous "mush" each day and night to insure against irritable bowel syndrome. "Keeping your bowels regular is a good preventive measure," says the 38-year-old homemaker. "I mix one part applesauce with one part miller's bran (wheat bran) and mix it with approximately one-half part prune juice," she says. "It makes a mush and is wonderful in helping regulate you."

Over-the-counter fiber treatments like Metamucil work because they contain digestible fiber, says Dr. Herrera. "Sometimes someone will get bloated on them, but most people do okay," he says. Between eating several servings of fiber a day—found in raw fruits and vegetables—and a single scoop of Metamucil, you could take in 25 to 30 grams of fiber a day, a dose that will not only keep you regular but may also reduce your risk for colon cancer, he says.

ENZYMES EASE HER SYMPTOMS

Miriam's pain started eight years ago. After eating at a questionable fast-food restaurant for lunch and having an improperly cooked dinner, she found herself in the hospital that very night.

Then, over the years, came the tests, the stomach pumpings and the diagnosis: irritable bowel syndrome. The retired Thomson, Georgia, resident tried to avoid spicy and Italian food, all the while wondering whether having her gallbladder out contributed to the problem.

But the pain never changed. "I've never had children, but I'm sure childbirth couldn't have been much worse," she says. "When I had an attack, this would go on for five, six, eight hours. My husband would draw up in fear when it would start, because he knew all he could do was put a cool cloth on my head and wait till it was over." She stopped going to hospitals. "The treatment was worse than the disease," she says.

But while she suffered, Miriam also searched for a cure, reading as much as possible about IBS. About a year ago, she ran across a story that described something called pancreatic enzymes—an over-the-counter supplement sold in most health-food stores designed to help your body digest food.

At the insistence of her chiropractor, Miriam gave the capsules a try, swallowing at least one before every meal. Remarkably, she claims she hasn't had a single digestive pain since. "I'm still cautious about what I eat to some degree, but it's been a miracle," she says. "To think that those doctors never suggested this is beyond me. But I knew I wasn't digesting my food right."

Exotic as they may sound, swallowing pancreatic enzymes can be helpful—if you have a deficiency. "Your pancreas produces over a thousand times the amount of enzymes you need for digestion," says Dr. Herrera. "As a matter of fact, for a person with pancreatic disease to develop a deficiency of pancreatic enzymes, over 90 percent of the pancreas has to be destroyed before he actually develops a deficiency. But if you have this problem, taking pancreatic enzymes might just work."

ACUPRESSURE AIDS HIM

John, a dentist who's studied healing all over the world, says somewhere along the way he learned an acupressure technique to cure a spastic colon that bothered him for decades. The 67-year-old Virginia man simply wraps four fingers around his belt and then gently presses his thumb into the area just above his navel called the solar plexus. "If I have the slightest indication of stomach problems, I just press that button and it goes away," he says. "You'd be amazed at what it will do for you; if you have any pressure, it will be relieved—coming out as gas or a belch."

Could hitting this sweet spot when your IBS erupts provide relief? It's hard to knock success, says Dr. Herrera. "I don't know enough about acupressure to say why techniques like this seem to work—except there are some nerves located in that area that could be stimulated by touch."

But there's also very good scientific evidence that shows relaxation techniques help IBS, he says. "When the attack starts, it's good to take a deep breath, try to control yourself and realize this isn't going to snowball into an incredible situation. You can control it. Just do whatever you're supposed to do and think about something else. A lot of people get too agitated, too excited, too preoccupied when the symptoms start, and it just feeds on itself. That's why they get into these one- or two-day-long episodes where they are incapacitated. It's uncomfortable, but it's not going to kill you or even get any worse."

Itching

Skin-Soothing Suggestions

They've endured mosquito bites, flea bites, welts, hives, rashes, measles, chicken pox, poison ivy and plain old dry skin. Some even suffer from something called dermographism—an allergic condition that makes skin wheal up from even gentle scratching. Leonard Grayson, M.D., chief of the Department of Allergy and Dermatology at Quincy Medical Group in Quincy, Illinois, is one such sufferer. "If I use a backscratcher, it looks like I've been whipped, the welts are so big," says Dr. Grayson, who, fortunately, happens to be a skin allergy specialist.

In their quest for itch-stopping relief, our survey takers report they've applied ice, baking soda, oatmeal, aloe vera, vitamin E, moisturizing lotions, antihistamines and steroids. If those things aren't handy, they'll grab whatever's around—toothpaste, Listerine mouthwash, lemon juice, vitamins, hydrogen peroxide, ammonia, chlorine bleach, milkweed juice, witch hazel, egg whites, salt—even, we are distressed to report, kerosene. ("That's something you absolutely don't want to use," emphasizes Arthur Jacknowitz, Pharm.D., professor and chairman of the Department of Clinical Pharmacy at West Virginia University School of Pharmacy in Morgantown. Kerosene vapors can damage the heart, lungs and nerves and cause seizures and coma.)

In fact, inhalation can cause toxicity similar to that experienced by people who actually ingest kerosene. Plus, it's highly flammable.

For those who stick with safe solutions, persistence and experimentation pay off. Here's what our 71 survey takers who answered this question say eases their itching.

TOPS AGAIN—BAKING SODA

What would our survey participants do without their baking soda? Well, they'd be scratching like monkeys, for one thing. Some 20 percent say baking soda is their emollient of choice for stopping itching.

"I have used baking soda paste for insect bites, chicken pox or just about anything that itches. It always helps," says Vera, 61, a Denver grandmother and sewing fanatic. In fact, she recalls her grandmother dabbing the white stuff on her chicken pox spots and leaving a little bowl of paste by the bed for her to use. "It helped keep me from scratching, which keeps the itch from getting worse," she says.

A few go in for total body immersion—a baking soda shower—for chicken pox or heat rash. "After you've wet your body, just pour the soda out in your hand and rub it on. Then, let it stay on for about five minutes before you rinse off," suggests Patricia, a long-time home remedies fan from Fargo, Georgia. "Unless it's a severe case, one bath does the trick."

"Baking soda is perfectly safe, and it may help relieve itching by temporarily changing the pH of the skin from acid to alkaline," says Dr. Grayson.

He suggests, if you can tolerate it, taking a cool, rather than warm, bath. Heat increases blood circulation to the skin and can aggravate itchiness.

OATMEAL SOOTHES THEIR SKIN

"I developed a weepy, raw rash on my legs from wearing rubber boots on a hot day," says Ann, 34, of Kent, Connecticut. The cortisone cream her doctor recommended didn't help.

"My cousin's wife suggested I take oatmeal baths. I put regular Quaker oatmeal in fine netting, suspended it in the bathtub, and soaked in the tub for at least a half-hour. One bath and I felt a lot better. A few days of baths and my legs were healed. I had no more itching."

Almost 20 percent of survey participants couldn't agree more. They use oatmeal baths for relief from chicken pox, poison ivy, sunburn and allergic reactions.

Rather than oatmeal, many use finely ground oats, called colloidal oatmeal. One popular colloidal oatmeal product, Aveeno, is available nationally. This product disperses through the water and forms a thin, water-holding coating on your skin.

In a study, researchers found that colloidal oatmeal baths taken twice daily helped relieve contact dermatitis, prickly heat, eczema and other itchy skin conditions. For best results, experts suggest sprinkling in the oatmeal as the tub is filling, soaking for about 20 minutes, then patting the skin dry with a clean, soft towel.

GLYCERIN WORKS FOR HER

"I tried just about everything, including a few creams recommended by my doctor, for my itching ears," says Virginia, 66, a retired pharmacy assistant from Ramsey, Illinois. She finally decided to try pure glycerin for her problem. "It worked better than anything else I'd tried," she says.

THEY CHILL OUT

Ice or cold water is a top-choice itch stopper for a few brave souls. "If I've been outside picking corn or strawberries, I'll run my hands and arms under cold water when I come inside to stop the itch from pollen and contact with the plant leaves," reports Marie, a retired teacher from Potlatch, Idaho. Other people rub ice cubes over insect bites or endure cool showers or baths to tone down heat rash or other prickly nuisances.

"Chilling relieves itching by temporarily reducing blood circulation to an area, which reduces swelling and inflammation and calms jumpy nerves," Dr. Grayson explains.

FLAXSEED "COCKTAIL" STOPS HER SCRATCHING

Dorothy, 90, of Silver Spring, Maryland, heard about this treatment on a cable network health show and decided to try it herself for dry, itchy skin she'd had for some time. She took a few teaspoons of ground flaxseeds, mixed in with dried fruit and nuts. "I can't say for sure that it worked, but I know that within a few weeks of beginning to take it, my skin had improved 100 percent," she says. She continues to eat this concoction daily.

It turns out flaxseed has been used for hundreds of years to improve the shine on animal coats, including mink and show dogs, reports Jack Carter, Ph.D., president of the Flax Institute in Fargo, North Dakota. "It's also added to animal feed to treat skin conditions and is even fed to elephants and rhinoceros in some zoos to maintain healthy skin."

Flaxseed poultices have a long history of use for a variety of skin problems, and Dr. Carter says he has gotten many case reports from people saying that taking ground flaxseed or flaxseed oil has improved the itch of psoriasis. "Flax oil is a rich source of alpha linolenic acid, which is essential for healthy skin," he says. People who use it for skin conditions generally take about one tablespoon of oil a day or three heaping teaspoons of ground seeds, he says. Flaxseed oil is available at most health-food stores.

EDITOR'S NOTE: Consult your doctor before taking flax oil if you are already taking an anticlotting agent, including high doses of aspirin. Flax may reduce the stickiness of blood platelets and cause increased bleeding.

ANOTHER EXCUSE TO GO TO THE BEACH

"As far as I'm concerned, the biggest free cure you can find for any kind of skin ailment is ocean water," says John, 56, a diver from Pembroke, Massachusetts. "I've used it to treat all sorts of itchy problems, including rashes, poison ivy and athlete's foot. I just get in the water and rub my skin down."

Salt water can help kill itchy fungus, such as yeast and athlete's foot, and dry up blisters from poison ivy or oak, says Glenn Copeland, D.P.M., podiatrist for the Toronto Blue Jays and author of *The Foot Doctor*. If you're landlocked, try using about two teaspoons of table salt per pint of warm water, and soak for five to ten minutes at a time, repeating often until the condition clears.

MOISTURIZERS GET SOME VOTES

Skin moisturizers are also popular itch stoppers with our survey takers. They say that regular use of these creams helps to keep skin not just smooth, but soothed as well.

"My doctor said my itching was simply due to dry skin and recommended an over-the-counter moisturizer, Vaseline Intensive Care," says Carole, 38, of Media, Pennsylvania. Her skin is especially dry because she swims regularly for exercise. "I apply moisturizer after showers," she says.

Moisturizers work best if they are applied to skin that is still moist, after a bath or shower, Dr. Grayson agrees.

One woman, Joanne, 53, a K Mart department manager from Sprakers, New York, has used a popular moisturizer, Avon's Skin-So-Soft, in a novel way. At her veterinarian's suggestion, she applied it to "hot spots" on her dog, Ruffles, during a time when the long-haired pup was suffering from flea allergies. "It was soothing, and she did scratch less when I did this."

Some of our survey takers said that moisturizing soaps such as Dove or Neutrogena work well enough that there is no need to slather on any kind of goop after bathing. "I'm glad to have air conditioning during the summer and heat during winter, but both can be very drying," says Dorothy, of Silver Spring. Dove moisturizing soap is one of several things she uses to keep her skin supple and itch-free. "People are surprised to find out how old I am," she says. "My skin certainly doesn't reflect my age."

CREAMS EASE THEIR ITCH

Some 15 percent of our participants say over-the-counter aids help stop itching. They use topical anesthetics such as Lanacane, topical antihistamines such as Caladryl, and hydrocortisone (steroid) creams such as Cortizone-10.

"I use a cream called Cortizone-10 on any little spot—you know, the embarrassing little places you don't want to be scratching all the time," says Jennie, 56, of Mattoon, Indiana.

"My hands seem to be sensitive to lots of things—they'll get red and itch like mad. And my doctor recommended an over-the-counter cortisone cream, which does help," says Laura, 24, a secretary from Sacramento, California.

EDITOR'S NOTE: "Any of these creams will help, but I suggest you not use them over large areas, or for more than a few days, without seeing a doctor, especially if your skin is raw and blistered," Dr. Grayson says. Sometimes, sensitive skin becomes even more irritated by a product meant to promote healing.

"I often recommend plain, old-fashioned milk of magnesia," Dr. Grayson says. "Just dab it on with a cotton ball. It is very soothing for itching conditions like chicken pox and measles and, unlike calamine lotion, doesn't form a thick coat."

A LITTLE "WITCH" STOPS HER ITCH

"Witch hazel is always in my medicine cabinet and has never failed to stop the itching from fly and mosquito bites," says Anne, 55, a sales representative from Boca Raton, Florida. "I just dab it on a few times, and there's no need for scratching."

Several other people say this simple, all-purpose old-fashioned product soothes all sorts of itches and irritations. Made with the aromatic oil extracted from the bark of the witch hazel shrub, this mildly astringent lotion contains tannins, chemicals that constrict the tiny blood vessels below the skin surface. That action helps to reduce swelling and itching.

VITAMINS AND MINERALS HELP SOME

A few people tell us that taking vitamin C supplements helps to relieve itching due to allergies or, in one case, to hepatitis.

"For hay fever, I increase my vitamin C dosage to 3,000 to 4,000 milligrams per day," reports another participant. "This helps the itching, tearing and sneezing."

Two separate studies demonstrate that blood levels of histamine—a biochemical that causes inflammation, redness and itching—rise when vitamin C intake is low. Studies also suggest that vitamin C supplements lower blood histamine levels.

"I was doing a lot of sitting around, and my feet, ankles and the lower part of my legs itched terribly for a few weeks," says Joyce, of Spokane, Washington. "Because I had hepatitis, I couldn't take anything for it. I'd read that vitamin C sometimes helps, and so I started taking about 1,000 milligrams a day. I don't know for sure if it helped, but within a few days my itching had subsided." She continued to take the vitamin for several weeks.

Two people say that vitamin E applied to the skin or taken orally helps to stop the torment of bug bites or hemorrhoids.

"I took vitamin E for a bad case of chigger bites, and it seemed to help relieve the itching enough so I didn't need to scratch," says Barbara, 58, a legal transcriber from Virginia Beach, Virginia. Her bites, mostly around her midsection, itched so much they were waking her up at night. "I took it orally, a couple of 400 IU (international units) capsules at a time for several days," she says. "I didn't even think to try applying it directly, but maybe that would have worked, too."

Like vitamin C, vitamin E may have some antihistamine properties. Histamines, released in the body as part of an allergic reaction, cause itching.

John, 55, of Pembroke, Massachusetts, believes that taking extra amounts of zinc, a mineral essential for healthy skin and immune response, relieved a problem he'd had for about 45 years.

"My skin itched so much that I used to scratch the back of my arms raw," he says. Within a week of starting to take 25 milligrams of zinc daily, his itching was gone. "I stopped taking the zinc after about two months, and the itching never did return," he says.

Research suggests that people with chemical sensitivities, which can include symptoms of itching, sometimes have low blood levels of zinc. In one case, a woman who had multiple symptoms, apparently from exposure at work to plastic fumes, became less sensitive after zinc supplements restored her body levels of this nutrient to normal.

EDITOR'S NOTE: Although vitamins C and E are considered to be quite safe, even in large amounts, experts suggest taking no more than 1,000 milligrams of vitamin C and 400 IU of vitamin E without medical supervision. In large amounts, the mineral zinc can interfere with the body's ability to absorb copper. Most experts suggest you stick with no more than 15 milligrams a day without medical supervision, and make sure you're getting 1 milligram of copper for each 10 milligrams of zinc.

Also, there is no research to support the use of vitamin C to relieve the itch that sometimes accompanies hepatitis.

Jet Lag

Time Travel Made Tolerable

The tattered, yellowed annals of folk remedies passed down through generations contain antidotes for virtually every health problem known to humanity. Sadly, however, there's no mention of jet lag in these tomes, mainly because the closest thing to a jet in generations past was a souped-up Conestoga wagon.

But here's where our survey takers take over. Those few who have mastered time-zone travel offer their suggestions for making it tolerable.

SUNSHINE GROUNDS THEIR JET LAG

After years of reading about sunshine's role in beating jet lag, Sharon put her knowledge to the test during a trip she and her husband took to Australia. "When we arrived, we didn't have any choice but to sit in the sun by the pool for several hours until our room was ready," says the 43-year-old Bethlehem, Pennsylvania, resident.

Once snug in their room, Sharon and her husband snoozed until 3:00 A.M., awoke briefly to raid the mini-bar for snacks and went back to sleep until morning. Body clocks reset and refreshed from their rest, the couple spent the next three weeks sightseeing in the outback and scuba diving in the shimmering Coral Sea.

Jeff has a similar success story. A 33-year-old former flight attendant from Kennesaw, Georgia, Jeff worked 24 hours straight one particularly nasty shift called the red-eye turn—Atlanta to Los Angeles and back! He was so tired when he arrived back in Atlanta, he was barely able to drive home from the airport. Once there, however, Jeff pulled a chaise lounge to a big window and snoozed for six hours in the sun. When he awoke, it was as if he'd never made the trip in the first place. No jet lag. "When I was with the airline, they told us that bright light of any kind would help us overcome jet lag," he says. "And for some reason, it works."

Both travelers are right on track, says James D. Frost, Jr., M.D., professor of neurology at Baylor College of Medicine and director of the

Methodist Hospital Sleep Laboratories, both in Houston, Texas. "These are good suggestions. We know that bright light will help reset your circadian rhythm—the internal clock that regulates your bodily functions," he says, "although you should stay awake during this time for best results. I tell people they should try to spend a few hours outside the first day or two they are in a new location. If they can't do that, they should probably try to spend some time in an indoor environment where they have very bright lights."

SHE KNOWS WHEN TO NAP

After several trips to the Philippines, Virginia says she's learned how to master the 17-hour plane ride without succumbing to jet lag. "What I do is to keep myself from sleeping when I reach the United States and wait for the evening to really sleep it out. The next day, I'm on the right track," says the Los Angeles resident.

Virginia has found the correct approach in timing her sleep to avoid jet lag, says Dr. Frost. "A lot of people will get on a plane no matter what time of day it is and do an awful lot of sleeping," he says. "But it's actually better to gear your sleep to the time of day of the new location. So if the new location is in the middle of the day when you get on the plane, then you should try to stay awake. The worst thing you can do is sleep a lot while it's day where you're going. You won't be able to sleep that night. It's better to be a little sleep-deprived than to sleep too much. Your body clock will be more quickly reset if you are deprived of sleep when you get there. You might not feel so great the first day you're there, but you'll sleep great that night."

Taking sleeping pills to force sleep, particularly if you don't normally use them, is also a no-no, says Dr. Frost. "Some people think taking sleeping pills will help them get resynchronized to the new time zone," he says. "It does help them get to sleep, but they get up the next morning usually feeling pretty bad. They're sort of groggy the next day, and they have trouble the next night. It's my observation that taking sleeping pills seems to prolong the adaptation process rather than help it along."

THEY CHOOSE BEVERAGES WITH CARE

Mary, a somewhat frequent flier to Yugoslavia (she has family and property there), says she drinks fresh fruit and vegetable juice 24 hours straight after a transcontinental flight to beat jet lag. "I know it gives you immediate energy," says the 78-year-old Lockport, Illinois, resident.

Bobbie, 55, of Rosenthal, Texas, says avoiding caffeine during air travel helps her reduce the effects of jet lag.

While the merits of juicing to defeat jet lag are debatable, Dr. Frost says there's no question that avoiding caffeine and alcohol will help. "Caffeine is a drug, a stimulant, and it will interfere with your sleeping patterns," he says. "You shouldn't use caffeine or alcohol while on the plane or during the first few days you are there except at levels you are accustomed to while you're at home. The tendency when you get on a plane is to drink much more caffeine and alcohol than you are used to. Both of them interfere with your sleep mechanism, and that works against getting your circadian clock synchronized to your new location."

EXERCISE IMPROVES HIS CONDITION

Jeremiah, 53, of Redmond, Washington, endorses moderate exercise upon arrival as his preferred therapy for jet lag.

If exercise is part of your regular schedule, make sure to get some in, says Dr. Frost. "If it's your habit to have activity during the day, it would be important to continue the same activity at your destination," he says. "So if you exercise in the evening, you ought to be exercising in the evening at your new location. I think it would useful in the sense that your body gets used to cues that tell it what time it is."

One study done at the University of Toronto on laboratory animals shows that exercise may actually help the body readjust more quickly.

Kidney Stones

Ways to Bypass Pain

There's no doubt about it. Kidney stones hurt. "It was the worst pain I'd ever had in my life, and after it was over, I said, 'I never want to go through that again.' " Those words from Claude, a resident of Springfield, Louisiana, are typical of the 22 survey takers who responded to our request for home remedies for kidney stones. The pain of passing one of these sharp crystals is enough to send anyone scrambling for ways to avoid a recurrence.

Those known as a former—meaning they have passed one stone and are at risk for another—say they were able to break a medical rule of thumb regarding kidney stones: "Once a former, always a former." Several of our survey participants passed dozens of stones over several decades before they finally hit on a solution that stopped their stones permanently.

"Keep in mind that kidney stones form when minerals such as calcium or phosphates, or other compounds such as uric acid, crystallize in the urine," says Peter Fugelso, M.D., medical director of the Kidney Stone Department at the Hospital of the Good Samaritan in Los Angeles.

That's likely to happen one of two ways: when concentrations of minerals or uric acid get too high in the urine, or when the composition of the urine itself changes to allow stone formation at normal concentrations. Urine pH—or acid-alkaline balance—helps determine how much calcium or uric acid urine can "hold" before crystals start forming. Those hard crystals are usually too big to pass through the tiny tubes through which urine exits the body. When they exit anyway, you're the first to know.

Here's how our survey takers reduce their risk for a recurrence.

SHE DRINKS WATER TO STAY SOLVENT

"I love water, so I have no problem drinking lots of it," explains Margaret, 74, of Washington, D.C. "I have 16-ounce glasses, and I simply drink four a day." Her kidney stones are mostly small—almost like sand, she says, and usually pass easily. "I've only had one bad case, about 15 years ago."

Half a dozen survey participants do the same, many at their doctor's advice. "When you've had pain as bad as I have, you do what the doctor says, even if he tells you to stand on your head," explains one.

Increasing water intake is a universal admonishment from kidney specialists, Dr. Fugelso says. "It's simple," he says. "The more fluid that passes through your kidneys, the more diluted the elements that can cause stones remain, so they are less likely to become concentrated and form the crystals that lead to stones." That holds for all types of kidney stones.

Dr. Fugelso likes his patients to measure their urine output for a few days, to see how much they need to drink to be urinating two quarts a day. "Some people who sweat a lot and live in hot, dry environments are surprised by how much water they need to drink to maintain this output," he says. They may need to take in three or four quarts a day. If measuring urine isn't your idea of a fun time, check urine color, he suggests. If you're adequately "watered," your urine should be almost clear, not dark.

THEY'LL DRINK TO THIS

In addition to water, people say they drink cranberry juice, vegetable juice cocktail, herb teas, mineral water, water mixed with vinegar, even beer, to prevent or flush out kidney stones.

"I decided to start drinking cranberry juice soon after I had a CAT scan that showed I had crystals in my kidneys," says Pamela, 45, of Mansfield, Massachusetts. Her self-designed regimen: an eight-ounce glass of water every half-hour and three small glasses of cranberry juice a day for ten days. "My pain was gone after about a week," she remembers. "My doctor and I were waiting to see if it got worse, but it disappeared. I never did go back for another CAT scan, but I am always aware of how much I drink each day and try to drink lots of fluids."

In Texas, it's well known that tomato juice or vegetable juice cocktail (V8 Juice) can prevent kidney stones, contends Phyllis, 63, of Ira, Texas. "We started on this soon after my husband passed a particularly painful stone," she says. They don't drink as much of it now as they did initially. "He might have two small cans of low-sodium juice a week. But we also started eating more vegetables. We try for five servings a day," she says. Thirty years of veggie drinking has had its benefits: no kidney stones.

Besides providing fluid, do any of these drinks have additional beneficial effects? "These juices do acidify the urine, and the most common type of kidney stones—calcium stones—can dissolve with urine acidification," says Dr. Fugelso. Acidic urine also causes less discomfort than alkaline urine as it passes through the bladder. That translates into less burning if you have a bladder infection.

Beer, while it's not acidic, does temporarily increase fluid flow through the kidneys, Dr. Fugelso adds. "Some people do use it to help flush out a stone."

And what about all those vegetables? Do they help prevent kidney stones?

Several studies indicate that people who follow a vegetarian diet are less likely to form stones than those who eat meat. "And even among meat eaters, studies show that those eating higher amounts of fresh fruit and vegetables have a lower incidence of stone formation," says Joseph Pizzorno, Jr., N.D., a naturopathic physician and founding president of Bastyr University in Seattle. The high protein intake associated with a meat-based diet apparently increases calcium and uric acid levels in the urine. Both calcium and uric acid are involved in stone formation.

HE TOUTS BAKING SODA

Some say they use baking soda dissolved in water as both a cure and a preventive for kidney stones. That may seem odd, since baking soda is alkaline, and we just found out that acidic substances can dissolve stones.

But for two types of kidney stones—uric acid and cystine—making urine more alkaline does help dissolve the stones, Dr. Fugelso says.

"We use this all the time for uric acid or cystine stones, but it is not good for calcium stones," he says. (Your doctor can help you figure out what kind you have.) Dr. Fugelso recommends taking a heaping teaspoon of baking soda four times a day, in eight ounces of water, for a week to ten days. "It's important that you take it about every six hours," he says.

EDITOR'S NOTE: Baking soda does contain large amounts of sodium, so if you have high blood pressure, you should use this treatment only under medical supervision, Dr. Fugelso points out. "Still, in my opinion, the benefits outweigh the risks, even in people with high blood pressure," he says.

MAGNESIUM STOPS THEIR STONES

Three of our survey takers report using supplements of an essential mineral, magnesium, alone or in combination with vitamin B_6, to prevent a recurrence of kidney stones. This is a remedy that has been around for quite a while, but with little current scientific study to back it up.

All three magnesium users were men who'd had impressive numbers of kidney stones. The two taking magnesium and vitamin B_6 said this combination of supplements had completely eliminated their stone-forming problem. The one person taking only magnesium said his number of stone-forming episodes had been greatly reduced.

Eddie, a tax preparer from Griffin, Georgia, says he has gotten calls from people all over the country since he reported in *Prevention* magazine that he'd completely eliminated the tendency for kidney stones that he'd had for 33 years by taking 400 milligrams of magnesium and 100 milligrams of vitamin B_6 a day.

"I had over 100 stones, was in the hospital 27 times, had 22 cystoscopies and five operations," he says. (A cystoscopy is a procedure that involves viewing the urinary tract through a special device.) Eddie started taking supplements in 1988 at the suggestion of one of his wife's beauty shop customers, who said she'd read about it in a magazine.

Claude, 72, of Springfield, Louisiana, had three episodes of kidney stones, even though he did everything his doctor ordered, including drinking lots of fluids. "After the last one in 1980, when I spent three days in the hospital, doubled up, waiting for that thing to work its way out, I said, 'I never want to go through that again,' " he explains. Just by luck, about that same time, he happened to read about a study that found magnesium and B_6 effective for calcium stones. He takes 500 milligrams of magnesium and 80 milligrams of B_6 a day. "On days when I eat a lot of calcium-containing foods, I'll take a bit more magnesium to balance things out," he adds. He hasn't had a stone since.

Richard, 71, a retired assembly plant worker from Long Island, New York, has been taking 500 milligrams of magnesium a day since 1970, when he read about it in a magazine. "I used to have two or three stones, twice a year, and this reduced it to one or two small, passable stones every five years or so," he says. He considers himself way ahead of the doctors who treat him. "They just laugh about this. They are just beginning to figure out for themselves that it does work," he says.

In studies done with laboratory animals, a diet deficient in magnesium accelerates the deposit of calcium in kidneys, Dr. Pizzorno says. "Supplementation with magnesium alone has been shown to be effective in preventing recurrences of calcium kidney stones, and to be even more effective when used along with vitamin B_6," he says.

"This is not nonsense," Dr. Fugelso agrees. "Doctors who treat kidney stones are just starting to catch on to this." Although there have been no reports of adverse effects with this treatment, he recommends trying it only under medical supervision.

EDITOR'S NOTE: Dr. Pizzorno recommends 600 milligrams of magnesium and 25 milligrams of B_6 a day. Vitamin B_6 can be toxic in large amounts. If you decide to take B_6, magnesium, or both, discuss it first with your doctor to make sure your kidneys can handle it, and so that you both can be alert for potential side effects. People with impaired kidneys should always consult their doctor before taking magnesium supplements.

Leg Cramps

Unclenching the Sudden Spasm

There's no convenient time to suffer a leg cramp. But isn't it a bit strange that most people suffer involuntary contractions of their leg muscles while flat on their backs in bed—rather than when waltzing with Matilda or actually using their legs in some way?

Medical experts still aren't sure just what causes nighttime leg cramps. Daytime leg cramps, like those suffered by runners, are easier to explain: Vigorous exercise and heat deplete your body's stores of water, sodium, potassium, magnesium and calcium. These nutrients are essential for carrying the electrical charges to the nerves that control your muscles' contraction and relaxation impulses.

If you regularly suffer from crampy pain in your legs while you're walking, however, you might be suffering from a circulatory problem known as intermittent claudication. Just as chest pains can be a symptom of heart disease, these pains can be a sign of arterial disease of the legs. This kind of cramp is a good reason to visit a doctor.

Some of our survey takers have learned how to deal with leg cramps. Here are several techniques that they recommend to end the ache.

THEY'RE PRESSING THE POINT

Maybe you've heard of a lip-lock—slang in some parts for smooching. Well, when our survey takers apply a lip-lock, they're not trying to get extra friendly. They're trying to relieve a leg cramp.

Take Margaret. Any time she gets a leg cramp in bed, she sits up, grabs her top lip and starts to squeeze. "I know it sounds strange, but it works," says the 46-year-old homemaker. "If the cramp has just started, it works really quick. If it's going full blast, it takes a little longer."

Back when she was a waitress in college, Elizabeth used to massage her calves at night, trying to soothe the cramps that sometimes troubled her at the end of her shift. Nothing, though, worked quite as well at relieving the pain as biting her upper lip. "I was amazed it was so simple," says the 37-year-old Phoenix, New York, librarian. "I would just bite down on my upper lip—not hard enough to draw blood or anything. The most practical solution is always the best."

Will a lip-lock stop a leg cramp? Or are these folks just paying lip service to their favorite remedy? Not according to Michael Reed Gach, Ph.D., author of *Acupressure's Potent Points* and founder and director of the Acupressure Institute in Berkeley, California. "Midway between your upper lip and your nose is an antispasmodic trigger point in traditional Chinese medicine. One 30-second squeeze with the thumb and forefinger often stops any leg cramp," says Dr. Gach.

Two other acupressure techniques for leg cramps include gradually pressing deeply into the heart of the cramped muscle for two to three minutes or pressing on the top of your foot in the valley between your first and second toe, also for two to three minutes, according to Dr. Gach.

SHE COUNTERS CRAMPS WITH A STRETCH

Jeanne never had a job that kept her on her feet for extended periods of time. And her retirement hasn't been any different. But until the 65-year-old Dallas resident taught herself a calf-stretching technique, she suffered through painful nighttime leg cramps that occurred every few months. "I've found that when that warning twinge hits just seconds before the cramp, if I immediately bend my foot upward so that my toes try to touch my shinbone, the cramp is averted," Jeanne says. "I've done this over and over. I think it stretches that calf muscle in some way that stops the cramp before it starts."

Stretching a potentially crampy muscle into gear just before the pain sets in can help prevent a cramp, agrees Morris Mellion, M.D., past president of the American Academy of Family Physicians and a clinical associate professor of family practice and orthopedic surgery (sports medicine) at the University of Nebraska Medical Center in Omaha. "Once a cramp is full-blown, simply stretching has some benefit," he says, "but a lot less than if you stop what you're doing and stretch when you have that vague feeling that your muscle is about to tighten. Contracting the opposing muscle sends an inhibitory signal to the muscle that's cramping. This is an excellent technique."

If you can't contract the opposing muscle yourself, press against a wall or have someone push against the stubborn muscle for you, he says. Kneading the crampy muscle with your hands is one of the most effective techniques of all, he says.

SHE TOUTS CALCIUM AND MAGNESIUM

Mary Jane suffered from nighttime leg cramps for years. She tried taking calcium supplements to ease the pain—without success. But the Larkspur, California, resident reports that once she added magnesium to the mix, her leg cramps disappeared. "My gynecologist suggested I begin taking calcium with magnesium," she says. "It worked, and now I take both daily. I only wish I had known about this before."

In fact, calcium and magnesium have emerged as the dynamic duo of leg cramp treatments, says Lorraine Brilla, Ph.D., associate professor of exercise physiology at Western Washington University in Bellingham. "There are a lot of studies that show magnesium helps leg cramps or spasms by acting as a powerful muscle relaxant," she says. "Magnesium helps pump the sodium and potassium your cells need through the cell wall. Calcium by itself may not have much benefit, but calcium helps magnesium absorption. You're going to absorb more of both if they are taken together."

Because many older adults don't eat enough food, many probably don't get enough calcium or magnesium in their diets, she says. Green leafy vegetables and grains are common sources of magnesium, while calcium is found in dairy products like skim milk and low-fat yogurt.

VITAMIN E ENDED THEIR PAIN

A former statistician at the U.S. Department of Commerce, John knows his way around numbers. And for him, 800 IU (international units) of vitamin E a day has added up to nearly a decade of cramp-free legs.

It wasn't always that way. The 76-year-old Forestville, Maryland, resident says he used to suffer from leg cramps so severe they'd wake him from a sound sleep. "I was practically paralyzed from pain it would hurt so bad," John says.

After reading about the vitamin's purported merits for treating leg cramps—he was already taking 400 IU a day—he doubled his dose, with good results. "Vitamin E is definitely underrated," he says. "It generally seems to help the whole circulatory system. That's my experience. I swear by it."

A retired home health care nurse, Freida fell in love with vitamins when they helped her cut the amount of prescription drugs she was taking for seizures. The appreciation only deepened, she says, when taking vitamin E allowed her to store her support hose in an old sock drawer. For good. "I used to have so many leg cramps, and especially at night," says the 76-year-old Mount Carmel, Illinois, resident. "Now I take 200 IU of vitamin E daily, no longer wear support hose and have no cramps."

Like magnesium, vitamin E may help end leg cramps by providing energy for the mini-nutrient pump located in each of your body's cells, says Dr. Brilla. "Vitamin E has been shown to be somewhat helpful in preventing leg cramps, and that may be because it also helps distribute nutrients throughout the cell," she says.

Whatever's at work, it seems to work well. In one study of 125 people who suffered from night leg and foot cramps for over five years, 103 reported relief after taking vitamin E. Of those taking the supplement, half felt relief with 300 IU or less a day, while the rest used 400 IU or more.

EDITOR'S NOTE: The recommended Daily Value for vitamin E is 30 IU. Although taking 600 IU a day is considered safe, most experts recommend taking no more than 400 IU daily.

QUININE WORKS FINE FOR THEM

Many of our survey takers said quinine helps ease their leg cramps—even though it was originally a prescription drug used to treat malaria.

"Sometimes when I've been mowing the grass and cleaning the yard and taking care of the horses, I'll just be walking along and a cramp will catch me just right," says Sammie, a resident of Ralls, Texas. "You take a little bit of quinine, and it eases up real quick." His wife, Billie, says she uses it, too, when she overexercises or overdoes it.

Quinine is a good treatment for night cramps in the leg, says Dr. Mellion. "That's been a tried and true remedy for years," he says. "When taken as directed, it's a benign medicine." Quinine is now available without a prescription at most drugstores.

SHE SOCKS IT TO HIM

Who needs an alarm clock? For years, Louise was repeatedly awakened from her slumber by a husband who bolted out of bed with leg cramps. "I've known him to actually jump out of bed during deep sleep," says the 92-year-old Salisbury, Maryland, resident.

But the time was right for a solution, and Louise says she came up with just the approach: wearing wool socks to bed. "I figured leg cramps are caused by poor circulation and if you're not circulating your blood right, the warmth in the socks creates more circulation," she says.

The result: "From then on, no more leg cramps. I've followed the same remedy, as many of my friends do, and for years it has worked."

While socks may help a circulatory problem, they probably won't prevent a cramp, says Dr. Mellion.

If wearing socks to bed makes you feel better, however, go ahead. At the very least, your feet will stay nice and warm.

Low Blood Pressure

Getting Those Numbers Up

Low blood pressure? Although low blood pressure—or *hypoten-sion*—does not carry the same serious risk of stroke or heart attack as its high-pressure counterpart, people who have this condition do not get off lightly. Low blood pressure can cause faintness and is a major cause of falls in older people. It can also leave you feeling like some limp, gray, unidentifiable object the cat dragged in.

"I was faint a lot of the time and had no energy. I just wanted to lie in bed. It was almost like a depression," says Barbara, a Gulfport, Mississippi, housewife whose blood pressure was once so low—90/60—that she was rejected as a Red Cross blood donor.

"Doctors distinguish between chronic low blood pressure—the type Barbara had—and brief episodes of low blood pressure," explains Scott L. Mader, M.D., assistant professor of geriatric medicine at Case Western Reserve University in Cleveland. "Chronic low blood pressure can be normal, can be the result of overtreatment with high blood pressure drugs, or it can be symptomatic of a weak heart."

Chronic low blood pressure can also occur for no apparent reason, as in Barbara's case. "My doctors never figured out what was causing it," she says.

Brief episodes of low blood pressure can also occur when you stand up suddenly, drink too much alcohol, suddenly stop vigorous exercise, even after a big meal. These spells usually do not cause symptoms in most people, says Dr. Mader.

Needless to say, it's important to get a medical evaluation for any episodes of dizziness or fainting. If your problem is low blood pressure, you may benefit from the experiences of our survey takers who answered this question. They offer suggestions for both chronic and occasional low blood pressure.

For one woman, avoiding the sauna or steam room at the Y soon after a vigorous workout was all that was needed. "I need to cool down for at least a half-hour before I can handle the heat," says Lisa, 40, an aerobics instructor from Tempe, Arizona.

For another, it's limiting alcoholic drinks to no more than two on any one night and having a tall glass of water or orange juice before retiring for the night. "I guess I'm just sensitive to alcohol, but as long as I follow this routine, I don't wake up in the morning with that weak, headachy feeling that's associated with low blood pressure," says Anne, 37, a waitress from Boston.

Here are several other things that our survey takers do to keep their blood pressure normal.

WALKING GIVES HER A LIFT

Barbara, the Mississippi housewife who was rejected as a blood donor, reports that a suggestion from a Red Cross volunteer brought her blood pressure back up to normal. "I was told to get some exercise, so I started walking a mile or two every other day," she says. "As long as I do this, my blood pressure stays normal, and I have a lot more energy as well. That's all I need to do." Others also report that they walk to improve their problem.

"People with little muscle mass tend to have low blood pressure," Dr. Mader agrees. "Muscle tone in your legs, especially, helps to put pressure on the veins, which transport blood back to the heart. So good muscle tone should help prevent blood from pooling in the legs, which can cause low blood pressure."

HE DRINKS PLENTY OF WATER

"My tendency was to feel faint after I'd exercised outdoors for a while," says Frank, 64, a postal worker from Riverside, California. The combination of heat and sweat caught up with him, creating a fluid deficit that reduced his blood pressure. "A tennis coach insisted that I drink water regularly while I played, even if I wasn't thirsty," he says. "As long as I do that, I have plenty of energy and no faintness."

Dehydration reduces blood volume, which can lead to a drop in blood pressure. Most doctors suggest drinking eight eight-ounce glasses of water a day, or more. Note that you don't have to sweat to become dehydrated, Dr. Mader says. Cold, dry air and the low humidity common on airplanes can also dry you out, he warns.

A PINCH OF SALT SUITS SOME

"I was limiting my salt, because I thought it was good for me, and my husband was told to do so, but after a few episodes of low blood pressure, my doctor said I should salt my food, especially during the hot summer months," says Alma, 68, of Fort Worth, Texas. Three other people also suggest adding a bit more salt to the diet to counteract low blood pressure.

"A low-salt diet isn't necessary for everyone, particularly older people who've always had normal blood pressure," Dr. Mader says. "Unless you've been diagnosed with high blood pressure and your doctor advises you to do so, avoiding all salt may not be good for you either."

EDITOR'S NOTE: If you have been diagnosed with high blood pressure and seem to have symptoms of low blood pressure, don't raise your salt intake without getting a doctor's evaluation. Ask your doctor to check your blood pressure while standing; if it is lower than when you are seated, chances are you could be on too high a dosage of your blood pressure medication, Dr. Mader says.

Memory Problems

Cutting through the Mental Fog

Y ou forget people's names. You forget where you put your car keys. Heck, sometimes you even forget where you put your car and spend long, uncomfortable moments at the mall trying to remember whether it was this week or last week that you parked in aisle Q.

A certain amount of short-term memory loss is natural and very, very common. Our survey takers have lots of experience with trying to jog the old gray matter into action. Here are their suggestions.

SHE SNIFFS HER WAY THROUGH

Ever catch a whiff of perfume that brought back a powerful mental picture of a long-lost loved one?

Claudia, a resident of Puerto Rico, applies the same principle with what she calls a memory recipe. Her recipe, she claims, actually helped a friend pass her bar exam following law school. Here's Claudia's secret for passing exams:

"Certain odors remind us of past events and people. With this in mind, when you have to study for an exam, select a perfume that you don't regularly use, such as rose, lemon or lavender or a fragrant herb such as cinnamon, rosemary or sage, and smell it periodically while you are studying. Then when test day arrives, put some of the perfume on the back of your hand or carry a bit of the herb in a handkerchief and smell it before and during the test. The familiar 'study scent' that you selected previously will bring to mind what you studied."

Psychologists call this aromatic approach contextual reinstatement, says Denise Park, Ph.D., director of the Center for Applied Cognitive Aging Research at the University of Georgia in Athens. "Being in a distinctive context—in this case inhaling something while studying—learning the information under those circumstances, and then recreating the environment is based on sound memory principle," she says. "It works."

SHE WINS THE NAME GAME

Karen, of Shelby, Ohio, relies on this trick to remember names: "When meeting someone new and wanting to remember his name, associate the name with someone you already know by the same name."

This approach is actually Dr. Park's favorite for remembering names. "Say I meet a Catherine. Well, I already know a Catherine or two, and for me I might picture this new Catherine standing next to the old Catherine," she explains. "I can see the two of them together. I'll have a set of Jennifers, Lisas or Christies. It works for me."

This technique will only work if you pay attention to the person's name when you first hear it, Dr. Park adds. "You have to be disciplined and controlled enough to direct your attention towards the information," she says. "Let's say we are at a party, and you are being introduced to bunches of new people. A lot of your mental energy will be focused on who is at this party, do I look okay, what should I say, things like that. You produce a fairly automatic response when someone says, 'Hello, this is Mary,' and you say, 'Hello, Mary, I'm delighted to meet you,' and shake Mary's hand. This response is so automatized that you may not realize that you didn't even process her name because you gave it so little attention. You do not know her name. You have not forgotten it. You never encoded it. You never devoted enough attention to learn the name in the first place. People who are very good at learning people's names and things of that sort are very good at focusing their mental energy and their processing resources on learning the name."

SHE AVOIDS ALUMINUM

One woman says her fears about aluminum's possible link to Alzheimer's disease have led her to avoid the metal. She doesn't use aluminum kitchen utensils, and she won't use any deodorant that has aluminum mentioned on the label.

There has been a lot of controversy in the past few decades over whether aluminum plays any role in the development of Alzheimer's. Scientific studies have come down on both sides of the question. Until this debate is settled once and for all, there's no harm in avoiding aluminum, says Dr. Park.

"It's absolutely unclear what the cause and effect is," she says. "Personally, although I seriously doubt there is a connection, I nevertheless threw out my aluminum pans. I really doubt that people are ingesting aluminum and they are getting Alzheimer's from this, but on the other hand, what if that is the case?"

B_{12} GIVES HER A BOOST

Valeta, 69, began taking vitamin B_{12} for anemia years ago when she was pregnant. But the Manhattan, Kansas, resident didn't forget her supplements after her babies were born—she still uses them to keep sharp and prevent depression. "They make me more alert," she says.

Whether B_{12} beats memory loss may be open to debate, but damage to the nervous system, deterioration of mental abilities and certain psychological problems have all been linked to B_{12} deficiencies.

In fact, it may be one of the reasons some older people seem confused, less alert and not well coordinated.

Studies show that older people tend to be deficient in B_{12} and that the lack of this nutrient is linked to nerve damage resulting in symptoms which can range from unsteadiness to depression.

Menopause

Tips for Smoother Sailing

For most women, estrogen levels start to drop at around age 40 as their ovaries' production of this hormone slows down. Over the next decade, their menstrual periods gradually become irregular. Eventually, estrogen levels become so low that periods stop altogether. For most women, this occurs around age 52.

The women we talked with about menopause range in age from 45 to 72. Many advocate just about everything "natural" they can to minimize unpleasant symptoms associated with menopause. They recommend exercise, vitamins, stress reduction and herbs.

Several say they prefer these treatments because they have strong reservations about taking estrogen replacement therapy. Some who tried alternative therapies, however, say they found that these things simply didn't do enough to relieve severe symptoms and they ultimately required estrogen.

"Estrogen has been a miracle drug for me," says Jean, a retired assistant elementary school principal from San Diego. A hysterectomy at age 55—even though her ovaries were spared—sent her estrogen levels into a nosedive. "My mother had ten long years of terrible symptoms, and I just didn't want to have to go through the same," she says.

Here, then, is what our survey participants do to keep pace with "the change."

VITAMIN E EASES THEIR HOT FLASHES

Tops on our survey takers' list of menopause symptom relievers? Vitamin E, with about one-third saying they use this essential nutrient to help relieve hot flashes.

"I worked in a health-food store, so I tried just about everything for my hot flashes," says Melrose, 72, of Tehachapi, California. No herbs or other vitamins worked as well as vitamin E for her. However, she did need to take large amounts.

"I worked my way up to 1,600 IU (international units) , increasing by 400 IU each week, before my hot flashes stopped completely," she says. She continued this amount for three or four years, with no adverse side effects, then cut back to her present dosage of 400 IU daily.

Other women say they take from 400 to 1,200 IU of vitamin E daily. Several get their vitamin E in multivitamin/mineral formulas designed specifically for women going through menopause. These include Change-O-Life vitamins from Nature's Way Products.

"Vitamin E often does a commendable job of relieving the severity and frequency of hot flashes," says Lila E. Nachtigall, M.D., associate professor of obstetrics and gynecology at New York University School of Medicine in New York City. She suggests starting with 400 IU twice a day (a total of 800 IU).

EDITOR'S NOTE: Vitamin E is considered to be safe, even in these large amounts. However, it's best to check with your doctor before beginning vitamin E supplementation. It can have a blood-thinning effect.

MANY TAKE OTHER NUTRIENTS

Vitamin E is just one of many vitamins and minerals our survey takers say they use. B-complex, calcium and magnesium are also popular, and a fair number make sure they get the full array of essential nutrients. "I've been taking a multivitamin/mineral formula for years, not just for menopause. And I believe the vitamins, along with a good diet, have helped me to stay as fit and healthy as I am," says Elena, 67, a retired nurse from Flagstaff, Arizona.

"Optimal intake of vitamins and minerals is extremely important during the menopause and postmenopausal years," agrees Susan Lark, M.D., director of the PMS and Menopause Self-Help Center in Los Altos, California, and author of *The Menopause Self-Help Book.*

"As women lose their hormonal support and the body's metabolism and chemical reactions become less efficient with age, an adequate intake of essential building blocks is critical to support repair, regeneration and maintenance of our cells," says Dr. Lark. "A good supplement program can even help to relieve and prevent many of the symptoms of menopause."

SHE ADDS BIOFLAVONOIDS

As a result of reading an article by Dr. Lark in a magazine, one of our survey participants started taking both vitamin E and bioflavonoids. Bioflavonoids are nutrients found in vegetables, grains and fruits—especially citrus fruits.

"I had surgical menopause five years ago, at the age of 39, and I seemed to need a large amount of estrogen—4 milligrams a day—to feel right," says Cheryl, a nurse from Alto, Michigan. Attempts to cut back on the amount didn't succeed until she started taking daily doses of 1,000 IU of vitamin E and 2,000 milligrams of citrus bioflavonoids. "I was then able to reduce my dose of estrogen down to its current level of 3.4 to 3.7 milligrams," she says. Her doctor approves of her regimen of nutrients and hormone replacement, she says, and even asked her for literature on the use of these nutrients.

"Bioflavonoids are one of the most important nutrients for women with menopause. In fact, along with vitamin E, bioflavonoids could be called the menopause vitamin," Dr. Lark says. "Bioflavonoids have chemical activity similar to estrogen and can be used as an estrogen substitute. Clinical studies have shown the remarkable ability of bioflavonoids to control hot flashes and the psychological symptoms of menopause. Many women with anxiety, irritability and menopause-related mood swings noted considerable relief of their symptoms while taking bioflavonoids." Dr. Lark recommends taking 700 to 2,000 milligrams of bioflavonoids daily.

THEY GET UP AND GO

Several of our survey participants say that regular exercise has helped them get through menopause more easily.

"Getting out every day, huffing and puffing and sweating, working my muscles, staying fit, staying strong, helped to minimize all my symptoms and keep me from focusing on the negatives," explains Roberta, 54, a credit union manager from Brooklyn, New York. Instead of losing muscle and gaining fat—a common scenario as we age—she has gained muscle and lost fat. "For the first time in years, I can actually lift my carry-on luggage up into the overhead compartment of an airplane," she explains.

Exercise is often recommended as a way to relieve the hot flashes, insomnia and weight gain that are sometimes associated with menopause. An added bonus: Regular physical activity helps ward off osteoporosis and heart disease, conditions more likely to occur in women after menopause.

Experts think exercise helps because it raises blood levels of endorphins. These "feel-good" biochemicals drop off when estrogen is low. Endorphins also play a role in the body's ability to regulate temperature. Regular physical exercise may increase endorphin activity and so diminish the frequency of hot flashes. In one Swedish study, severe hot flashes and night sweats were only half as common among women past the age of menopause who were physically active.

WATER DOUSES HER FLAMES

"I drink plenty of water—eight glasses a day," says Rosalee, 54, a housewife from Grass Valley, California. "I measure it out and keep it in my refrigerator. Believe me, you have to work to get that much down."

Drinking plenty of fluids is important, especially after exercising, experts agree. Being properly hydrated helps keep body temperature in check.

THEY TAKE TIME TO RELAX

Several women say they were able to temper hot flashes, anxiety and insomnia by doing meditation or yoga. Several, in fact, have been involved in these disciplines for years.

"I do a lot of meditation and have strong beliefs in a higher power," says Jean, of San Diego. "I have inner peace and am happy and content for what I have. I feel it's paid off for me—I am in pretty good health."

Yoga poses and some types of meditation include breath control. In one study, women who were experiencing frequent hot flashes were trained to slowly breathe in and out six to eight times for two minutes during each episode. They had fewer hot flashes than women trained to use either muscle relaxation or biofeedback.

Menstrual Problems

Put the Crimp on Cramps and Bloating

In old-time folk remedy books, menstrual cramps, irregular bleeding and breast tenderness are quaintly referred to as female concerns. Times—and treatments—have changed considerably since then, but menstrual discomfort still causes a lot of concern.

Our survey takers recommend a wide array of remedies—over-the-counter drugs, herbs, vitamins and minerals, and applications of heat. Here again, the combination approach works best for many women. "I fooled around with a lot of different things—PMS tea, vitamin B_6, exercise—and found that a combination of things helps me the most," says Diane, 42, a school bus driver from Wilmington, Delaware.

Here's what our survey takers say helps their menstrual problems.

THEY OPT FOR PAIN RELIEVERS

"My mother used to lie down with a heating pad and a cup of tea," recalls Pattie, 45, a schoolteacher from Ann Arbor, Michigan. "I think that's a nice idea, but I've got two kids and a full-time job, and I just don't have the time or inclination for it." Instead, she relies on one or two ibuprofen (Advil) when menstrual cramps or headache come on.

More than 50 percent of our survey takers say they take nonsteroidal anti-inflammatory medications such as ibuprofen and aspirin. Doctors say these drugs work best to relieve menstrual cramps—as well as the breast pain and diarrhea that sometimes go along with cramps—because they inhibit the formation of prostaglandins. Prostaglandins are chemicals that cause muscle spasms and pain.

THEY WALK AWAY FROM PAIN

Among our survey takers, exercise trails over-the-counter medications such as aspirin by only a nose for relieving menstrual pain. In fact, several women combine the two for what they say is quicker relief. "Two aspirin and a 20-minute walk, and I'm good for the rest of the day," says Joanna, 42, an apartment complex manager from Escondido, California.

For some, walking is the preferred activity during this time of month. "I run, swim and do a lot of other things, but for the first or second day of my period, which are always the worst days, I'm tired and achy, and too vigorous a workout wipes me out. So I stick with what feels good, and that's walking," says Melissa, 37, a cashier from Sudbury, Massachusetts.

Experts agree that exercise is one good way to take the edge off both premenstrual symptoms, such as bloating and anxiety, and menstrual symptoms, such as cramps.

HER EXERCISE ADDS A TWIST

"I use exercise positions that alleviate pressure on the uterus and so relieve menstrual cramps," says Linda, 44, a junior high school physical education teacher from Elyria, Ohio.

For one exercise, she positions herself on her knees and elbows, head lower than her hips, and either simply rests in that position or slowly extends each leg back and up. She also lies on her back and brings her knees up to her chest.

Both these positions are similar to the knee-to-chest or hands-and-knees positions recommended by yoga instructors to relieve menstrual cramps, says Susan Lark, M.D, director of the PMS and Menopause Self-Help Center in Los Altos, California, and author of *The Premenstrual Syndrome Self-Help Book*. Dr. Lark recommends a yoga posture called the child pose to relieve menstrual discomfort.

To get into this posture, sit on your heels with your arms relaxed at your sides. Slowly bend over until your forehead touches the floor. Make sure your spine is stretched and your body is totally relaxed. Close your eyes while breathing slowly and deeply. Hold this position for about a minute or for as long as you're comfortable.

SOME SEEK HEAT

Heating pads, hot water bottles and hot baths are all surefire cramp cures, our survey takers agree. "I can just feel my pain melt away if I lie down for a few minutes with a heating pad on my lower back," says cashier Melissa.

Heat helps to relax the muscle spasms that cause cramps, according to doctors.

THEY GIVE B VITAMINS AN A

When it comes to vitamins, the B-complex family tops our survey takers' list of female-friendly nutrients. "I start taking them about ten days before my period, and they have helped my premenstrual symptoms of irritability and bloating," says Diane, our Wilmington, Delaware, school bus driver.

The B vitamins are important because they perform a number of important functions that can help relieve symptoms, says Dr. Lark. Among other things, these important nutrients help the body use sugar, regulate estrogen and stabilize brain chemistry, she explains. Also, any kind of emotional stress causes the body to lose B vitamins, resulting in fatigue and irritability.

Dr. Lark suggests eating plenty of foods high in B vitamins—whole grains, brewer's yeast and beans—or taking a B-complex supplement.

SHE CHOOSES GINGER

"On the first day of my period, which is always the worst, I'll make up a pot of tea using grated fresh gingerroot soaked for ten minutes in hot water," says Michele, 23, a student from Madison, Wisconsin. She uses one heaping teaspoon of gingerroot per cup of tea. "It tastes good, it's soothing and it relieves my cramps and nausea," she says.

In fact, ginger contains ingredients with analgesic and antinausea actions, and it even has some fever-reducing properties, herb experts say.

You don't have to grate gingerroot to make a tea. You can make a ginger tea by pouring a cup of boiling water over two teaspoons of powdered ginger. And most health-food stores carry powdered ginger in capsule form.

SHE GETS HELP FROM CHINA

Linda, 45, a youth minister from Florissant, Missouri, was suffering from heavy bleeding and cramps so bad they confined her to bed each month. She consulted her gynecologist, who suggested she try birth control pills.

"I took them for three days and was so sick I thought I would die," says Linda. She refused a surgical procedure that involves scraping out the uterine lining and was terrified that she would ultimately face a hysterectomy.

Finally, someone in a health-food store told her to try dong quai—a Chinese herb.

"After one month of taking this herb, I had the first normal period I'd had in 18 years," says Linda. She continues to take the herb. "I did stop taking it for a while, to try something else I thought might work better. But my menstrual problems came back worse than ever, so I know I need to continue to take it."

EDITOR'S NOTE: Dong quai has been used in traditional Chinese medicine for thousands of years, mainly for female disorders. Many active substances have been isolated from dong quai, including anti-inflammatory, painkilling, muscle-relaxing and blood vessel–dilating compounds. Although this herb is considered relatively safe, it does contain compounds that prolong blood clotting time and cause sun sensitivity. So it's best used with medical supervision.

Prolonged or heavy menstrual bleeding during two or more periods warrants a doctor's evaluation. Hormonal imbalances, fibroid tumors, ovarian cysts, even endometrial cancer, can cause these symptoms.

Muscle Soreness

Simple Soothers

Whether you're a farmer working the fields or a weekend warrior hitting the weights, sore muscles come with the turf. Strenuous repetitive activity actually creates small tears in your muscles called micro tears. After the muscle heals, it's just a little bit stronger, but in the meantime, you have that achy, breaky feeling to contend with.

Muscle soreness almost always fades in a day or so on its own. But who wants to feel stiff when proven muscle soothers stand ready to help? Not our survey takers. Their methods may surprise you—wait until you read about Mary's cayenne pepper cure or the original Skinner's Salve—but all claim these remedies make them sore no more.

THEY SEASON THEIR BATHS WITH SALT

Good old Epsom salts—first identified in the mineral-rich waters of Epsom, England—is a leading treatment among our survey takers. But few had a need quite like Laurie's. During her brief career as a pro bowler, Laurie bowled as many as 12 games in one day. So after a hard day at the lanes, the Memphis, Tennessee, resident would come home, draw a hot bath, throw in a few cups of Epsom salts and soak her sore muscles.

"She said soaking in an Epsom salts bath takes out some of the soreness and relaxes her muscles," says her mother, Joe Ann, a retired medical technologist. "And she'd soak until the water got cold."

Liberally sprinkling Epsom salts in a warm bath is actually one of the best ways to beat muscle soreness for two reasons, says Ronald Lawrence, M.D., president of the American Medical Athletic Association and author of *Goodbye Pain.* "Epsom salts, which is basically magnesium, has a tremendous relaxant effect on muscles," he says. "Also, achy muscles are filled with fluid, and Epsom salts helps pull fluid out of the muscles. This stuff works great. I recommend it."

THE RUB THAT WORKS

As it turns out, Joan is both an aloe vera aficionado and a square dancing buff. Guess what she rubs on her body to treat muscle soreness after she's been out all night kicking up her cowboy boots? "When you've been dancing on concrete floors for several hours, you can feel it all the way into your thighs," says the 56-year-old San Jose, California, resident. "I rub some aloe vera on before I go to bed, and it relieves my stiffness, soreness and throbbing. Compared with other creams, it's cool and soothing and vibrant. Tingling. Fresh." To ensure good results, Joan says she buys only products that are primarily aloe vera. "Some will have aloe vera listed as the third or fourth ingredient, and that's not good enough for me," she says.

While aloe vera's role in treating muscle soreness needs further study, massage—which Joan gets when she rubs in the cream—is a proven healer, says Dr. Lawrence. "When someone massages you or you massage yourself, you increase venous blood circulation—meaning you increase blood flow back to your heart. It also stimulates lymph drainage, which is another way to clean the muscle of waste products, like lactic acid, that build up during exercise or activity."

But you—or your partner—don't have to be a graduate of a Swedish massage school to benefit. Simple fingertip pressure for 30 seconds to one minute at any tender point on a sore muscle is enough to trick your brain into relaxing the muscle. "The brain gets a message that there's too much tension in the muscle and then sends an order to the muscle to relax," Dr. Lawrence explains. "People use all kinds of devices to do this, too, like wooden rollers, or even lying on tennis balls."

HOT PEPPER EASES HER PAIN

As unexplained muscle soreness gripped her body, Mary grew increasingly worried. Although a test for lupus—a connective tissue disease—came up negative, her doctor insisted she might have it anyway. "I could hardly move," says the 72-year-old Kingman, Arizona, resident. "They had to set me up on a platform rocker just so I could stand up. I couldn't even turn my head."

About that time, a friend concerned about Mary's health called to suggest a remedy she had heard would help ease the pain: a mixture of cayenne pepper and baby oil.

Following her friend's directions, Mary remembers mixing oil and cayenne pepper in a quart jar and applying the hot stuff each night. "I mean I got rubbed from the top of my head to the bottom of my feet," she says. "And it does burn some."

Although the mixture did not provide instant relief, the applications seemed to gradually reduce muscle soreness and swelling. Within three weeks, her symptoms were gone. "I felt a little better after each time," she says. "I think the cayenne pepper had a lot to do with it, and I know the other people who have tried it for things like arthritis say they really like it."

Mary says she used old bedclothes while undergoing treatment to avoid staining her nice things.

Unbelievable as it may sound, Mary's remedy not only has an interesting past as a pain reliever, but an exciting future as well, says Dr. Lawrence. "They've been using something like this in Hungary for years. Paprika contains capsaicin—the same thing that's in cayenne pepper—and they mix it with some kind of vegetable oil," he says. "Capsaicin is the drug of the 1990s and the turn of the century. It works by reducing something called substance P in your tissues. You need substance P for pain transmission, for your body to register pain. Capsaicin doesn't take all your substance P away like anesthesia would, but it reduces the transmission of pain impulses to the spinal cord, and that means you feel less pain. And it increases circulation, which is good for healing."

Capsaicin works so well, in fact, that several over-the-counter pain relievers contain the same hot pepper ingredient.

EDITOR'S NOTE: Just as Mary described, capsaicin can cause burning, so you need to apply it carefully, and you should also wear rubber gloves while preparing and applying the mixture. Use ¼ to ½ teaspoon of pepper per cup of warm vegetable or mineral oil and rub it into the affected area. Be sure to avoid getting it anywhere near your eyes, mouth, nose or genitals. Also avoid contact with sores or open wounds.

WATER WASHES HER PAIN AWAY

After several near-fatal episodes with antibiotics and other drugs (she actually caught polio when she was vaccinated for the disease as a child), Bonnie says she now visits doctors only as a last resort.

Her reluctance to put her health in someone else's hands has caused her to develop several home remedies. Among them: a method for using a hot shower to treat muscle soreness.

Rather than simply jumping into a steaming shower, the 54-year-old Roy, Utah, resident says she slowly increases the temperature until the water is nearly as hot as she can stand. Bonnie also drapes a washcloth over the sore muscle, allowing the water to heat the cloth. "There's a double benefit in that. I minimize the pain of the water on full force, and I can get the water a lot hotter," she says. And to make sure the water hits the right spot, Bonnie says the family purchased a shower head that can both be held in hand and raised and lowered on a pole fixture.

Exposing your sore muscles to warm water gives your brain the green light to relax them, says Ben Benjamin, Ph.D., founder and executive director of the Muscular Therapy Institute in Cambridge, Massachusetts. "Heat activates the parasympathetic aspect of the autonomic nervous system, and when that happens, your body relaxes," he says.

On the other hand, an ice pack applied immediately after exercise for no more than 20 minutes at a time helps reduce inflammation and soreness, says Dr. Lawrence. "I know it's simplistic. But if I were to suggest something, ice would be near the top," he says.

THEY USE ASPIRIN AND WINTERGREEN

Corn and soybean farmers were always visiting Cain's Drugstore in Vandalia, Illinois. It was the only pharmacy for miles around and folks from all over stopped in to grab a soda from the fountain, pick up gifts and cosmetics and fill their prescriptions. Virginia remembers it well.

As a young pharmacist technician who also served as cashier from time to time, she couldn't figure out why the sun-baked, grizzled men who came to the counter all asked for the same thing: wintergreen rubbing alcohol and a bottle of the cheapest aspirin in the house.

Finally she got up enough courage to ask. "They'd dissolve the aspirin in the rubbing alcohol and rub it on sore muscles and arthritic joints," she says.

Although Virginia worked in the same store for 34½ years, she says she never tried the remedy. "But it was quite popular," she insists. "We had about 100 customers who used it."

In fact, this combination works so well that several over-the-counter drug manufacturers now offer similar topical products for muscle soreness, says Dr. Lawrence. "It's really an old remedy that's been incorporated into over-the-counter stuff," he explains. "The wintergreen acts as a solvent, delivering the aspirin into the skin, and the aspirin is an anti-inflammatory," he says.

EDITOR'S NOTE: If you are sensitive or allergic to aspirin, do not try this remedy; it could cause a reaction. Also, check with your doctor before using an over-the-counter remedy. Many of them contain compounds similar to aspirin that could also cause a reaction.

SKINNER'S SALVE SOOTHES THEIR SORENESS

Mabel calls it her miracle salve. And judging from the list of ailments she treats with Skinner's Salve, it's no wonder: stuffy nose, sore throats, even bruises (like when the 72-year-old New Haven, Indiana, resident smashed her foot on the steel edging surrounding her garden).

She also uses it to treat the muscle soreness she gets from walking three to four miles a day. "When my leg muscles get sore I can't be without it. I just think it's great," she says. "I've been using it for five years."

She began using Skinner's Salve after she tagged along on a friend's visit to a reflexologist who uses it in his practice. Now she buys three jars at a time. Her husband, Max, loves it too. "I'll tell you what, that stuff is really penetrating," he says.

Could something like Skinner's Salve provide relief from sore muscles? Certainly, says Dr. Lawrence. Like Vicks metholatum or sports rubs, Skinner's works as a counterirritant on the skin to provide relief, says Dr. Lawrence.

Skinner's Salve is not always easy to come by, however. Made for the past 50 years by the same company, Skinner's Salve is a combination of four different oils—eucalyptus, wintergreen, fir and camphor—in a petroleum jelly base, according to Greg Skinner, grandson of the late R. Lester Skinner, the originator of Skinner's Salve. Greg says his granddad originally created the salve to help heal his wife's respiratory ailments. When the salve worked, his neighbors clamored for a jar of their own. Word slowly spread, and last year the tiny family-run company sold 7,200 jars. (That's total national sales.)

Skinner's Salve can be purchased in some health-food stores and from some chiropractors or ordered directly from the company. The address is Skinner's Salve, 1055 West Elm Street, Lima, OH 45805. Prices vary, depending on the size of your order.

SHE STRETCHES FIRST

A sometime snow skier, Sharon has learned to stretch to avoid muscle soreness the day after. "I do a minimum of ten minutes of stretching before hitting the slopes, preferably after a hot shower. Twenty minutes is even better. This really helps," says the Bethlehem, Pennsylvania, resident.

Although a hot shower may not provide enough warm-up for a pre-ski stretching session, some light stretching will boost circulation to leg muscles, preparing them for strenuous activity, says Dr. Lawrence.

Nail Problems

Look Great Down to Your Fingertips

Fingernails take lots of abuse, no doubt about that. They are used in place of knives, tweezers, screwdrivers, scouring pads and staple removers. They are immersed in hot, soapy water and exposed to bleach, chemical solvents and soil. They are picked at, chewed on, buffed, polished, filed and glued. They are routinely smashed in accidents involving drawers, car doors and hammers. They are attacked by fungi and bacteria, discolored by illness and thickened by age.

Most people's fingernails survive these assaults, but not without dings and scuffs.

Our survey takers aren't interested in cultivating the long, perfectly polished nails of people who don't have to work with their hands. However, they are concerned about maintaining a well-kept appearance. They realize that hands and nails help present that image as much as face and hair. Here's how people who garden, wash dishes, clean their own houses and, yes, even occasionally miss the mark with a hammer keep their nails healthy and attractive.

MOISTURIZERS SAVE THEIR NAILS

People say the same creams and lotions that keep their hands soft and moist help to keep fingernails in good shape. "I try to keep my nails looking good because I wear lots of rings, and people are always looking at my hands," says Johanna, 77, a retired hairdresser living in Miami. "So I simply work some hand cream around my nails. I've been doing that for years."

Our survey takers also view petroleum jelly as strong medicine for nails that break easily, especially nails that are often exposed to water, detergents and bleach. "When my hands and nails get really bad, I keep a tube of petroleum jelly handy in my office and use it a few times a day," says Patty, 34, a New York City physical therapist who often spends part of her day in a swimming pool.

"Hard, brittle nails—often the result of aging, nail polish removers or detergents—do benefit from moisturizing creams," says C. Ralph Daniel III,

M.D., clinical professor of dermatology at the University of Mississippi Medical Center in Jackson. "If you have soft and brittle nails, however, a moisturizer will only make nails softer. You need to protect your nails from too much moisture."

HOOF HELPER KEEPS HER NAILS HARD

"Believe it or not, I use a veterinary product, Hoof Saver, on my nails, and I am very pleased with the results," says Carolyn, an adventuresome housewife from San Antonio, Texas. No, she doesn't own horses. "I heard about this on television and decided to try it," she explains. She doesn't mind shopping at the feed store for cosmetics, especially since this particular item costs only $7.99 for a two-pound container.

Hoof Saver contains animal collagen protein, glycerin, vegetable oils, allantoin and aloe vera gel—some of the same ingredients found in human hand creams.

"It's basically hand cream for horses, and the people around here who use it always say how nice it makes their hands feel," agrees Robert Sigafoos, the University of Pennsylvania Veterinary School of Medicine's farrier—horse shoer.

GLOVES SPARE HER NAILS

"My nails break easily, even when they are cut short, and they break too deeply to cut or file," says Rosetta, 75, of Seattle. "So I wear rubber gloves when cleaning with soap or other household cleaners in water and work gloves for other chores." A widow, she maintains a three-bedroom house (complete with two "live-in" sons) and a large yard. "I'm cleaning all the time, and the gloves do protect my hands and nails," she says.

EDITOR'S NOTE: If you have hand or nail problems, you could be sensitive to rubber gloves. So you should wear vinyl (not latex) gloves under them, Dr. Daniel says. They can be purchased at a drugstore. Rubber also makes you sweat more, which can also be irritating to the hands.

A VOTE FOR VINEGAR

Apple cider vinegar comes up so often as a home remedy for what-ails-you that a suspicious person might think the people who recommend it own stock in the companies that make it. But Martha, of Bayonet Point, Florida, insists her only interest is helping eliminate an ugly, stubborn nail problem—fungus.

"My family used apple cider vinegar for a number of medical problems, and so, when I developed a fungal infection in a fingernail and over-the-counter remedies didn't seem to help much, I decided to try vinegar," she explains. "I saturated a piece of cotton with straight vinegar, put it on the nail, and wrapped a bandage around the finger. I did that every few days for about a month until the nail started to show new, normal growth."

Fungus infections usually begin under the tip of a nail, as a distinct yellow or white spot, and then gradually spread, causing the nail to be raised up from its bed and become thickened, brittle, cracked or ragged-edged, Dr. Daniel explains. Fingernail infections seem to be more common among dishwashers, meat packers and bartenders, who frequently immerse their fingers in water. Using glue-on nails and cutting or pushing back cuticles also makes nails vulnerable to fungus infections, he says.

Abnormal nail growth can be caused by an array of microscopic organisms, Dr. Daniel says. "The best way to get effective treatment is to have the infection cultured (grown in a laboratory) and identified, then to use whatever drug your doctor recommends. And the sooner you have this done, the more likely you are to be cured," he says.

EDITOR'S NOTE: Dr. Daniel says vinegar can work for a nail problem caused by a bacterium called Pseudomonas, *which turns your nail green. But he doesn't believe it can cure a fungal infection.*

NAIL POLISH GETS SOME VOTES

Cruise the cosmetics aisle at any drugstore and you'll find plenty of shelf space devoted to products promising to keep nails long, strong and pretty. Our survey takers have tried perhaps more than their fair share of these products, with fair results. "If I have a splitting or peeling nail, I paint on clear nail polish to keep it from getting worse, and usually, it works," says Johanna, of Miami.

"I use a nail hardener before I apply my nail polish, and it seems to help keep my soft, thin nails from breaking," says Patty, the New York City physical therapist.

EDITOR'S NOTE: While these products can temporarily solve some nail problems, overuse of nail hardeners, nail polish and polish removers can cause problems, Dr. Daniel says. "These products tend to dry out nails," he says. "Formaldehyde, often an ingredient in nail hardeners, does help to harden nails, but can make them brittle. And some people develop a sensitivity to formaldehyde, which makes the area around their nails inflamed and makes their nail start to separate from its bed."

Nausea

Banishing That Queasy Feeling

Nausea—the sickening feeling that what's gone down is about to come up—strikes practically all of us at one time or another. An all-too-memorable boat ride, a careening taxicab, too much to eat or drink, the flu, extreme stress, even some medications, can cause a queasy stomach. For women in the early stages of pregnancy, just getting up in the morning can be enough to trigger nausea and vomiting.

The people who answered our survey question on nausea know all too well that their stomachs are the sensitive type. They've learned through trial and error what it takes to cajole a finicky stomach into compliance. And they're eager to share the remedies that worked. So if unsettled stomach is your problem, consider these solutions.

GINGER TAKES THE CAKE

A spice with a bite—ginger—tops our survey participants' list of stomach-settling remedies. Almost 70 percent of the people who responded to this question tell us ginger relieves their nausea. And the form the ginger comes in doesn't seem to matter: Ginger ale, gingersnap cookies, crystallized ginger, gingerroot and capsules of powdered ginger were all reported effective.

There's actually some good scientific evidence that ginger can prevent the nausea associated with motion sickness. In a study by British researchers, powdered ginger delayed the development of motion sickness better than Dramamine (a popular over-the-counter anti-motion-sickness medication).

A Danish study found that powdered ginger effectively reduced nausea and vomiting during pregnancy. This was among women whose symptoms had been severe enough to warrant hospitalization. And the powdered spice prevented the nausea that often follows major surgery just as well as the standard drug used for that purpose, British researchers found.

"Scientists don't know exactly how ginger works. But it seems to affect the stomach directly, rather than working through the central nervous system, as anti-motion-sickness drugs do," says Varro E. Tyler, Ph.D., a professor of pharmacognosy at the School of Pharmacy and Pharmacal Sciences at Purdue University in West Lafayette, Indiana, and author of *The Honest Herbal.*

Of the ginger remedies used by those who participated in our survey, ginger ale gets the most votes. Some insist flat, room-temperature ginger ale works best, but others say the cold, bubbly kind does just fine.

"The trick with ginger ale is to sip it slowly, not gulp it down," advises a Georgia homemaker who claims this remedy can abort even the stomach-churning effects of a hangover.

Others prefer their ginger with crunch instead of carbonation. "I'd read that ginger helped nausea, so when I was feeling a little queasy one day, I tried eating a handful of gingersnap cookies. They settled my stomach immediately," reports Diane, a Williamsburg, Pennsylvania, housewife and former nurse. "I've used the cookies several times since, and they always help. The brand that I feel has the strongest ginger flavor, Sunshine, seems to work best for me."

Some survey takers find relief with ginger capsules, sold in health-food stores. "We like to go scuba diving, but my husband had a problem with seasickness," says Arlene, 61, a Columbia Station, Ohio, church organist. "He couldn't take Dramamine because it made him drowsy. So he tried taking two ginger capsules about a half-hour before getting on the boat. And it proved to be a good alternative."

If the going gets really rough, her husband repeats the dosage as needed. "He hasn't had to 'hang over the side' since he's started using the ginger capsules," Arlene reports.

CRACKERS AT THE CRACK OF DAWN

More than 60 percent of our survey participants say that a bit of carbohydrate (sugar or starch) often placates a mildly belligerent belly. Crackers, candy and Coke were all reported to have a soothing effect.

Eating a few bland soda crackers can ease the nausea of morning sickness during pregnancy or calm a flu-stressed stomach, some people report.

"I had terrible morning sickness when I was pregnant," recalls Verna, a housewife in Lexington, Kentucky. "A friend suggested I try eating saltine crackers. I kept a box by the bed and would eat a few before I'd even stir in the morning. The crackers did ease my nausea most days. I've recommended this remedy to a few mothers-to-be, and they've told me it worked for them, too. It sure beats taking drugs when you're pregnant."

CANDY FOR CAR SICKNESS

A 49-year-old British native has clear memories of her childhood bouts with car sickness. Her mother would bring along a bag of barley sugar candy, an old-fashioned sweet, and dole it out during bumpy excursions. The candy did the trick.

"I often got sick to my stomach, so my mother would give all of us kids a piece of candy as soon as I complained of feeling the least bit nauseated," says Vivien, of Princeton, New Jersey. "It would calm down my stomach almost immediately."

Barley sugar candy is also sold in the United States. (Brock, a candy distributor, makes Barley Sweets, available at stores such as Wal-Mart.) Vivien's own children, however, never required the treat. "I don't recall any one of them getting carsick," she says.

FOR HER, THE REAL THING REALLY WORKS

One nausea remedy that's as handy as the nearest soda machine is Coca-Cola. Several survey participants say they drink Coke for medicinal purposes.

"When it comes to an upset stomach, Coca-Cola works for me," reports Marie from Miami. Like ginger ale, she says the potion must be sipped, not guzzled. "When I got sick in Mexico a few years ago, I survived on Coke."

Others say a teaspoon or so of cola syrup, available over the counter at drugstores, works as well as the soda.

EMETROL: HE WON'T LEAVE HOME WITHOUT IT

Boats, airplanes, cars, even elevators, can make Sammie, a retired store owner living in Ralls, Texas, turn greener than a parrot. That's why he carries with him a bottle of Emetrol, an over-the-counter nausea medication. With ingredients like glucose, fructose and phosphoric acid, Emetrol is similar in composition to cola syrup but contains no caffeine or cola flavoring.

"He tried Dramamine, but it made him shaky," his wife explains. "He does get sick a lot, so he's learned he needs to keep Emetrol with him. He'll take a swig before he gets in a car or on an elevator, and it keeps his stomach settled."

B_6 EASES THAT EMPTY FEELING

A housewife from Chillicothe, Illinois, has found that vitamin B_6 quiets her queasy stomach when she is dieting.

"I'd read that vitamin B_6 relieves morning sickness during pregnancy, and I know how bad that can be. So I thought I'd try it myself for other kinds of stomach upset. I am sometimes bothered by nausea if I haven't eaten for a few hours. Of course, my first inclination is to grab a snack to settle my empty stomach. But that adds calories I don't want or need. So I take a 100-milligram tablet of vitamin B$_6$, along with water or fruit juice, and my nausea disappears within a half-hour."

Several studies in the 1940s suggested that vitamin B$_6$ was an effective treatment for morning sickness. A much more recent study, involving 59 pregnant women with nausea and vomiting problems, confirmed its effectiveness. Half the women took 25 milligrams of vitamin B$_6$ every eight hours for three days. The other half took placebos (blank pills). At the end of the study, only 8 of the women in the vitamin B$_6$ group were still vomiting, compared with 15 in the placebo group. Vitamin B$_6$ proved most effective for those women who were having the most severe problems—vomiting more than seven times a day.

EDITOR'S NOTE: Very high doses of vitamin B$_6$ can be harmful. Long-term use of high doses has been associated with nerve damage. Most doctors recommend that you take no more than 50 milligrams a day of vitamin B$_6$ without medical supervision.

PEPPERMINT UNDER THE TONGUE

A breath-freshening remedy handed down in her family over the generations also eases nausea, says Carol, a massage therapist from Howell, Michigan. "I put a few drops of tincture of peppermint, available at some health-food stores, under my tongue. It calms my stomach within minutes. I'll use this if I get carsick or airsick. I'll also use it if I simply feel queasy after missing a meal. If I don't happen to have the peppermint with me, I'll stop and buy one of those big peppermint patties. They work well, too."

Other survey takers say peppermint tea or hard peppermint candies soothe the stomach, too.

Peppermint is an antispasmodic (muscle relaxer), medical experts say. Its main constituent, menthol, relaxes the circular muscle at the base of the esophagus, allowing gas to escape from the stomach. In other words, it promotes burping. And peppermint also calms agitated stomach muscles in the throes of indigestion.

CHAMOMILE TEA LIKE MOTHER MADE

Paul, a retired machinist from Little Rock, Arkansas, recalls that his mother made chamomile tea when she felt under the weather. She often made it for him, too, when he was a child. "I'd sip it, and before long, I'd feel better," he says.

Years later as an adult, Paul made himself a cup of chamomile tea when he had an upset stomach. He found it worked as well as he had remembered. "I wasn't real sick, but my stomach was a little upset, and the tea made it ease up a bit," he says.

Chamomile is an herb with a long tradition as a digestive aid, and scientific studies support its use. Several chemicals in chamomile oil appear to relax the muscles of the stomach and intestinal wall.

You can buy chamomile herbal tea at the supermarket or health-food store. Or to make your own from scratch, try adding two or three heaping teaspoons of pulverized dry chamomile flower heads to a cup of boiling water. Steep for 10 to 20 minutes.

EDITOR'S NOTE: Chamomile is a member of the daisy family and can trigger an allergic reaction in people sensitive to ragweed, aster or chrysanthemums.

BONINE SAVED HIS VACATION

Getting ill while you're on the road is no picnic. And the worst is getting sick on vacation.

Mort, a retired executive from Green Valley, Arizona, was into the sixth day of a three-week vacation in the Smoky Mountains when he became "violently ill," as he puts it. "I don't know what I had, but I was throwing up nonstop, and I ached all over." He'd been retching for two or three hours when the motel owner brought in the doctor. "He gave me Bonine, an over-the-counter chewable tablet that's used for motion sickness and other kinds of nausea. Within a few minutes, it stopped my vomiting," Mort says. His achiness improved, too. "I was fine within a day and was happy to continue my vacation."

EDITOR'S NOTE: Although over-the-counter drugs may help control the condition, severe vomiting requires a doctor's evaluation and treatment. It can be a symptom of serious illness.

Nosebleeds

Stemming the Flow

History does not record the date of the first nosebleed. With a little imagination, however, you can picture the moment: two guys dressed in animal skins slugging it out over a mastodon steak.

Nosebleeds have been around a long, long time, so it's no surprise that there are quite a few home remedies to stem the flow. After years of suffering spontaneous bleeds or helping those who have fielded line drives with their faces, our survey takers have plenty of recommendations.

THEY KEEP A STIFF UPPER LIP

Several people say they stuff something between their top lip and gum to stop a nosebleed. Just to clarify: That's inside the mouth, not outside.

Edith, a 54-year-old Taylorsville, Kentucky, resident has been forced to learn about nosebleeds from long experience. Since age four, Edith has suffered from unexplained bleeding that sometimes lasts as long as 45 minutes. "Sometimes I'm just walking down the street and my nose will start bleeding, and I won't even know it," she says.

In search of a cure, Edith has seen doctors and tried all kinds of remedies that she's heard about, including putting ice on the back of her neck—all without success. But so far, tightly rolling an inch-wide strip of tissue paper into a small wad and placing it between her top lip and gum actually works best. "If I do this, usually the bleeding will stop in about ten minutes," she says.

Joy has since had the blood vessels in her nose cauterized—a simple procedure that sears them closed. But when she was young, she would place a small piece of rolled-up paper bag between her top lip and gum to stop recurrent nosebleeds. "I don't know where my mother learned it, but she was of German descent, and it may have been something she learned from her mother," says the 72-year-old Warrior, Alabama, resident.

Instead of paper, Pam, of Maine, says she presses a piece of gauze between her gum and top lip. Another woman claims that tucking a copper penny in there also works well.

There's plenty of evidence that paper or gauze placed between your top lip and gum will slow a nosebleed, says Sanford Archer, M.D., assistant professor in the Department of Surgery, Otolaryngology Division, at the University of Kentucky Chandler Medical Center in Lexington. "I know this works, because I grew up with it," he says. "It's not the main artery to your face, but there is a significant blood vessel that travels under your upper lip and into the area of your nose that bleeds most often. By putting something under there, you're actually putting pressure on the blood vessels, and that can diminish bleeding."

THEY PRESS FOR RELIEF

As a school guidance counselor, Laurie sees almost as many nosebleeds as she does class troublemakers. But the Girard, Pennsylvania, resident says she's found a remedy that's "safe and never seems to fail."

First, she cuts a piece of light cardboard into a strip one inch long and half an inch wide. Next, she places the cardboard against the outside of her upper lip just under the nose and presses.

"In my experience, this stops a nosebleed in less than three minutes," she says.

As far as Betty remembers, her kids never had bloody noses. Betty's sister Kitty, however, was forced to cope with a brood that frequently seemed to have them—just like Mom herself. "I guess they just have sensitive noses," says Betty, a 67-year-old Fort Worth, Texas, resident.

Whatever the cause, Kitty came up with a cure that Betty still brags about. "She'd tear a strip of paper off a newspaper and press it on the spot between her upper lip and nose," she says. Soon the bleeding would stop. "I don't know where she got the idea; I don't remember Mom using it when she was alive. But Kitty says it works."

These techniques differ slightly from the ancient Chinese cure still used by acupressurists today, but they should work, says Michael Reed Gach, Ph.D., author of *Acupressure's Potent Points* and the founder and director of the Acupressure Institute in Berkeley, California. Your top lip and the fleshy area just above it is considered a crucial acupressure point in traditional Chinese medicine. Holding for a one-minute squeeze with the thumb and forefinger while breathing slowly and deeply should stop any nosebleed, he says. Or try pressing on your lip like Betty did, he says.

POLLY PREFERS PINCHING

Her children grown and with kids of their own, Polly hasn't treated a nosebleed in years. But the 69-year-old New Rochelle, New York, resident is ready with a remedy just in case. "What I used to do is put a tissue in the nostril and hold it closed for a few minutes and keep the head back. In just a couple of minutes, the bleeding stops," she says.

Of all the techniques for stopping a nosebleed, compression works best, says Charles P. Kimmelman, M.D., a professor of otolaryngology at New York Medical College in Valhalla and attending physician at Manhattan Eye, Ear and Throat Hospital in New York City. "When you pinch the nose, you're actually closing off the blood vessels in the front part of the nose, which shuts off the bleeding and allows a clot to form in the vessel," he says. "In about three to five minutes, the bleeding should stop."

EDITOR'S NOTE: *"You have to be careful about inserting any foreign material into the nose, however," says Dr. Kimmelman. "It may irritate or cut the delicate lining, making the bleeding worse or even causing an infection."*

THEY LEAN AND PINCH

Even though she has four kids—Tracy, Tony, Troy and Terry, Jr.—Janis has only treated two nosebleeds. But so far, this 44-year-old Champaign, Illinois, homemaker reports complete success.

In one mishap, Tracy broke her nose against the back of Troy's head while the two were horsing around. As the blood began to spill, Troy sat his sister down in the bathroom and went to tell Mom. When she arrived, Janis told Tracy to lean her head forward, hold a cold washcloth over the bridge of her nose and pinch her nose shut. Within just a few minutes, the bleeding stopped, she says.

And when Terry, Jr., mysteriously developed a nosebleed at age five, Janis applied the same technique with the same quick results.

"My daughter's studying nursing and they told her that's the best way to treat a nosebleed. If you tilt your head up, the blood runs down the back of your throat and that's not good," she says. "Keeping your head down allows the blood to coagulate."

"How you tilt your head doesn't really matter just as long as you keep it above your heart," says Dr. Kimmelman. "You do not want to put your head between your legs as some people suggest." Leaning your head back will cause blood to flow down the back of your throat, however, which can lead to an upset stomach in some, he says.

THEY GO FOR THE NECK

After suffering a stroke and recuperating in the hospital, Dorothy's husband was placed on the usual blood-thinning drugs and sent home. Before long, however, Dorothy discovered that the slightest aggravation made her husband's nose bleed.

To help stem the flow, Dorothy would soak towels in cold water and place them on the back of her husband's neck. Within minutes, the bleeding would stop. And once it did, the 83-year-old Pensacola, Florida, resident says she would gently place small pieces of tissue in her husband's nostrils. "I told the doctor that's how I was dealing with his nosebleeds, and he said that was fine," she says.

The coach of a girls' softball team, John tries to teach the youngsters how to use a glove to field a fly ball instead of their faces. It doesn't always work, though. "We get two or three hit in the face a season," says the 45-year-old Wellsville, Utah, resident. "One girl caught a line drive in her face last season and it knocked her flat."

When such collisions occur, John says he places an ice pack on the back of the child's neck to stop the bleeding. "Actually, my wife told me about it," he says, "but it seems to help."

Although placing something cold on the back of the neck to stop nosebleeds has a long history in folk medicine (some people even suggest using metal keys or scissors), science cannot yet provide an explanation of why it may work. "Ice does take some of the stress off the back muscles and relaxes the body, but I'm not sure there's any exact physiologic mechanism. There are no blood vessels on the back of the neck involved in nosebleeds, per se," says Dr. Archer.

EDITOR'S NOTE: "I don't like the idea of placing anything in the nose," says Dr. Kimmelman. "But cold compresses on the back of the neck may cause a reflex blood vessel spasm in the nose and help stop the bleeding. If a person has repetitive nosebleed, especially when blood-thinning medication is taken, a doctor familiar with nasal problems should be consulted."

Osteoporosis

Building Rock-Solid Bones

When illness strikes close to home, it often leaves powerful images. That's certainly the case for Lorraine, 55, a Minneapolis phone service manager. Both her mother and grandmother suffered from osteoporosis—literally, porous bones—and Lorraine watched them crumple.

"My grandmother, especially, was terribly hunched over and looked like she was in pain a lot of the time," Lorraine says. Years ago, she adds, doctors seemed to think this condition was an inevitable consequence of old age. "I don't recall my grandmother, or my mother, being treated for this problem," she admits.

Today, Lorraine realizes that she, too, runs a risk of developing osteoporosis. "I'm small-boned and thin like them, and I don't want to go that course," she says. So she's taking calcium supplements and walking, and after discussing it with her doctor, she's also decided to take estrogen replacement therapy.

Lorraine is typical of many of the people who answered our survey question about osteoporosis. She's an older woman, at risk for this condition, and doing a number of things, both medical and self-care, to keep her bones rock hard. Here's what our survey takers do.

MOST BANK ON CALCIUM

More than two-thirds of the people who responded to this question say they make sure they get plenty of calcium to help keep their bones strong. That makes sense to anyone who knows even the least bit about bones. Although the initial framework of bones is a protein-based fiber called collagen, it's crystals of calcium phosphate laid down on this fiber that provide bones with their exceptional hardness.

"My doctor has prescribed 1,800 milligrams of calcium a day," says Mary Alice, 75, of Pinellas Park, Florida. "I had been having pain in my hip, which my doctor said was due to osteoporosis, and within a few weeks of starting on calcium, the pain went away, and it has not returned."

The amount of calcium she is taking is more than most doctors recommend. Experts suggest you aim for 1,000 milligrams of calcium a day, even if you haven't reached menopause. And they push it to between 1,200 and 1,500 milligrams a day for women past the age of menopause who are not getting estrogen replacement therapy.

SHE OPTS FOR VITAMIN D

"I know from the reading I've done that people need vitamin D to be able to absorb calcium. That's why milk is fortified with vitamin D," says Barbara, 54, of Dorchester, Massachusetts. Since she relies on supplements, not milk, as her main calcium source, and because she doesn't get much sun (another source of vitamin D), she takes a supplement that gives her 200 IU (international units), the equivalent of the Recommended Dietary Allowance (RDA) of vitamin D for a woman her age.

"That's a smart move," says Robert P. Heaney, M.D., a leading osteoporosis researcher and professor of medicine at Creighton University School of Medicine in Omaha, Nebraska. One study showed that 400 IU (international units) of vitamin D a day helped to prevent wintertime bone loss in women past the age of menopause. Levels of vitamin D are likely to be lowest in winter, when people are least likely to be baring their hides to the sun.

EDITOR'S NOTE: A cup of milk contains about 100 IU of vitamin D. But don't count on other dairy products, such as cheese, yogurt or ice cream, to fulfill your vitamin D needs. Unlike milk, these foods are not fortified with vitamin D. "If you do take supplements, stick with no more than 800 IU a day," Dr. Heaney advises. Large amounts of vitamin D can be toxic and can lead to deposits of calcium in soft tissues where it doesn't belong—leading to kidney and heart damage. Use vitamin D supplements only under a doctor's supervision.

SOME ADD EXTRA MINERALS

A small but vocal minority of our survey takers believe that, while upping calcium intake is important, it is only one part of the nutritional picture when it comes to building or maintaining strong bones. They take an array of minerals.

"I use a nutritional supplement called Bone-Builder, made by Ethical," says Geraldene, 58, a retired accountant from Lebanon, Ohio, who says she started learning about nutrition more than 30 years ago after a series of illnesses left her wondering whether she'd live to see middle age. "I feel better now than I did in my twenties," she says. Both she and her 83-year-old mother take this product. "And neither of us has any apparent bone deterioration," she says.

This particular product contains a special form of calcium called microcrystalline hydroxyapatite—whole bone extract that its manufacturer says is better absorbed than calcium gluconate, a calcium compound found in some supplements.

"The chemical nature of a calcium compound is less crucial to absorption than its pharmaceutical formulation," Dr. Heaney says. "In other words, if a pill is put together badly, the pill won't break up and be absorbed, no matter what kind of calcium is being used." He tells his patients that it's enough to pick a name-brand calcium supplement or a chewable product.

In addition to calcium, Bone-Builder contains trace minerals such as phosphorus, fluoride, magnesium, iron, zinc, copper and manganese—minerals its manufacturer says are essential to bone health.

"It would be hard to argue against the benefits of these minerals. Certainly, there is much evidence to indicate that these minerals are essential when it comes to bone health in growing animals, but when it comes to postmenopausal women, more research needs to be done," Dr. Heaney says.

The bottom line, he believes, is that there is currently not enough evidence to recommend trace mineral supplementation to prevent osteoporosis. "I'd try to get these nutrients from a varied diet that contains shellfish, beans, nuts, seeds and whole grains," he says.

THEY SHAKE A LEG TO SAVE BONE

Most of our survey participants realize that bone strength depends as much on regular exercise as it does on good nutrition. Some 25 percent of our participants say they get some sort of regular physical activity to shore up their bones, with walking by far the most popular bone-boosting workout.

"I walk about 3½ miles a day, for a total of about 25 miles a week, and I find it has helped relieve the pain I've had in my neck and shoulders," says Kathleen, 42, of Roseville, Minnesota. She has what her doctor calls brittle bones—the result of early menopause and taking steroid drugs for rheumatoid arthritis.

Experts agree that physical activity—particularly weight-bearing exercises such as walking and running, which force the skeleton to support the weight of the body—is an essential element for growing strong bones. The more you engage in this kind of exercise, the more calcium you deposit in your bones, making them stronger and thicker. Exercise seems to be especially helpful in preventing bone loss in the spine.

EDITOR'S NOTE: If you already have osteoporosis, consult with a health professional with expertise in exercise physiology before starting an exercise program. Sudden movement, too much strain or pounding could cause fractures.

If you've already had a fracture or two, your best choice of exercise may be walking in chest-deep water, working up to 30 minutes at least three times a week, suggests Sydney Lou Bonnick, M.D., director of Osteoporosis Services at the Cooper Clinic in Dallas. The water will help support your body weight and take stress off bones and joints.

SHE PASSES ON POP

"I used to drink a lot of diet sodas, sometimes as many as half a dozen cans a day," says Elaine, 49, a data processor from Virginia Beach, Virginia. "It just got to be a habit, a way for me to try to stop eating or drinking stuff with calories."

Her dieting strategy wasn't working too well, though, and when she consulted a dietitian, she discovered she was getting less than half the RDA of calcium. "To correct that, I agreed to drink two glasses of skim milk a day," Elaine says. Once she started doing that, she lost her taste for diet soda. "And the milk helped to control my appetite better, too," she adds.

Colas and some other carbonated soft drinks get their sharp taste from phosphoric acid, which contains phosphorus. Too much phosphorus in the diet can interfere with calcium absorption, so if you're an inveterate soda guzzler, you may want to cut back on your intake.

"The big problem with soda, especially for children, is that they choose it over milk, which is their main source of calcium," Dr. Heaney says.

Panic Attacks

Facing Down the Fear

These are the times that try men's (and women's) nerves: Your boss calls on you to speak at a crucial corporate meeting or your child wanders away from your side at the shopping mall. Panicky moments for sure. But is a panicky moment a panic attack?

Not really, experts say. For one thing, shear fear, while plenty uncomfortable, isn't quite bad enough to qualify, says Robert D. Kerns, Ph.D., chief of psychology services at the Department of Veterans Affairs Medical Center in West Haven, Connecticut. In fact, he says, you must actually suffer from four or more of the following symptoms to be diagnosed with a true panic attack: dizziness, shortness of breath, heart palpitations, trembling, sweating, choking, nausea, numbness, chest pain, fear of dying or fear of going crazy.

What's more, these symptoms must come on unexpectedly, seemingly without being sparked by a troubling incident. "The experience is literally out of the blue," he says. "There's really no reasonable explanation for why the attack is happening."

Finally, before you're diagnosed with panic attacks, you must have at least four episodes over a four-week period. (Whew!) While our survey takers say they've undergone some pretty stressful events, only a handful actually have panic attacks. Here's what they do.

SHE BREATHES DEEPLY

A veteran police dispatcher, Dee suffered her first panic attack while driving home from a successful evening shift at work. "At first I thought I was having a heart attack or a stroke," says the 41-year-old Nederland, Texas, resident. The pain was so intense, she says she felt like the character Fred Sanford from the television show *Sanford and Son*: "Here I come, Elizabeth; I'm a comin'," she says, laughing.

The attack subsided about five minutes after she started breathing deeply through her nose and exhaling through her mouth. "Now when I feel one coming on, I breathe deeply, and it subsides before becoming a full-blown attack," she says.

Dee's technique and rapid response are key tactics for helping control and prevent panic attacks, says Dr. Kerns. "Using deep breathing to relax decreases your body's arousal and, perhaps most importantly, helps you gain control of your body," he says. "That shifting of belief from helplessness to one of being in control may be the key. It may not be the physiologic changes per se, but it may be just thinking, 'I'm going to control my body,' that helps you get over the panic or prevent it in the future."

Another important coping strategy involves identifying your thoughts the moment you begin to have a panic attack, says Dr. Kerns. "Suddenly you have a thought that is catastrophizing about something," he explains. "It might even be a thought of having a panic attack. In a sense, that thinking causes some arousal—fear, panic—and that brings on your symptoms."

SHE CALLS ON THE DOG

Madeline doesn't own a St. Bernard. But like the dogs originally trained to pull stranded travelers from the Swiss Alps, her pooch, a half chow/half German shepherd named Peaches, comes to the rescue when she's having a panic attack.

"You can try a lot of things: nerve pills, go see a psychiatrist . . . but I guarantee spending some time with my pets calms me down. They don't talk back to you. They love you no matter what," says the 46-year-old Halfway, Missouri, farmer's wife. "Petting dogs and looking at them has always been soothing to me."

Is Madeline barking up the wrong tree? Or can pets help treat a panic attack? Don't rush to the nearest kennel, but there may be something to her approach, says Dr. Kerns. "The specific thing about a dog is you are getting out of yourself by focusing your attention on another object, in this case, a pet. If she were my patient, I'd be reinforcing the heck out of this and maybe even getting her to think through what she thinks is effective about it, and see if there aren't similar things that she can do in other situations where the dog isn't available," he says.

PERFECTION WAS HER PROBLEM

Linda says she had her first panic attack when she was down with the flu and had a high temperature.

"Later, while perfectly healthy, I had another attack. Only then did I realize how serious this could be," says the Southgate, Minnesota, resident. "I was determined to beat it. Now, rather than be a perfectionist, I let minor problems slide and encourage my family to lend a hand. I no longer try to be Supermom. I have since read that illness, stress, caffeine, alcohol, even prescription drugs, can cause anxiety that leads to panic attacks."

While you may be more likely to suffer a panic attack if your personality is rigid, a counselor or a psychologist is better suited to say whether that trait is contributing to your problem, says Dr. Kerns.

THE DOCTOR'S ADVICE

Avoiding stimulants like caffeine, depressants like alcohol and prescription drugs when possible may be a good idea if you're prone to panic attacks, says Dr. Kerns. "These can raise your level of arousal," he explains. "Someone who is prone to panic and fear might be set up to have a reaction. Alcohol can act the same way. People drink to control these symptoms, but when the alcohol wears off, they may be where they were to begin with, or they may have a rebound."

Phlebitis

Clot-Stopping Strategies

The pain feels like a hard, painful knot or a sore, bruised spot, but for the life of you, you can't remember how it happened.

"I thought I'd bumped my leg or pulled a muscle, but I couldn't recall having done that." That reaction, from Anthony, 60, a retired printer from Norristown, Pennsylvania, appears to be typical of first-time phlebitis sufferers.

In fact, that sore area is a blood clot that has developed in a vein, usually in a leg. The clot blocks the vein, stopping blood flow and causing inflammation—pain, redness, swelling, a lump and heat. Often the clot occurs in a varicose vein near the surface of the skin, and the results are visible.

"My vein swelled up to the thickness of my thumb, and I could feel it through my skin," Anthony explains. He also developed a red streak under his skin. "My wife, a nurse, took one look at it and said, 'That looks like phlebitis.' "

Even though the less serious, superficial forms of phlebitis respond to home remedies, you'll want to see a doctor to make sure that's really what you have. If you have deep-vein phlebitis—the risky variety—you may need some downtime in the hospital while doctors give you blood-thinning drugs. The risk with deep-vein phlebitis is that the clot can dislodge and travel through your bloodstream to your lungs or heart, causing blockage and tissue damage there. (In superficial phlebitis, the clot becomes fibrosed—fixed in place by scar tissue.)

The survey takers who answered our question about phlebitis are all under a doctor's care. Here's what they—and their doctors—recommend to reduce the chances of having another bout with this problem.

THEY TAKE A LOAD OFF

A number of people suggest elevating the legs. That's also the number one piece of advice from doctors to prevent another attack. They suggest that, whenever you can, you keep your legs raised 6 to 12 inches above the level of your heart.

Elevating your legs counteracts the effects of gravity and so helps to prevent blood from stagnating in your veins and forming clots, explains Michael Silane, M.D., chief of the Division of Vascular Surgery at New York Hospital–Cornell Medical Center in New York City.

THEY KEEP ON MOVING

A number of survey participants say they rely on regular physical activity to keep phlebitis at bay.

"I walk a couple of miles most days, and my doctor says it's done a lot to prevent a recurrence," says Margaret, 67, a grandmother from Toledo, Ohio, who's had phlebitis off and on since the birth of her second child, back in 1951.

Dr. Silane puts physical activity at the very top of his list of treatment measures. "Lots of doctors tell their patients with superficial phlebitis to get off their feet," he says. "I encourage them to stay as active as they can and avoid long periods of standing or sitting, and I think they do a lot better when they follow that advice."

Exercise that builds up calf muscles may provide additional benefits for prevention, he adds. "The toned muscles keep continuous pressure on the veins in the calves, just as a pressure stocking would. This squeezes blood upward in the veins, helps to prevent veins from becoming dilated, and improves the function of valves in the veins that keep blood from flowing backwards."

THEY SHAKE A LEG

Our buddy Anthony can tell you exactly what brought on his first case of phlebitis some 20 years ago—a long road trip to Alaska, when he logged almost 12,000 miles in six weeks. "I could drive for as long as 36 hours without stopping," he says, not without some pride. Now he knows better than to do that.

If you've had one bout of phlebitis, you can help prevent another one by taking frequent breaks from driving, taking an aisle seat on planes or trains, and getting up to walk around every hour or so, says Dr. Silane. If you're really stuck in your seat, it helps to pump the calf muscles by flexing the ankles up and down, he adds.

SOME SOCK IT TO THEMSELVES

A couple of people say that surgical pressure stockings help their problems with phlebitis. These stockings squeeze your legs tightly at the bottom, with gradually less pressure farther up your leg. Not everyone has had good experiences with them, however. "I wore them when I first started back to work and needed to stand for long hours at a time, but they were so hot and heavy, I soon stopped wearing them," Anthony says.

"Compression stockings can be a nuisance," Dr. Silane agrees. Fortunately, lighter-weight compression stockings are now available for both men and women. (One brand, Jobst, is sold through surgical supply stores.) "If a man needs a stocking, I'd rather have him wear a knee-length compression sock than prescribe a full-leg stocking that I know he will not wear for long," says Dr. Silane.

EDITOR'S NOTE: Although several people mentioned over-the-counter support hose as helpful, Dr. Silane says this sort of hosiery may be counterproductive for people with phlebitis. That's because these stockings sometimes apply more pressure at the top than the bottom of the leg.

ASPIRIN EASES THEIR ACHE

Three people in our survey say that taking one aspirin a day has prevented a recurrence of their phlebitis. "I started doing this, at my doctor's suggestion, after I had bypass surgery, not to prevent phlebitis but to help prevent heart disease," says Anthony. "But I haven't had phlebitis since." He takes a single enteric-coated aspirin a day.

Besides reducing pain and easing inflammation, aspirin has blood-thinning properties, so it may reduce phlebitis by preventing rapid clot formation. For best results, experts recommend taking aspirin before prolonged periods of bed rest or travel, which are the times when your circulation is most sluggish.

HEAT HELPS SOME

Four respondents say they apply a heating pad or a warm, moist towel to an aching leg, usually while elevating it. "My doctor told me to do this twice a day for about 20 minutes, and it certainly does make my leg feel better," says Margaret.

"Heat is a traditional treatment, and it may increase blood circulation to an area, helping it heal but, to be honest with you, I don't recommend it to my patients, and I don't know that it really does much of anything," Dr. Silane says. As long as you don't also have poor circulation from blocked arteries, and if it makes you feel more comfortable, it's certainly okay to apply heat.

Phobias

Fighting Back the Fear

Whether it's hairy, long-legged spiders, flying on airplanes or being enclosed in small spaces, nearly everyone's got a secret fear. But when that fear is irrational and actually prevents you from getting on an airplane or venturing into a crowd or working in the garden, then you've got a phobia, says clinical social worker Jerilyn Ross, L.I.C.S.W., president of the Anxiety Disorders Association of America and author of *Triumph over Fear: Help and Hope for People with Anxiety, Panic and Phobias.*

Fortunately, phobias are nearly always treatable—a fact our survey takers attest to with their stories of personal triumph.

SHE STARTED OUT SMALL

For the longest time, heights frightened Evalee—especially elevators and airplanes. "I had such fear when I flew it was white knuckle all the way," says the 57-year-old Mount Pleasant, Iowa, resident. "Once, my husband had to take a ski lift to the top of Mount Hood by himself because I couldn't bring myself to go."

Since then, however, Evalee has forced herself to ride elevators and take plane trips, gradually increasing the distance. But the big test came one summer when her women's group took a trip to Chicago and the Sears Tower, the world's tallest building.

Her husband, now deceased, would have been proud. Evalee rode the elevator all the way to the top, stood next to the edge and even peered at the city below. She's also planning a plane trip to London. "I'm not ready for sky diving—I still have a certain amount of fear of these things," she says. "But I just decided I was just going to do this. I'm going to try to enjoy the things that I missed out on by facing the fear. I thought, it's just silly to miss out."

Evalee's methodical approach is similar to a preferred technique for treating phobias called systematic desensitization, says Marilyn Gellis, Ph.D., founder and director of the Institute for Phobic Awareness: Phobics Anonymous in Palm Springs, California, and author of *From Anxiety Addict to Seren-*

ity Seeker. If you're afraid of dogs, for example, a counselor might show you a picture of a dog. Next you'd be instructed to put the picture where you might see it often during the day. "Then they move the picture a little closer and a little closer, and then they introduce a stuffed animal . . . until finally you are comfortable holding a stuffed animal," explains Dr. Gellis. "The exposure moves slowly, one step at a time, until you are no longer troubled by whatever is causing the problem." There's probably no danger in trying this technique on your own, but, says Dr. Gellis, it might be best to enlist a support person to help you through the situation.

SHE USES VITAMIN B$_{12}$

Dee, of Wilmington, Delaware, says she often couldn't bear to be around other people—until she discovered vitamin B$_{12}$. "As long as I take vitamin B$_{12}$, I'm symptom-free," she says. "If I forget to take the nutrient or reduce the dose, the symptoms slowly return. And when I resume the right dose, the symptoms gradually disappear."

While further research is needed to determine whether B$_{12}$ supplements are an effective treatment for phobias, there's probably no harm in taking some, says Ross. "If people find that taking a vitamin such as B$_{12}$ helps them, they should do it. I wouldn't recommend it as a treatment of choice, but there are enough people who have had positive experiences that it wouldn't hurt someone to try."

Because B$_{12}$ deficiencies have been linked to psychiatric disorders and a decline in mental functioning, some experts believe that taking B$_{12}$ supplements can be of benefit. In a study of 39 people with B$_{12}$ deficiencies who were suffering from symptoms like psychiatric disorders and memory loss, all improved after taking B$_{12}$.

Vitamin B$_{12}$ is abundant in meats, fish, dairy products and eggs.

SHE'S WALKING AWAY FROM HER PHOBIA

Walking changed Dana's life. Until she discovered the merits of foot travel, the Clovis, California, resident had an anxiety disorder so severe that she was mentally and physically immobile.

"My doctor recommended I start an exercise program, but I was so tired all the time I couldn't muster up enough energy," she remembers. "While waiting in the doctor's office, I picked up a magazine and found an article on walking. I read that it could relieve stress, anxiety and depression. I've been walking two miles four to five times a week ever since. I've lost 20 pounds, feel wonderful, sleep better, and best of all, have been medication-free for over ten months. I've been back to work for eight months and credit the article with helping me turn my life around."

Starting a walking program can be a step toward getting over depression and anxiety, says Ross. "For many people with anxiety disorder, walking and other forms of exercise are very helpful components to their recovery," she says.

PRACTICE BEATS HER PROBLEM

Some folks' phobias make them gasp in horror. Lori's fear gripped her fingers. What's worse, her terror always struck while she was playing the piano at recitals. "It's pretty hard to hit the right note when your hands are shaking," says the Oak Brook, Illinois, resident.

Rather than trying to convince herself not to be afraid the day of a recital, Lori began working on relaxation during her daily practice.

"I think through the points in the melodies where I need to breathe and program in places where I know I'm going to have to relax—like fast runs with a lot of notes," she explains. "Where I'd ordinarily say, 'Oh, no! Here are a lot of notes,' now I say, 'This is a wonderful opportunity to show off.' I relax into it."

The techniques must have worked: Having gone back to college for a music degree, Lori now teaches music in her home.

Lori's program is music to Ross's ears. "What she's doing is just fine," he says. "Rather than fighting the phobia's symptoms, you want to go with it. If you have butterflies in your stomach, picture them flying in formation. That way you're taking what's a negative symptom and turning it into a positive. If your heart is pounding, give it a rhythm. As soon as you try to stop your symptoms and exaggerate the focus, they get worse. You want to accept that this is how your body acts when it gets stressed and then go on to focusing on the present."

If you're phobic about public speaking, touch the podium, feel the surface of the wood and notice the color or texture of the grain, says Ross. "The more focused you are on your environment, rather than your anxiety," she says, "the more your anxiety will abate."

Poison Ivy and Oak

Stopping the Itch

Most people avoid poison ivy like the plague. But not Jim Meuninck. A botanist, author of *The Basic Essentials of Edible Wild Plants* and producer of several health videos, Meuninck actually (shudder!) rubbed his body with the problem plant.

"We were doing a video on Native American medicine, so I took poison ivy, crushed it up and rubbed it all over my body—I was in a bathing suit and this was on camera. I just rubbed it all over me, and then I took the juice of the jewelweed plant and washed myself off. Jewelweed holds a lot of water, and I used that as a wash and never got any poison ivy, even though I'm what you call allergic. I've used jewelweed for many years, and I've found it's a good antidote."

Although none of our survey takers deliberately turned themselves into human guinea pigs to test their remedies for poison ivy and oak, all claim some level of success against the itching, swelling, redness and pustules. Here's what they recommend.

SOAP'S SUDS PREVENT THEIR ITCH

Fels-Naptha supporters worked themselves into a lather touting the benefits of their favorite soap for treating poison oak and ivy.

Ruby became a lifelong Fels-Naptha user after a brush with poison ivy so severe she was hospitalized for a week. Unwilling to give up her beloved walks in the woods, she consulted her doctor on how to avoid further outbreaks. Her doctor suggested scrubbing with Fels-Naptha soap both before and after any woodland jaunts. "I still use Fels-Naptha, and I haven't had a problem for years," says the 66-year-old Mahtomedi, Minnesota, resident.

Pauline, an 84-year-old Boyertown, Pennsylvania, resident, also touts

Fels-Naptha. Before she and her sister went outside to play, her grand-mother always had the kids wash their arms, legs and feet with Fels-Naptha soap and let it dry there as a preventive. "I can still hear her now," recalls Pauline. "She and her husband were tenant farmers, and they used things like that."

While just about any soap could help remove the resin in poison ivy and oak that causes you to break out in a rash if it's left on the skin, few serve as well as Fels-Naptha, says William Forgey, M.D., a Merrillville, Indiana, general practitioner and author of *Wilderness Medicine*. "The best idea is to get that resin off as fast as possible. A lot of backpackers don't carry those old-fashioned soaps because of the phosphate content and their concern for the environment," he says. "They use the biodegradable, nonphosphate detergents, and those are fine in a pinch. But soaps like Fels-Naptha are the ones that have been used for years and probably are the most effective against the poisonous resin of these plants. It's going to take something strong, capable of dissolving the resin and washing it away. It wouldn't hurt to carry a sliver in your backpack and have some on hand just in case."

Thoroughly washing in just about anything within two hours of being exposed to the resin in poison ivy or oak is usually enough to prevent a problem, says Meuninck. "I would say the best antidote is soap and water or just water," he says.

First introduced in Philadelphia in 1894, Fels-Naptha Bar Soap was created when entrepreneur Lazarus Fels combined his soap with a powerful dirt-loosening ingredient called naptha. Although the Dial Corporation made some changes when the company bought Fels-Naptha soap in 1985, most of the original ingredients remain. Among them is mineral spirits—a solvent that may be responsible for the soap's success against poison ivy, says Mary Beth Finkey, Dial's manager of bar soap product development and former manager of clinical research and product evaluation. "We haven't tested Fels for poison ivy or advised people to use it that way, but over the years we have heard that many do use it for that purpose," she says.

OATMEAL BATH EASES HER ITCH

Franceline loved picking strawberries and dewberries with her father when the family lived in Arkansas and Louisiana. Dad did most of the picking—it was Franceline's job to hold a rifle and shoot any snakes that meandered across their path. Invariably, however, Franceline would suffer from poison ivy or oak. "He never seemed to get it," recalls the 77-year-old West Branch, Michigan, resident. "But I would."

When her face started itching, Franceline's parents were quick to pack some tepid oatmeal onto the rash. And when a rash covered her body, they had her bathe in the mushy stuff. About three-quarters of a box of oatmeal would do the job if the tub was filled waist-high with water, she says. "It probably doesn't stop the itching as well as some things that are out now, but it will do if you don't have anything else to put on it," she says.

Although he's never used oatmeal for poison ivy or oak, oatmeal works so well for itchy outbreaks like chicken pox that it ought to be great, says Dr. Forgey. "For chicken pox, you fill a sock with oatmeal, and you make something like a big tea bag out of it and swirl it in water that's tepid," he says. "Use warm, not hot water, because hot water makes any rash itch worse. But you just swirl that big, old sock around, and it turns the water very milky, and then you dip in it. You don't have to soak in it very long because before you know it, you'll be covered with white oatmeal powder. Don't wash it off when it dries either; that really takes care of the itch. I've never heard of oatmeal used against poison ivy, but it makes sense. Just don't fall in the tub—the oatmeal can make it slippery."

Oatmeal may also contain ingredients that help draw poisons like the resin in poison ivy away from the skin, says Meuninck. "It draws the moisture toward the surface of the skin," he says. "Now, will this draw the resin out of the skin and into the oatmeal? Could be."

HE GIVES GOLDENSEAL A GOLD STAR

His face and arms badly swollen, Clifford leafed through the pages of his herb books searching for a cure for poison ivy. When one recommended the herb goldenseal, the 65-year-old retired high school teacher hopped in his car and drove to his local health-food store.

After finding goldenseal in liquid and capsule form, Clifford picked up both and groped to the counter. "At this point my eyes were almost shut," he says. "I could just barely see daylight."

Clifford took the goldenseal capsules as directed and rubbed some of the liquid on his arm. "It was drying up within an hour or two," he recalls. "Now I swear by it."

About a year later, the minister of a church he was attending mentioned he wouldn't be shaking anyone's hand after the service. It seems he encountered some poison ivy and didn't want to pass the rash to the congregation. On his way out, Clifford told him about goldenseal, and the pastor vowed to go buy some. Within a few hours after he tried it, the pastor was also singing hosannas to the herb. "He made a point to tell me later that it worked," says Clifford.

Clifford and his pastor aren't the only ones to give goldenseal a gold star. This herb's powerful anti-inflammatory and anti-infection properties are well documented, says Meuninck. "If you apply it to the pustules of poison ivy, it may dry them since goldenseal is a very drying agent when mixed with water, but I've never tried it myself," he says.

THEY FIGHT POISON IVY WITH PLANTS

Several survey takers cite jewelweed, also known as impatiens and touch-me-nots, for their role in preventing poison ivy rashes. The first few times Stephanie's kids wandered into poison ivy while the family lived in Bellows Falls, Vermont, she would lather on the calamine. The lotion was messy, however, and, frankly, didn't help much, says the 72-year-old Llano, Texas, resident.

Then she heard about jewelweed—a bushy plant with salmon-colored flowers that often grows near poison ivy and oak. After collecting some jewelweed, she boiled the plant in a gallon of water and strained off the vegetable matter. The next time one of her children strayed into a poison ivy patch, Stephanie was prepared.

"Jewelweed works much better than calamine. It absolutely stops the itching," she says.

Linda, a 43-year-old Elyria, Ohio, physical education teacher, has never encountered poison oak or ivy herself. But when she brought her survey to school with her, she received a suggestion that she didn't hesitate to write down. Another teacher told the story of having his poison ivy or oak relieved after rubbing his hands with leaves from an impatiens plant. "I can't say I've ever done it, but it worked for him," she says. "Teachers are always ready to give you their opinion."

Jewelweed is called different things in different parts of the country. In clinical trials of its effect on poison ivy, jewelweed worked just as well as prescription cortisone creams, according to Varro E. Tyler, Ph.D., professor of pharmacognosy at the School of Pharmacy and Pharmacal Sciences at Purdue University in West Lafayette, Indiana, and author of *The Honest Herbal*.

TECNU IS TOPS TO THEM

Their children grown, Jack and his wife thought their poison ivy and oak days were all but behind them. Then they adopted a son named Chuck. Now the retired Sandoval, Illinois, couple keeps a bottle of Tecnu Poison Oak-N-Ivy Cleansing Treatment handy just in case.

"My wife and I were at the Woolworth's, and I was just nosing around for some bug bite stuff 'cause I'm in the yard a good bit," says the 72-year-old retired salesman. "And I saw this, and I said to my wife, 'I think I'm going to get this for Chucky.' "

Now when Chuck gets into either plant, Jack applies Tecnu as directed to relieve the itch and prevent it from spreading. "It says on the label that it removes poison oils and decontaminates clothes, too," says Jack. "It's the best stuff we've used."

Made by Tec Laboratories of Albany, Oregon, Tecnu contains ingredients that probably would be effective against poison ivy and oak, says Dr. Forgey. "Propylene glycol is an organic solvent, and that would absorb the resin, and I imagine that the other ingredients help soothe the itch and irritation," he says. "I could see how their formula might work."

THEY BOAST ABOUT BLEACH

Household bleach also has a sparkling reputation among our survey takers for both removing poison ivy and oak resin and treating the rash they cause.

June, a 68-year-old Dover, Delaware, resident, is so allergic that poison ivy burning nearby is enough to cause an itchy rash on her exposed skin. She says that once she's been exposed to the weed, she first scrubs with a soap like Fels-Naptha. Then she dabs the area with a cotton ball soaked in a half water/half bleach mixture. "If you use it the first time the blisters appear three times that day, by the next day the rash should be gone," she says. "My mother was a nurse, and I'm sure she didn't learn about this in nursing school, but she's the one who told me about it. And I still use it."

EDITOR'S NOTE: *Rather than putting bleach on your skin, which can cause irritation, Dr. Forgey suggests applying a warm, wet compress. "When you have the actual lesions, make a wet compress with a piece of gauze or a washcloth, a little table salt or Epsom salts and apply that for 30 minutes. That will help dry it," he says. "That's a home remedy that works."*

Premenstrual Syndrome

Strategies for Ending Discomfort

Ever since premenstrual syndrome was given an official psychiatric label in 1987—late luteal phase dysphoric disorder—women around the world have been wondering: "Am I nuts?" For our survey participants, the answer is a reassuring "Nah." But several of them admit it's still best to tread lightly in their presence for certain days of the month.

"It's kind of a joke around our house, but my husband, bless his heart, has learned the hard way—by having an entire Easter ham thrown at him—that I can be impossible," says Diane, 37, a school bus driver from Wilmington, Delaware. She's had premenstrual syndrome (PMS) since the birth of her first child seven years ago.

Up to 90 percent of all women have some premenstrual symptoms, such as depression, irritability, mood swings, anxiety, decreased energy, insomnia, food cravings, headache and breast tenderness during the 7 to 14 days prior to beginning menstruation.

But studies indicate that only 20 percent of women who complain of PMS actually have symptoms severe enough to interfere with their lives, points out psychiatrist Leslie Hartley Gise, M.D., director of the Premenstrual Syndromes Program at Mount Sinai Medical Center in New York City.

Most doctors believe PMS is a result of hormonal shifts that occur during the second half of the menstrual cycle, although exactly what hormonal changes are responsible for symptoms has yet to be determined. Nor has much research been done to pinpoint what treatments really help PMS.

"Most doctors initially suggest lifestyle and eating changes, exercise and stress control, thinking these are treatments that will do no harm," Dr. Gise says. And doctors are often surprised when their patients report these simple things work wonders to minimize their symptoms, she adds.

Our survey takers are frank about what bothers them most about PMS: the psychological symptoms. Snapping out, withdrawing, feeling mean and unlovable cause a lot more pain than headaches or breast tenderness. They also report that a little TLC from family members goes a long way to relieve that pain.

"I know it sounds corny, but the more despicable you are, the more you need someone to walk up to you and give you a hug," says Marge, 47, a greeting card employee from Chicopee, Massachusetts, who says she had PMS long before it became trendy. Her advice to friends and families of PMS sufferers: "Don't take the 'Get lost' seriously. Show you care."

For pain and discomfort, then, both physical and psychic, here's what our survey takers do.

THEY KEEP MOVING

Exercise is tops, with one-third of our survey participants reporting that getting out and about eases their PMS symptoms.

"I walk at least mile a day, every day of the month, to help me calm down and relax," says Diane, of Wilmington. "If something happens that I can't exercise for a few days before my period, I notice that I am really irritable and edgy. Exercise is important to me. I can't stress that enough."

She needs to exercise, she says, because PMS medications make her drowsy. "You can't drive a school bus with 60 kids in it when you're dopey," she explains.

"I exercise regularly, but I also plan ahead during the week before my period, to make sure I am doing at least a half-hour of something physically active every day," says Laura, 41, a textiles marketer from Essex, Massachusetts. Planning ahead, and then sticking with it, is important for her. "I tend to get lazy and discouraged during this time—moody and prone to procrastinate. I retain more energy and feel better mentally if I 'just do it' and don't give in to my mood," she explains.

"I recommend regular aerobic exercise, ideally 20 minutes a day, or, second choice, 30 minutes three times a week," Dr. Gise says. "Whether it's through the release of endorphins, which are the body's natural opiates, whether it's the concept that women are taking time out for themselves, whether it's stress relieving or specific to PMS, nobody knows. But I do know from the experience of the hundreds of women who come to me that it is helpful."

MINERALS HELP SOME

Both calcium and magnesium are popular PMS-fighting minerals with our survey takers.

Diane says she gets her calcium by eating dairy foods. "I buy low-fat

Swiss cheese, one percent milk and frozen yogurt, and when I feel tense and uptight, I eat this stuff and feel better," she says.

A couple of studies support the use of calcium and magnesium supplements for PMS symptoms. One study showed that women who received 1,000 milligrams of calcium a day for three months had fewer PMS symptoms. And in two studies, women with PMS who took 360 milligrams of magnesium daily had a reduction in symptoms, including premenstrual headaches.

"The original recommendation for PMS was to limit your calcium intake and to get more magnesium," Dr. Gise says. Until more research clarifies matters, she suggests you simply try to get the Daily Value of magnesium—400 milligrams. Food sources of magnesium include beans, greens, whole grains, shrimp, salmon and nuts.

B VITAMINS ARE FEEL-BETTER FAVORITES

About one-third of our survey takers take vitamin B_6 or B-complex vitamins to alleviate their PMS symptoms.

"I am hyper to begin with, and I find that these vitamins help soothe the jitters, the nerves," says Marge.

"I found that taking B-complex vitamins worked like a charm for me," says Carolyn, a Medford, Oregon, woman who says her major symptom is anger fits. "I tested it several times to see if it really was the vitamin B complex or my imagination, and it didn't take long for both my husband and me to notice the difference."

"There's some evidence that vitamin B_6 has a mild, positive effect on mood throughout the menstrual cycle, although there's no evidence that it has a specific premenstrual effect," Dr. Gise says. For mild cases of PMS, she suggests trying 25 to 100 milligrams of vitamin B_6 a day, along with a multivitamin that offers the Daily Value of the other B vitamins: thiamine, riboflavin, niacin, folate and B_{12}.

EDITOR'S NOTE: The Daily Value of Vitamin B_6 is 2 milligrams. Vitamin B_6 can be toxic in large amounts. Long-term use has been linked with nerve damage. To date, there have been no reports of problems in dosages up to 50 milligrams a day. But because everyone is different, you should undergo vitamin therapy only under the supervision of your doctor.

SHE PUTS SALTY FOODS OFF LIMITS

"Salt is an absolute killer for me. I crave it, but if I get it, I am like Dr. Jekyll and Mr. Hyde, it's that bad," says Diane. Even a single bag of salted popcorn can cause monstrous transformations. "There is some fluid retention, yes, but the worst of it is, all of a sudden I am just snapping out," she says.

There are a couple of scientific studies that show a reduction in fluid retention in women who follow a low-fat or low-salt diet. (No word in yet on whether such a diet helps eliminate Mr. Hyde behavior, however.)

Diet Cleanup Helps Them

Good nutrition seems to provide both physical and psychological benefits when it comes to relieving PMS symptoms, but several of our survey takers say it's darn hard to stick with healthful foods when every potato chip and chocolate bar in sight has their name on it.

"If I can stick with good foods, I don't get that totally out-of-control feeling," Marge says. "Unfortunately, I am weak, and I usually end up eating junk and drinking more alcohol than I'd like during this time. And it just makes things worse."

Some studies indicate that women who eat diets high in fat, sugar, salt, caffeine or alcohol are more likely to have PMS symptoms. "I don't know how it works, but being in control by eating normally—three balanced meals a day—is related to feeling better," Dr. Gise says. "It gives women a more stable, balanced feeling."

And if a woman's healthful-eating plan excludes caffeine and alcohol, the positive effects on PMS are even more pronounced, Dr. Gise says.

"Alcohol abuse is a big problem that most women don't admit to themselves or their doctors, and this really affects their moods up and down," Dr. Gise says. "If you add a menstrual cycle on top of that, these people go off the wall, so getting on top of alcohol abuse is important."

Caffeine, too, affects mood, and she finds that women who are able to wean themselves off it have a reduction in symptoms of irritability.

They Put Stress on Hold

"When I have PMS, I go out of my way to avoid doing things I know will put me on edge," says Diane. "When I don't have PMS, I can do these things and enjoy them."

Stress makes any kind of physical ailment worse, and that goes for PMS, too, Dr. Gise says. Women frequently are aware that they are operating on overload, she explains. "They just need some confidence to say, 'Yes, I am not a superwoman; I can't do all these things. I will get help. I will give that up.' Tackling a physical problem such as PMS often gives them the incentive to do just that," she says.

Psoriasis

Ways to Stop the Flaking

Normally, a skin cell takes about 28 days to grow from the bottom to the top of your skin. If you have psoriasis, the itchy, red, non-contagious patches on your body make that journey in just 4 or 5 days.

"It really is amazing. People can take their clothes off, and they will literally have a small pile of dead skin at their feet," says Michael Zanolli, M.D., director of clinical dermatology services in the Department of Medicine at Vanderbilt University Medical Center in Nashville and a spokesman for the National Psoriasis Foundation.

While researchers are still tracking the cause of psoriasis, our survey takers say they've found ways to fight back—and win—on their own.

COD LIVER OIL IS THEIR SALVATION

During and just after college, Paulette's scalp had large, itchy, flaky patches that refused to respond to any number of shampoos and treatments. "I tried everything," says the 36-year-old Rockford, Illinois, mom.

Then she read a letter to a magazine written by a doctor who claimed to have successfully treated his psoriasis patients with cod liver oil capsules. Paulette began taking a cod liver oil capsule a day, sometimes two when her symptoms were bad. A month passed. And then Paulette noticed the change. "It's like it just went into remission," she says. "It was really weird."

Paulette continued to take cod liver oil for the next several years, and as far as she can remember, her symptoms all but ended. She stopped taking the capsules when she became pregnant and has not used them since.

Today, she suffers from minor scalp irritation that her doctor describes as seborrhea. Did she cure herself of psoriasis with cod liver oil? "To be truthful, I don't know. But something helped me," she says.

Helen, a resident of La Salle, Illinois, is confident that cod liver and linseed oils keep her psoriasis at bay. After spending her childhood and more than half of her adult life with psoriasis on her arms, lower back, knees and scalp, Helen read that cod liver and linseed oil capsules help in some cases. So she decided to give them a try.

About 14 weeks later, she began to notice improvement. And within five months, she was nearly free of psoriasis for the first time in her life.

Helen says she keeps her psoriasis at bay by taking two capsules of each just before bed every night. A recent trip out West reminded her of what happens when she doesn't take them: Within a few weeks, her arms and lower back again were red and scaly. "It was severe," she says, "but when I got back on schedule, within two months it was under control."

Are these fish stories—or could cod liver or linseed oil help some cases of psoriasis? In fact, Dr. Zanolli actually recommends fish oil supplements for some of his patients. "There's some evidence that the fatty acids in fish oil may help decrease the inflammation and redness of psoriasis," he says. "As long as you don't overdo it, supplementing your diet with fish oils is a recognized adjunct for overall care of your psoriasis."

In one study, 28 people with chronic psoriasis were given either ten capsules daily containing a total of 1.8 grams of refined omega-3 fatty acids or vegetable oil look-alike capsules for eight weeks. Researchers soon found those who took the fish oil capsules experienced a "significant lessening" of their itching and scaling. Even the size of their psoriasis patches seemed to shrink!

EDITOR'S NOTE: Cod liver oil, fish oil and linseed oil are available at most health-food stores. (If you want linseed oil, these days you'll have to ask for "flaxseed oil.") Although you should probably consult your doctor before taking fish oil supplements, there's no harm in getting them from the source: fish. A seven-ounce serving of salmon contains 2.4 grams of beneficial fatty acids.

CREAMS KEEP HIM LUBED

One morning in the early 1980s, Delbert woke up with psoriasis on one of his knees. "It seems kind of funny it just kind of showed up there," says the retired Zanesville, Ohio, resident.

Fortunately, the psoriasis hasn't spread to any other parts of his body. To keep his knee from becoming itchy and red and the scales from piling up, Delbert rotates applying Blue Star ointment, Cortizone-10 cream and vitamin E cream. "I'll put one of these on every two or three days while sitting in the evening watching TV," he says. "It doesn't completely cure it, but it keeps it from getting any worse."

All three of these topicals may be of some benefit, says Dr. Zanolli, but you may be better off using Vaseline or mineral oil. "You need things on the skin that can help restore some sort of protective barrier and preserve moisture within the skin," he says. "These will help keep the patches of psoriasis softer. They'll be less likely to crack and bleed. I've found that plain mineral oil or Vaseline is the least expensive and can be very helpful massaged on at night, especially on places like the elbows, knees and hands."

Moisturizing soaps, like those containing lanolin, vitamin E and aloe vera, work best for showers and daily skin care, says Dr. Zanolli. "I generally recommend a very gentle, mild soap with additional moisturizers within the soap. I don't recommend harsh deodorant soaps or those with fragrances for my patients," he says. Any of the over-the-counter dandruff shampoos containing cold tar—though messy—or selenium should also help, he says.

HE QUITS CAFFEINE

David, of Jamison, Pennsylvania, says quitting caffeine helps his psoriasis. "The psoriasis completely disappears upon elimination of all sources of caffeine," he maintains. "If I ingest caffeine only once after weeks of abstinence, there is little or no problem, but ingesting caffeine more than once results in a full-blown flare-up."

Although he's unaware of a caffeine-psoriasis connection, "I would encourage that guy to continue," says Dr. Zanolli. "When people come and tell me that they are doing something to help their psoriasis, I encourage it, and especially something that would be of overall good without doing themselves any harm."

Moderating your alcohol intake can also have big benefits, he says. "Here's my guideline for alcohol intake: one beer or one six- or eight-ounce glass of wine or a mixed drink. You have to wait at least a couple of hours between drinks," he says. "If you drink excessive amounts of alcohol, you can absolutely make it easier to treat your psoriasis by modifying or moderating your alcohol intake."

In fact, studies have shown a possible link between psoriasis and both alcohol and caffeine. Five out of six people improved in one study when they avoided acidic foods like coffee, tomato, soda and pineapple. And in a study of 160 people, severe psoriasis was more common in those who were heavy drinkers.

FIGHTING FAT HELPS HER

Marjorie, of Billings, Montana, says eliminating some fat from her diet has improved her psoriasis.

"About two years after my psoriasis was diagnosed, I read that during World War II, German citizens ate a low-fat diet because of food shortages and that, coincidentally, psoriasis disappeared from the population," she recalls. "So I eliminated butter from my diet, and this brought my psoriasis under control."

A variety of studies have shown at least some benefit of a low-fat diet for people with psoriasis. In perhaps the largest and the oldest, 140 people were placed on vegetarian diets. In many cases, the eruptions steadily faded and actually disappeared.

Rashes

How to Make Your Skin Behave

Whether you've got a maddening itch, unsightly redness, or both, a rash can make you consider some pretty ... well, rash behavior to stop your symptoms.

Don't feel like you're alone. Our survey takers say they routinely raid the kitchen to come up with antirash formulas.

OATMEAL SOOTHES THEIR SKIN

Ann started sowing her bath with oats after she developed a weepy, raw rash on her legs from wearing rubber boots on a hot day.

"My cousin's wife suggested I take oatmeal baths," says the 34-year-old Kent, Connecticut, resident. "I put regular Quaker Oats in fine netting, suspended it in the bathtub, and soaked in the tub for at least a half-hour. One bath and I felt a lot better. A few days of baths and my legs were healed. I had no more itching."

Rather than oat flakes, many people use finely ground oats, called colloidal oatmeal. One popular colloidal oatmeal product, Aveeno, is available nationally. This product disperses through the water and forms a thin, water-holding coating on your skin, says Dr. Jerome Z. Litt, M.D., a Cleveland dermatologist and author of *Your Skin: From Acne to Zits*.

In one study, researchers found that colloidal oatmeal baths taken twice daily helped relieve contact dermatitis, prickly heat, eczema and other itchy skin conditions. For best results, experts suggest sprinkling in the oatmeal as the tub is filling, soaking for about 20 minutes, then patting the skin dry with a clean, soft towel. Be careful though; oatmeal can make your tub slippery.

SHE GIVES APPLE CIDER VINEGAR AN A

Katherine splashes apple cider vinegar on her skin for everything from poison ivy to sunburn. She even uses it as a skin toner. That's why the 56-year-old Chicago legal secretary reached for apple cider vinegar when she developed a mysterious rash while working in a "sick" office high-rise building.

"It was one of these buildings that was designed for energy efficiency," she recalls. "The air was filtered through miles of duct work, and there was one air supply for seven floors. We never got any fresh air. I was itching constantly."

When she got home each day, Katherine says she got out her gallon jug of apple cider vinegar and commenced treatment. "It didn't make the rash go away, but it sure made it feel better," she says. "It's very cooling."

Possibly the first antibiotic, apple cider vinegar has been used throughout the ages to treat such skin conditions as impetigo, ringworm and poison ivy. Experts say apple cider vinegar apparently can kill some bacteria.

SHE RELISHES MUSTARD

A Cleveland Browns fan, Janet hasn't had much to cheer about for the last few seasons. But she's still a booster of her favorite remedy for rashes: dry mustard.

"When I was a kid and I had a rash, like the measles or prickly heat, my mom would put a few tablespoons of dry mustard in a warm bath," says the 51-year-old Cleveland resident. "And I used it on my kids. I don't recall that it made the rash go away, but it was very soothing. It would help the itching." And once the kids stopped itching, the rash seemed to vanish, she says.

Dry mustard may work for some, but Cortaid cream—an over-the-counter anti-itch product—or baby powder may be even better. "Just a light application or dusting should help," says Dr. Litt.

SHE'S SWEET ON HONEY

Margaret has never rubbed honey on a rash, but when she was talking about home remedies with her son's girlfriend, the young woman gave it high marks. "Anything soft, creamy or oily like that seems like it should soothe a rash," says the 76-year-old La Puente, California, resident. "Unless you're allergic to honey."

Historically, honey has been thought to have anti-infection and wound-healing properties. And these may all contribute to the successful treatment of a rash.

CORNSTARCH SOOTHES HER ITCH

Marie, a 58-year-old Potlatch, Idaho, resident, says her mother used to grab cornstarch to treat heat-related rashes. "It would probably help dry up moisture," she says.

EDITOR'S NOTE: Cornstarch will help a rash, but be careful if you're prone to yeast infections. "Yeast thrive on that; they love cornstarch," says Dr. Litt.

SHE SAYS NO TO DETERGENTS

The rash on Connie's hands was so bad that her skin would rip open if she merely closed her fingers. So for a while, the 44-year-old Romulus, Michigan, resident would simply spread on some doctor-prescribed cream and hope for the best. Then she learned her dishwashing liquid might be to blame and switched to a nonallergenic version she bought from Shaklee. In a few days, her rash went away and her hands healed. "If I'm at my sister's and wash dishes for a couple days, it starts breaking out again," she says.

While there are literally thousands of products that can cause rashes, things like detergents and rubber gloves are notorious for it, says Dr. Litt. "Fabric softening pads that you toss in the dryer are another common cause," he says.

If you suspect a cleaning solution is giving you a rash, avoid it for several weeks, says Dr. Litt. Then try using it again. If the rash recurs, you have your culprit, he says. Or simply switch to detergents like Cheer-Free or Oxydol or soaps like Lux or Ivory, which seem to be less allergenic, he says.

Restless Legs Syndrome

Calming the Relentless Urge

P eople with restless legs syndrome struggle to find the right words to describe the sensations associated with this curious but not so uncommon disorder. Some say it feels like tingling; others says it resembles a deep itch or crawling sensation. One says it's worse than any kind of pain. And more than a few say it practically drives them crazy!

Although restless legs syndrome has been around for quite some time—it was first described in the seventeenth century—it remains something of a medical mystery, says Lawrence Z. Stern, M.D., professor of neurology and director of the Muscular Dystrophy Association's Mucio F. Delgado Clinic for Neuromuscular Disorders at the University of Arizona Health Sciences Center in Tucson. "People say it happens to them in bed at night or while sitting for long periods of time, that it's a sensation that amounts to pain, and that it leads to the irresistible desire to get up and move," he says. Bouts typically last a half-hour to two hours.

Just what causes restless legs remains unknown, and there may be more than one cause, Dr. Stern says. Some medical experts have speculated that prolonged muscle contraction may play a role. Others think imbalances in brain chemicals that send nerve signals are involved, and that is why antidepressants relieve symptoms in some people. Symptoms have also been associated with nutritional deficiencies. And the condition definitely runs in families.

Most people don't need medical treatment for this condition, however, Dr. Stern says. Here's what our survey takers do instead.

THEY SHAKE THE SENSATION

The urge to move is so strong with this condition that people get out of bed at night to haunt the hallways, pace the parlor, even kick the walls. And in fact, movement does alleviate symptoms, at least temporarily.

"For me, it feels like a drawing or pulling movement deep inside my legs," says Lori, 47, a piano teacher from Oak Brook, Illinois. Her mother also had this problem, and Lori remembers, as a child, on long car rides her mother would plead until her husband stopped the car and let her out. "We'd park while she walked a mile or two down the road," Lori remembers. "Then, we'd drive along until we saw her and pick her up."

These days, Lori doesn't insist on curbside service. Instead, she simply stops her car at the nearest rest stop and moves around for a few minutes until her legs feel normal again.

If the urge to move strikes during the night, Lori shakes and beats her legs against the carpeted floor. "Sometimes I simply stretch my legs out straight and shake them around," she says.

"I get up and walk around, literally shake a leg, go up and down the stairs, get a drink of water, do some leg stretches, whatever it takes," says Carole, 49, a nurse from Akron, Ohio. Her episodes usually last 15 minutes to a half-hour and seldom occur more than once a month. "I find that, if I get out and walk for at least a half-hour every day, I am less likely to have even my occasional problem with this," she adds.

Several people say that regular exercise during the day helps them avoid restless legs at night.

"Exercise does help, and it's something I recommend to all my patients," Dr. Stern says. For best results, he suggests aerobic exercise—such as walking—regularly at any time of the day that's best for you, and, if necessary, add on a leisurely walk as close to bedtime as possible.

THEY KNEAD THEIR LEGS

Just as exercise seems to relieve these exasperating symptoms, so does stimulation. People rub their legs together like crickets, drag them back and forth across the bedsheets, and massage them to stop the creepy-crawling feeling. Unfortunately, relief is usually short-lived.

"I'll sometimes massage my legs first, hoping I won't have to get up out of my warm bed and walk around, but usually that's still what I end up doing," says Monica, 47, a catering service employee from Fort Wayne, Indiana, who's had this problem for about 20 years.

"People do whatever it takes, and what works for one person doesn't necessarily work for another," Dr. Stern says. All these techniques provide messages to the nervous system, which can compete with and temporarily override those messages causing the bothersome symptoms, he explains.

IRON SOOTHES HER SYMPTOMS

One woman says her restless legs problems ended, at least for a time, when she was diagnosed as having anemia and treated with iron supplements. "I never really recovered my strength after the birth of my last child, and for months I had been having trouble sleeping because of problems with my legs," says Imogene, 61, a housewife from Alvin, Texas. "I would drift off to sleep but awaken moments later with involuntary movements of my legs."

Several studies have shown that iron deficiency can trigger restless legs syndrome symptoms, Dr. Stern explains. "It's a good idea to have blood tests to check for this deficiency," he says.

EDITOR'S NOTE: If you are iron deficient, you may need to take an iron supplement. You should discuss it with your doctor, however. Your doctor will want to determine the cause of the deficiency.

SHE TAKES POTASSIUM

Imogene's leg problem returned about three years ago after she started taking a diuretic for high blood pressure. "It was so bad I'd wake up because the bed was shaking," she says. She was still taking iron tablets, so she didn't believe iron deficiency was involved. She was also taking one 600 milligram potassium supplement a day, to make up for the urinary loss of potassium caused by her diuretic.

"I did some reading and some figuring and decided to increase my potassium intake," she says. When she finally got up to six 600-milligram potassium chloride tablets a day, her restless legs stopped completely. "Yes, I did tell my doctor about this," she says.

EDITOR'S NOTE: It's true that potassium deficiency can cause muscle cramps, which are sometimes found along with restless legs or mistaken for restless legs, Dr. Stern says. "It's important for a doctor to check someone with restless legs for potassium and other nutrient deficiencies," he says. Such deficiencies can be caused by diuretics or other medication.

You can boost your intake of potassium with baked potatoes, prune juice, avocados and bananas. High-dose potassium supplements are available only by prescription, with good reason. They should be taken only under medical supervision and only in the dosages prescribed.

Scarring

Smoothing the Way for Better Healing

Your skin tells the story of your life. Once you've inhabited it for a few decades, it becomes a *tableau vivant*—a living slate. Scars punctuate that story, often evoking strong memories. Our survey takers can trace on their skin encounters with hot stoves, sharp rocks, barbed wire and surgeon's knives, among other dermis-damaging objects.

While it's true that scars can add character to an otherwise plain face, most people prefer to do without them or, at least, to keep them to a minimum.

Here's what our survey takers suggest to keep scrapes, burns and gashes from becoming a permanent part of your epidermis epic.

ALOE VERA EARNS THEIR PRAISE

Gloria, 50, of Houston, Texas, makes no bones about expressing her opinion of the healing powers of aloe vera: "It's one of God's miracles as far as I'm concerned."

In fact, the spiky succulent with thick, fleshy leaves is so well-known as a burn remedy that it also is commonly called the burn plant. People who use the gel inside the plant's leaves claim that it works so well it often prevents burn scars.

"I keep it around the house and find it very helpful for minor burns," says Connie, 76, of Voluntown, Connecticut. "So when my neighbor was suffering from radiation burns from cancer treatment to his throat, I offered to let him try it. He tried it first on one side of his throat for three days, and it worked so well, he started using it on the other side, too."

Those who swear by aloe vera use it mostly one way: straight from the plant. "I've never found any aloe product that heals as well as fresh gel," says Gloria from Houston.

There are good reasons aloe vera gel is helpful for burns, says Varro E. Tyler, Ph.D., professor of pharmacognosy at the School of Pharmacy and

Pharmacal Sciences at Purdue University, West Lafayette, Indiana, and author of *The Honest Herbal.* "Aloe gel contains a substance that reduces inflammation and swelling and that inhibits the action of bradykinin, a peptide that produces pain in injuries like burns," he says. It also inhibits the formation of thromboxane, a chemical detrimental to wound healing.

THEY RUB IN MOISTURIZER

Our survey takers massage all kinds of moisturizers into their skin to reduce scar formation. They recommend cocoa butter, almond oil, baby oil or any other emollient.

"I did this on a Caesarean section incision, and it seemed to help keep the area flexible and smooth," says Marcia, 46, a government worker from Princeton, New Jersey.

In fact, massaging the healed skin with moisturizer is one of the most effective things you can do to eliminate or reduce the size of a scar, says Stephen M. Purcell, D.O., chairman of the Division of Dermatology at Philadelphia College of Osteopathic Medicine and assistant clinical professor at Hahnemann University School of Medicine, also in Philadelphia. "Massaging improves blood flow to that area and encourages more even distribution of collagen, which results in a less thickened scar," he explains. (Collagen is a fibrous substance that forms a support structure just under the skin.)

SHE BELIEVES IN GOOD NUTRITION

"If you want to avoid problems in the first place, eat well."

These words, from a survey participant who also happens to be a nutritionist, have a sound basis in scientific fact. A wound that heals quickly and neatly is less likely to develop a scar than a wound that festers and takes forever to mend. And a wound is more likely to heal quickly if your skin cells have all the ingredients they need to manufacture new cells: those include protein, vitamin C and zinc, not to mention the 20 or so other essential nutrients we all need.

THEY SMEAR ON VITAMIN E

A full two-thirds of our survey takers recommend vitamin E as a scar minimizer. And several believe they have dramatic evidence that it works.

"I used vitamin E on surgical incisions from a hysterectomy, and I saw a big difference in the speed of healing and size and color of the scar," says Kathy, a nutritionist from McKinleyville, California. "The scar is the same color as my skin, not red, and it is relatively narrow." It did really well compared with another surgical scar she had on her abdomen that she did not treat with vitamin E, she explains.

She started using vitamin E two days after the surgery, as soon as she got home, simply breaking open and applying the contents of capsules of vitamin E oil. "I used it about three times a day until the incision was healed, applying lots of it over the stitches and then, when the stitches were out, massaging it into the area," she says. After the incision healed, she continued for three months to massage the scar with vitamin E every few days.

Another woman, Sandi, 50, of Chillicothe, Illinois, has also used vitamin E on surgical incisions. "I've had surgery several times, and I really believe the incisions healed a lot faster, with less scar tissue, during the times I used vitamin E," she says.

She used the vitamin on her neck following surgery on her thyroid gland. "I saw another woman who'd had the same surgery, and she had bad scars," Sandi says. "I started using vitamin E on the incision as soon as I got home, and I really noticed a difference. There was no redness, the incision remained pliable, and the scar is barely visible. She says she used it three times a day, each time massaging in the contents of a vitamin E oil capsule.

There are decades' worth of such anecdotal evidence that vitamin E used topically helps to reduce scarring and improve wound healing, and some surgeons recommend it to their patients, says Jeffrey Blumberg, Ph.D., chief of the Antioxidants Research Laboratory at the U.S. Department of Agriculture Human Nutrition Research Center on Aging at Tufts University, Boston. There are, however, no well-controlled scientific studies to support this use for vitamin E, he says.

EDITOR'S NOTE: Dr. Purcell notes that vitamin E may cause allergic reactions. And, he says, "I would not advise using it on a fresh incision." Rubbing a fresh incision may hamper healing, and you have no guarantee that the vitamin E is sterile. "If you must use vitamin E, wait until the incision is fully healed," advises Dr. Purcell.

Shinsplints

Pain-Stopping Tactics

Shinsplints are usually the result of overuse or abuse—too much running or walking, especially on hills or uneven surfaces or in worn-out or ill-fitting shoes. They develop when the connective sheath attached to the muscles and bone of your lower front leg become irritated. The result is razor-sharp pain in your lower leg along the side of your shinbone.

Our survey takers who suffer from shinsplints fit a certain mold: Whether it's work or play, they know how to overdo it! "I was working two jobs, one as a waitress and the other as a chambermaid, and was on my feet for about 12 hours a day when I developed this problem," says Michele, 34, of Yonkers, New York.

"I had started running about a year earlier and was increasing my mileage to train for my first race—a half-marathon (13 miles)—when I started to develop pain in the fronts of my legs," says Mike, 40, a government contractor from East Stroudsburg, Pennsylvania. "From talking with other runners, I figured it was shinsplints."

Taking a break from the offending activity is the treatment of choice for people with this condition, says Jennifer Stone, A.T.C., head athletic trainer at the U.S. Olympic Training Center in Colorado Springs. Here's how our survey takers squeeze in that downtime, along with other shin-soothing suggestions.

THEY'D RATHER SWITCH THAN HURT

"I eventually gave up my waitressing job, and, luckily, I found an evening job as a cashier, where I could sit," Michele says.

Mike continued to train for his race, but when it was over, he decided to diversify. "I found I could stay in just as good shape by alternating biking and running," he says. "In fact, not only are my shinsplints gone as a result of this, but some knee and back pain, as well."

"Our athletes don't stop exercising, but they do rest the muscles causing the pain," Stone says. Biking and swimming are both good activities to maintain cardiovascular fitness without aggravating shinsplints, she says. "When your legs start feeling better during normal, everyday activities, you can generally work your way back slowly into your regular exercise routine," she advises.

ICE SOOTHES HER SORE SHIN

"My boys and I were all running, and all of us got shinsplints," says Pamela, 44, a rental property manager from Mansfield, Massachusetts. "I learned from my sons' coach what to do—ice, rest and stretches. Those three things combined did help."

To chill her aching shin, she props her leg up on a chair and applies an ice pack on and off every few minutes for about 30 minutes. "I usually do this in the evening, when I have the time," she says.

"The best way to ice shinsplints, if you can stand it, is to stand for about 15 minutes in a tub of ice water up past wherever it hurts," Stone says.

For less hardy souls, ice massage is a good option, she says. Freeze water-filled paper cups, then peel away enough of the paper to expose an inch or so of ice and rub over the painful area for 15 or 20 minutes.

THEY WARM UP FIRST

"I used to think that I was warming up, but, in fact, I was impatient and wasn't taking enough time to really warm up right," Mike says. It wasn't until he started to hurt, and was trying to figure out what was wrong, that he learned how to warm up properly—by breaking a sweat.

"Your body is not warmed up until you start sweating," Stone explains. "Start out gradually, walking, slow biking or a light jog, and keep at it until you break a sweat." Then, she suggests, stop for a few light stretches before moving on to the harder part of your workout.

THEY SAVE SERIOUS STRETCHING FOR LAST

Pamela and Mike both learned that they need to stretch their leg muscles to prevent a recurrence of shinsplints. They stretch both the front and back—the calf muscles, in the front of the shin, quads and hamstring muscles.

"The best time to work on flexibility problems that can cause shinsplints is when you're finished exercising and as warmed up as you're going to get," Stone says.

To keep hamstrings loose, she recommends the hurdler's stretch. Sit on the ground, extend your right leg forward and place the bottom of your left foot on the inside of your right leg so you're making a P with your legs. Slowly lean forward from the waist, keeping your back straight and reaching your hands to your right foot for a count of ten. Switch legs and repeat.

Stretching the calf and Achilles tendon—the tendon that joins your calf muscles to your heel—also helps you avoid shinsplints. Face a wall and lean against it with your hands pressed against it, legs shoulder-width apart. Move your right leg forward while keeping your left leg straight. Gently lean toward the wall until you can feel the stretch on the back of your left leg, and hold for a slow count of ten. Bend your left knee slightly and hold for another count of ten. Repeat both straight and bent-knee versions with the other leg.

To stretch the muscles on the front of your calves, simply straighten your legs and point your toes, Stone adds.

Side Stitches

Stopping the Painful Stab

You don't get a lot of complaints from your diaphragm—the dome-shaped muscle located just under your lungs that helps you breathe and holds your abdominal organs in place. In fact, you hardly even know it's there. But when you're exercising intensely and your diaphragm goes into spasm, the resulting pain—known as a side stitch—is impossible to ignore.

Our survey takers say they've come up with several ways to banish this aggravating pain. Here's what they do.

SHE GETS BENT OUT OF SHAPE

Stephanie, a 72-year-old Llano, Texas, resident enjoyed hiking in the Massachusetts woods when she was a child. Whenever she felt a side stitch, she used a technique she learned from her teacher. "You were to remain standing, bend down, grab behind your knees and squeeze your body, doubling up as hard as you could for about 20 seconds," she recalls. "I haven't had any side stitches in recent memory, but I'm sure it worked."

Although he's never tried Stephanie's technique, there's good reason to believe it would work, says Owen Anderson, Ph.D, editor of *Running Research News* in Lansing, Michigan. "One theory we have about side stitches is that the diaphragm holds some of the internal organs in place with ligaments like puppets on a string," he says. "And, as a result, downward pressure caused by running pulls the diaphragm. Doubling up as she suggests would relieve that pressure."

SHE KNOWS WHEN TO RUN

It was the same scene every day: School officials played a John Philip Sousa march on an old Victrola to announce lunch, and Dorothy and her brothers raced home a quarter mile through the hilly streets of Port Jefferson, New York, ate lunch and raced back—all within an hour. Invariably, this led to side stitches and Dorothy's remedy. "Don't run after eating," says the 72-year-old. "Side stitches are very painful. I always seemed to get mine on my right side."

Dorothy learned her lesson well, says Dr. Anderson. "When you eat, you've taken a fairly empty, light stomach and added bulk. Sometimes you've eaten quickly because you know you have to get somewhere fast afterward. Sometimes your food is not mechanically digested; you've chewed it up quickly, so it's just kind of lying there. And I think that increased weight seems to add just enough weight to create a greater strain on the diaphragm."

If you eat moderate amounts of foods high in carbohydrates and low in fat—foods like pasta, toast and jelly or mashed potatoes without a lot of butter—you could run within an 1½ to 2 hours after eating, says Dr. Anderson. Eating a meal high in protein or fat, like a hamburger with french fries, could sideline you for as many as 4 hours, he says.

STRETCHING IS HER SOLUTION

A physical education teacher for seventh and eighth graders, Linda has had to deal with her share of side stitches. But it wasn't until she quizzed a track coach that she came up with a solid solution. "I don't have track kids; I have regular kids, but I tell them to lift their hand over their head and then lean away from the side that's hurting until the pain goes away," says the 44-year-old Elyria, Ohio, resident. "If it works for the track kids and they're running all the time, then it ought to work for someone who doesn't run all the time."

Sounds like a winner! Stretching will often take the edge off a side stitch, says Dr. Anderson.

LYING DOWN DOES IT FOR HER

Never underestimate the power of inactivity—so says Margaret, of Colorado, who recommends lying flat on your back when a side stitch starts.

This technique is usually an instant success, says Dr. Anderson. "You should get relief almost as soon as you lie down," he says. "Lying flat on your back works well, especially if you lie flat on your back and pull your knees toward your chest."

Sinusitis

Draining Away the Pain

It feels like a burning, boring or pounding pain on the front of your face—across your forehead, behind or between your eyes, around your cheeks or ears.

"I call it a splitting headache, because the pain goes down the center of my face, making my head feel like it's being split in half," says Louise, 49, a veterinarian's assistant from Toledo, Ohio. Like some of our other survey participants, she says her sinus pain is linked to changes in the weather. "When the pain starts up, I can be sure a storm is on the way," she says.

Fluctuations in barometric pressure can play a role in sinus pain, says Michael Borts, M.D., codirector of the Comprehensive Sinus Clinic at St. Louis University School of Medicine in Missouri. So can a lot of other things.

Most often, it's related to an upper respiratory tract virus infection—a head cold. The virus irritates mucous membranes in the nose and sinuses, making them swell and closing off the sinuses' tiny openings into the nose. That results in a painful vacuum. If the openings stay closed for long, the sinuses can fill with fluid and become infected. When that happens, antibiotics are in order, Dr. Borts says.

"Infected sinuses are not something you want to fool around with," he warns. "Fever, pain that persists for more than two days, or green or yellow nasal or postnasal discharge are signs that it's time to see a doctor."

Chronic sinus problems can be due to allergies, which swell mucous membranes, or to an obstruction of the sinus opening (such as a nasal polyp).

Whether it's an occasional or frequent problem, here's what the people who suffer from sinusitis do to clear their heads and turn down the pressure.

THEY GET ALL STEAMED UP

Some hit the steam room or opt for a hot shower or a pan of steaming water. Others stick their noses over a cup of hot tea or soup.

"I head for the steam room at the health club the minute my sinuses start acting up, and I usually can prevent a little problem from becoming a big one," says Michael, 68, a retired businessman from Morton Grove, Illinois.

"We've tried a variety of teas over the years, but when it comes to sinus congestion, we always go back to chamomile," says Clarence, 65, of Urbana, Illinois. "It's fragrant and soothing, and it does clear out your nose." He uses about two heaping teaspoons in a small electric steaming pot, using a bath towel to create a steam tent.

"Inhaling steam gets moisture into your nose, where it helps to liquify secretions that are blocking the openings to the sinuses," Dr. Borts explains. That helps the cilia (microscopic hairs on the mucous membrane) to move the mucus out of your nose.

SHE RECOMMENDS EUCALYPTUS

"I add a few drops of eucalyptus oil to a pot of steaming water and hang my head over it for a few minutes," says Sarah, 36, a nurse's aide from Burlington, Vermont. "I like the way it smells, and it does seem to work better at clearing my head than steam alone."

Eucalyptus oil, available at some health-food stores, contains a chemical that loosens mucus, making it easier to blow out. Some cough drops are flavored with it.

EDITOR'S NOTE: Although it is safe to inhale its vapors, eucalyptus oil is highly poisonous when taken internally. Fatalities have been reported from ingestion of as little as a teaspoon.

SHE FLUSHES OUT WITH PIZZA HERB

Margaret, 54, an assistant shipping manager from Corpus Christi, Texas, says oregano is very effective at clearing congestion.

"I use it as a hot tea, steeping one or two teaspoons of oregano in a cup of boiling water," she says. "Soon after I start drinking it, my nose starts to run, and I can blow out the mucus, or cough it out." As for the taste, she says, "it's not particularly pleasant—it tastes kind of medicinal—but I figure it's worth tolerating for the beneficial effect."

Traditional herbalists have long used oregano to treat colds, flu and chest congestion. And modern medical researchers have determined that it does, indeed, contain compounds that help to loosen phlegm and make it easier to cough up.

HEAT OFFERS THEM RELIEF

Heat also seems to offer people a fair amount of relief from sinus pain. People are most likely to apply warm washcloths to their faces, but one woman, Debra, 35, a computer operator from Shannon, Mississippi, prefers to get her whole body warmed up.

"I went to the gym to work out, but my sinuses hurt so bad I ended up simply sitting in the sauna for about ten minutes," she says. "When I left, my headache was gone, and I thought, 'This is great!' " Since then, any time she has sinus pain, she heads for the sauna.

EDITOR'S NOTE: "Heat packs on the face may relieve some muscle tension associated with sinus headache, and they may increase blood flow and so provide some beneficial effect," Dr. Borts says. However, he prefers a steam bath to the dry heat of a sauna. "Breathing in dry air will make the mucus in the nose thicker and harder than ever to move out," he says.

FRIGID AIR FREEZES HER PAIN

The exact opposite of heat—cold air—relieves sinus symptoms for some people.

"I heap ice cubes or cracked ice in a small, deep bowl and hold my face over the bowl so that I breathe the cold, moist air," says Dorothy, of Casselberry, Florida. "It will often stop an attack in its tracks and give hours of relief without pills or sprays."

Other people say that simply drinking cold water eases their sinus pain.

"Drinking cold fluids or inhaling cold air may provide some temporary relief from pain and inflammation, but I don't believe it is going to do much to relieve congestion or get mucus flowing," Dr. Borts says.

THEY GIVE THEIR NOSE A BATH

It doesn't sound like much fun—literally rinsing out your nose with salt water. But the people who rely on this remedy say it works wonders in relieving sinus congestion. And not one of them has come close to drowning.

"It's a remedy from back in the depression days," says Norma, 66, of Spanish Fork, Utah. She mixes up a pint of water with ½ teaspoon of salt and one teaspoon of witch hazel, puts just a few drops in the palm of her hand, and sniffs it up each nostril. "I'll do this a couple of times a day, if necessary, until my sinuses clear up," she says.

"I use a spray bottle that lets me drizzle a stream of salt water in one nostril and out the other," says Jean, 63, a Bloomington, Michigan, seniors' center employee who weaned herself away from a nasal spray habit by learning to do saline nasal rinse. "I simply tip my head sideways over the sink, put the nozzle of the bottle in my upper nostril, and spray until it runs out the other nostril for a while. I really do flush it. Then, I gently blow my nose."

It takes a while to master the technique, she admits. "But you'll feel better right away doing this. I used to have to sleep in a recliner chair, I was so stuffed up. Now I can sleep through the night with no problems."

"A saltwater rinse is helpful because it washes away any thick and dry mucus, and there are some studies that demonstrate that use of a saline nasal spray improves the flow of blood through the mucous membrane," Dr. Borts says. "It's possible this increased blood flow brings in additional cells to fight inflammation."

If you want to try a nasal wash, use just a pinch or two of salt in about ½ a cup of water, says Dr. Borts. If the solution stings your nose, it's too salty.

CULINARY COMBUSTIBLES UNCLOG THEIR NOSES

Some people take advantage of the mouth-watering, brow-beading properties of spicy hot foods such as chili peppers, ginger and horseradish. They eat these foods to clear out nasal congestion.

"As a result of a radio show, I started using about ten drops of Tabasco in ½ cup of water on mornings when I am congested, and I find it relieves my sinus congestion almost immediately," says Virginia, of Ramsey, Illinois.

"I use a stuffy nose as a good excuse to pig out on something I like," says Theresa, a day care center worker from Raceland, Louisiana. She buys a jar of hot salsa and a bag of corn chips, stuffs her face and *un*stuffs her nose.

"When you take a bite of something hot, it irritates and so stimulates glands in your nose, which then starts running," explains Gordon Raphael, M.D., associate clinical professor of medicine at George Washington University in Washington, D.C. In effect, a mouthful of salsa acts pretty much the same way as an over-the-counter expectorant might: It stimulates mucus secretion of the nose and throat, thins the mucus and makes it easier to clear out.

"Chemicals in red peppers also trigger the release of hormones which may help open nasal passageways," Dr. Raphael says. "And people may be right on the money when they say that a hot and spicy diet helps them avoid colds in the first place." That's because the mucus secreted by the cells lining the nose and throat contains antibacterial compounds—the body's first line of defense against the germs that cause sinus infections. "Increased mucus production washes incoming germs right back out," he says.

THEY PREFER A LITTLE PRESSURE

Facial massage or, better still, pressure applied with the fingertips to several appropriate spots over sinuses helps to relieve pain and promote draining, our survey takers report. Best spots: under the cheekbones, along the sides of the nose, and between the eyes at the bridge of the nose.

"My husband suffers terribly from chronic sinus problems, probably from a deviated septum, so I massage his face for him," says Jacqueline, 50, of Floral Park, New York. "I start at the middle of his forehead, right by the scalp, and, using both hands, go in small circles with my fingertips across the forehead, to both temples, which I massage in circles. I then apply continuous pressure for about 30 seconds. I do this across his whole face, applying pressure at the bridge and base of his nose, under his cheekbones, and then right underneath his ears. It helps him a lot. He sits up and everything is open. He can blow his nose and breathe better."

Facial massage and acupressure can help relieve the congestion and muscle tension that accompany and aggravate sinus pain, says David Nickel, O.M.D., doctor of oriental medicine and a certified acupuncturist in private practice in Santa Monica, California.

"You can't actually massage the sinuses, which are encased in bone," he explains. "However, applying pressure on top of or near the sinuses improves circulation of blood and lymphatic fluid through the sinuses, which is the key to healing." Blood supplies oxygen, which all tissues need to survive, while lymphatic fluid delivers white blood cells, part of the body's immune system.

MENTHOLATED VAPORS UNCLOG THEM

Fragrant menthol ointments, such as Vicks VapoRub and Ben-Gay, are popular nose openers for our survey participants.

"I use Vicks salve on my forehead, and it makes the pain and pressure go away," says Rose, 71, of Hurricane, West Virginia. "It's all I ever have to do."

"I rub in just a bit of hot original Ben-Gay on my temples, across my forehead, under my cheekbones, and on the bridge of my nose," says Merry, 43, of Pensacola, Florida. "This really loosens up and drains my head." Beware, though, she says. "I lie down and keep my eyes closed when I do this; otherwise my eyes will water. Don't get it in your eyes, and make sure you wipe your hands off afterward!"

These salves contain menthol, camphor and other strong-smelling chemicals that evaporate readily and impart a sensation of clearing the nose, says Alan R. Hirsch, M.D., director of the Smell and Taste Treatment and Research Foundation in Chicago. While these scents won't relieve the inflammation of a real case of sinusitis, they may relieve the pain of a migraine headache, which is sometimes mistaken for sinus pain, Dr. Hirsch says.

Inhaling menthol or any other strong odor irritates a major pain-conducting nerve—the trigeminal nerve—in your face, he explains. This stimulus overrides the pain message coming from other nerves, blocking your perception of pain while you inhale the strong smell and sometimes preventing a beginning headache from becoming a full-blown head cruncher.

Snoring

Getting a Little Peace

It vibrates. It buzzes. It honks. It sometimes rattles the rafters. Depending upon how loudly your spouse snores—and how sensitive a sleeper you are—normal snoring can be anything from a mild nuisance to a major relationship-threatening problem.

Most of the people who answered this survey question say their spouse is, at worst, a moderate snorer—someone who snores, but not constantly, perhaps only when he's on his back, when he has a cold or when he's particularly tired. (Most of the snorers in this survey are men . . . and most of the remedies come from their long-suffering wives.)

Serious snoring—the kind where the snorer stops breathing for seconds at a time—is known as sleep apnea. It warrants medical attention, the sooner the better, says Derek S. Lipman, M.D., a Portland, Oregon, ear, nose and throat specialist and author of *Stop Your Husband from Snoring*. Sleep apnea has been associated with high blood pressure and heart disease. In fact, a recent study showed that the worst snorers had a 23-fold increase in heart-attack risk.

For run-of-the-mill snoring, however, here are some sleep-saving tactics from our survey takers.

THEY MAKE HIM ROLL OVER

Heavy snorers can saw wood in just about any position, but moderate snorers do so only when they lie on their backs, which allows the tongue to fall back into the throat, obstructing the airway.

So it's no surprise that keeping a snorer on his side or stomach is a major noise-stifling strategy.

A couple of women say they've had good results by sewing a tennis or golf ball into a pocket between the shoulders of their husband's pajamas. "Of course, you have to get your husband to wear the pajamas," admits Sylvia, 34, a Hicksville, New York, marketing associate. "It did work, true, but after a few nights my husband refused to continue to use it. He said he liked to sleep on his back and that he would sleep in another room if his snoring bothered me so much. I decided it didn't bother me that much."

"This technique works because when you roll over and hit the tennis ball, you unconsciously roll off your back," Dr. Lipman explains.

SHE CUSHIONS HIM

"I tuck a pillow behind my husband's back so he can't easily roll over on his back," says Donna, 50, who runs a secretarial services business in Logan, Utah. "It does work, and it's a little bit easier on a marriage than a sharp elbow, I believe. Although if he does move, I have to readjust the pillow."

A well-placed pillow or two behind the back can help keep a snorer on his side, Dr. Lipman agrees.

SHE REACHES FOR A DECONGESTANT

"I've found I snore the worst when I have a cold or when, for some other reason, my nose is stuffed up," says Myra, 47, of Greensburg, Pennsylvania. "So I use a nasal decongestant spray. It helps me sleep better, too."

EDITOR'S NOTE: Nasal congestion can acctually cause or aggravate snoring, Dr. Lipman says. "Sprays open your nasal passages and allow you to breathe more easily for a while, but they can also lead to a rebound effect," he explains.

The chemicals in nose drops that relieve congestion do so by constricting the nasal blood vessels and shrinking the mucous membranes. Shortly after application, however, the vessels expand again and the mucous membranes begin to swell. With repeated use, the membranes lose their ability to react and may remain in a permanently swollen, congested state.

Dr. Lipman recommends, instead, using a simple saline spray—salt and water.

HEAD-HIGH ANGLE HELPS HIM

"My husband noticed he slept better in a reclining chair than in bed, and when he told our doctor about it, the doctor suggested we raise the head of the bed a bit," says Louise, 61, a housewife from Amarillo, Texas. They put a four-inch-thick brick under each of two bedposts. "It helped some, but the doctor also wanted my husband to use pressurized air, which he now does." With this treatment, you wear a mask over your nose and mouth that is connected to a pressurized air tank. The higher air pressure keeps your upper airway open. Her husband has also been told he needs to lose weight—"not just for his snoring, but for his heart," Louise says.

Elevating the head of your bed a bit may help to minimize airway obstruction, Dr. Lipman says. But don't rely on a stack of pillows to raise your head, he warns. Instead, elevate the head of the bed using bricks or blocks of wood. "A large pillow can put a kink in your neck, aggravating your snoring problem," he explains.

DROPPING POUNDS WORKS FOR SOME

Several of our survey takers say snorers in their families have been advised to lose weight.

"We were both restless, noisy sleepers for many years, and it was taking its toll on us with fatigue and lots of little aches and pains," says Marilyn, 53, a caterer's helper from Dayton, Ohio. Getting a bigger bed helped for a while, "but we both knew we needed to do something," she says. That "something" finally became a doctor-supervised exercise and weight-loss program. "It was the best thing we ever did for ourselves. It stopped the snoring and a lot of other health problems," she says.

Excessive pounds contribute to snoring problems in two ways, Dr. Lipman says. "The increased tissue bulk in the neck and throat of obese people, together with poor muscle tone, reduces the area of the upper air passage, making it more prone to obstruction," he says. "Plus, a large abdomen pressing on your diaphragm when you lie on your back increases the likelihood of sleep apnea by further decreasing the size of your lungs and the amount of air you obtain with each breath."

Sleep studies have shown that a weight loss of 10 to 25 percent can eliminate apnea or significantly reduce the number of times you stop breathing during the night, Dr. Lipman adds.

Sore Throat

So Many Soothers

A sore throat is one of those symptoms that cries out—in a scratchy, weak voice, of course—for home treatment. At least, that's the only conclusion possible after looking over the hundreds of suggestions we received from our survey takers.

Once these folks determine that they aren't suffering from something more serious—high fever, intense pain, bleeding and trouble breathing are among the most important symptoms that should send them to a doctor—they try everything from apple cider vinegar to cloves to ease the soreness. Here's what they say does the job.

SALT WATER WASHES AWAY THEIR PAIN

You could fill an ocean with all the warm saltwater solutions we received—easily the runaway favorite as a soother.

For Brenda, a 30-year-old Goldendale, Washington, resident, there's only one way: "Finger-test warm, slightly salty water, gargling every half-hour until the sore throat stops. I know that's not too scientific, but it's a home remedy. What can I say? It works. I've been using this method since I was 12 or 13."

Gerry, of Sterling Heights, Michigan, is less exacting, but just as insistent. "I just dump the salt into the glass—maybe a tablespoon at the most. If my throat hurts a lot, I gargle several times that night and it soothes. The salt is very healing."

Judy, a 52-year-old Goodland, Kansas, vocational high school food service manager, gargles with four ounces of water seasoned with a pinch of salt.

Warm salt water is actually one of the best treatments for a sore throat, according to Ronald Amedee, M.D., a spokesperson for the American Academy of Otolaryngology and Head and Neck Surgery and an associate professor at Tulane University School of Medicine in New Orleans. Bacteria make the throat more acidic, and salt water helps restore the natural acid balance, he explains.

Warmth provided by the gargle is also soothing to the soft tissues of the throat, says Dr. Amedee. "That's a large muscular wall, and it has the same benefit warmth would have to a sore muscle in any other part of the body," he explains. For the record, ¼ teaspoon of salt for each half cup of water gargled several times a day seems to work best, he says.

THEY THINK ZINC

Because it begins with a z, you'll find it at the bottom of the mineral charts. But zinc is tops with many of our survey takers for treating a sore throat.

Take Helen, for example. The 76-year-old Saddle Brook, New Jersey, resident has faithfully used vitamins since 1970, but it was her doctor who suggested she savor lemon-flavored zinc lozenges to help ease a sore throat. "What happens to me is, if I don't clear up the sore throat, I'll get a bad cough and cold in my chest," she says. "These lozenges soothe the sore throat and generally help prevent the cold from working its way down." Helen says she buys the zinc lozenges at her local health-food store and takes several a day when the pain starts.

Claudine has a tough time deciding which is more effective: an Old World potato poultice remedy passed down by her German grandparents or a New World remedy learned from a savvy surgeon who knows his vitamin and mineral supplements. But there's no question which one's easier: sucking on a zinc lozenge.

"My daughter, who's a registered nurse, was experimenting with different things and talked to this doctor who is as interested in alternative remedies as she is. And he said zinc is good for what ails you," says the 76-year-old Charleston, West Virginia, resident. "I won't use more than two or three zinc lozenges in a day because I don't like to overdo it, but in the morning my sore throat will be gone."

Some studies show zinc may actually help end your sore throat by knocking out your cold. A study by researchers at Dartmouth College found students who took zinc had colds that lasted less than five days, compared with the more usual nine days. They also had less severe nasal congestion, runny nose and coughing.

GIVE THEM THE SOUR STUFF

Ysleta, a 70-year-old Oklahoma City, Oklahoma, resident, is a big advocate of the healing powers of vinegar and water. "It's the best stuff I've ever used," she says. "It really cuts the mucus in the back of your throat."

Following a recipe recommended to her by a friend, Ysleta says she combines a tablespoon of apple cider vinegar in an eight-ounce glass of room temperature distilled water for use as a gargle. If she prefers to sip, she'll add a tablespoon of honey. It's so good for getting rid of a sore throat that she recommends it to all her friends.

"I have this little old 87-year-old neighbor, and she had the flu and a sore throat and didn't know what to do," says Ysleta. "I said, 'Let me fix you up some of my potion.' I made her a gallon, and she kept it by her bedside, and she said it helped her sore throat more than anything."

Taking apple cider vinegar for enhancing health has had many champions over the years, among them D. C. Jarvis, a Vermont M.D. who wrote a book published in 1958 called *Folk Medicine*. Based on his observations of nature (livestock, mostly) and his understanding of physiology, he decided that many health problems could be attributed to a lack of potassium—a deficiency he often corrected by recommending apple cider vinegar.

EDITOR'S NOTE: Although the acid in vinegar may help thin mucus that can cause a sore throat, it may also be irritating, says Charles P. Kimmelman, M.D., professor of otolaryngology at New York Medical College in Valhalla and attending physician at Manhattan Eye, Ear and Throat Hospital in New York City. If vinegar and water irritates your throat, don't use it.

THEY PREFER HYDROGEN PEROXIDE

While we're still talking gargles, we can't forget those who prefer hydrogen peroxide. Rita, a 56-year-old Texan, says gargling with a hydrogen peroxide solution three times a day does the trick. Another woman says she swabs her throat with hydrogen peroxide.

Gargling with a mild peroxide solution is like giving your throat a massage, says Dr. Kimmelman. "You get a release of bubbles, it's effervescent, it's soothing, it even takes away some of the bad odor by oxygenating the tissues, killing some of the bacteria," he says. "Use a three percent hydrogen peroxide solution mixed with water four times a day. Spit it right out."

SHE USES CLOVES

Ruby, a retired Mahtomedi, Minnesota, resident, sucks on a clove to stop a sore throat. "I'm sure I read about it in some old-fashioned remedy book somewhere," she says. "It's very hot, and you just kind of hold it in your mouth and it warms the throat—kind of numbs it." And if taken at the first sign of a sore throat, Ruby's noticed her clove cure seems to have the power to ward it off entirely.

So reliable is her remedy that she keeps several in a pill bottle at her bedside.

"I'll tell you how I think this may be working," says Dr. Amedee. "It's stimulating saliva flow. Many times sore throats are due to dryness. You've got to swallow. And bathing the dry tissues with excessive mucus generated by cloves makes quite good sense to me."

EDITOR'S NOTE: Cloves do have numbing properties. Dentists have used clove oil for years as an oral anesthetic. Sucking on a clove is okay, but don't try to treat a sore throat with clove oil. Swallowing it can cause upset stomach. (Swallowing the clove itself can also lead to upset.)

SHE LOVES HER HYSSOP

Back when she lived on Long Island, New York, Veronica often picked fresh hyssop from her half-acre herb garden to make tea to treat her family's sore throats and coughs. Now a Carpinteria, California, resident, she's had less success growing hyssop, but she still tries to find it in health-food stores if a sore throat threatens. "I had a friend from Germany, and she was into herbs in the early 1960s and she told me about it. She brought me some when I was sick, and it did help," says Veronica.

When she's got fresh hyssop on hand, Veronica says she steeps it longer but uses less because it's stronger. "Depending on how bad my sore throat is, I'll have one cup at a sitting morning, noon and night," says Veronica. "It seems to ease the symptoms, and if it's not too severe, it may go away." (You can make hyssop tea by pouring one cup of boiling water over two teaspoons of dried herb. Allow it to steep for ten minutes.)

Hyssop has a long history as a soothing herb—it even appears in the Bible. Modern herbal experts say that hyssop contains substances that can loosen phlegm and ease coughing, both of which can contribute to a sore throat.

THEY TAKE TIME FOR TEA

Brenda, one of our saltwater aficionados, serves her sons (ages three and five) Red Zinger tea, seasoned with lemon and sugar, when they have a sore throat. "It's got rosehips and licorice root in it, so you get some menthol action," she explains.

Hot tea probably provides relief for some of the same reasons as does warm salt water, says Dr. Amedee.

"Once again, we're coming back to moisturization. Just the act of swallowing stretches the musculature of the throat," he says. "Warm vapor is also soothing to the nose and enhances mucus flow. And guess what happens when you put lemon or honey in your mouth? It fills with saliva which, when swallowed, is soothing to your throat."

SHE SAYS GARLIC GETS IT

Remember saltwater Judy? She has no problem keeping her other sore throat remedy a secret. All she has to do is breathe. Her remedy: rubbing garlic oil on her neck. "You rub it on there just like you would with Vicks or some kind of mentholatum," she explains. "It's a little hard to find in a bottle with a dropper, but you can take apart liquid garlic capsules."

Judy says she tried garlic oil for a sore throat at the suggestion of an alternative medical practitioner and has been using it ever since.

Another woman suggests holding a clove of garlic in the mouth. "Follow by frequent use of breath mints," she adds. "It works even for strep."

Although he's never tried garlic for a sore throat, Dr. Amedee says he's had patients who claim success with the pungent bulb. "Winter, particularly, is associated with postnasal drip, but instead of running down the front of your nose, it runs down the back of your throat and collects, which causes you to clear your throat and forces it into spasm," he says. "I suspect the smell of garlic could open the sinuses a bit, and this may allow the mucus to flow more freely, key to relieving a sore throat."

And don't forget garlic's antiviral possibilities. A compound (called allicin) found in garlic has been shown to kill bacteria—even in extremely low concentrations.

SHE RELIES ON OVER-THE-COUNTER RELIEF

Stephanie's home remedy for sore throats originates at the drugstore, and she's never found anything better: Chloraseptic Sore Throat Spray. "I've used the spray and the lozenges, but the spray seems to work better and faster," says the Llano, Texas, resident.

Chloraseptic works fine for some, but you may also want to consider finding an over-the-counter sore throat spray containing dyclonine, says Dr. Amedee. "This ingredient is very fast acting and long lasting—it hangs around for several hours," he says. The only problem: It may cause too much numbness for some people, he says. Sucrets sells a sore throat spray containing dyclonine, and some supermarket brands have it, as well.

SHE USES A COLD COMPRESS

Fern, a Berrien Springs, Michigan, resident and former nurse, says that, whenever she has a sore throat, she wets a small cotton cloth with water, places it over her neck and then covers it with wool flannel. Two measurable things tell her when she can quit: Her throat feels better and the compress remains wet.

"I think the water is absorbed by your throat and when you've got enough, it doesn't absorb it any more," she says. "The compress does wonders. It's itchy, but it really works."

Fern's cold compress sounds a lot like a once-common throat soother called an ice collar, says Dr. Amedee. Doctors use to apply it the first 24 or 48 hours after a throat operation. "It has soothing properties, makes the blood vessels shrink and decreases swelling," he explains. "When you put ice on something, blood vessels tighten down and can't leak. And that's got to reduce inflammation."

SHE PEPPERS HER THROAT

You can appreciate her Southern hospitality, but be careful if Beth offers you a drink. The Athens, Georgia, resident recommends stirring cayenne pepper into ginger ale for soothing a sore throat.

While the taste of this mixture may leave something (okay, a lot) to be desired, Dr. Amedee says that Beth's beverage may actually be beneficial. "Cayenne will cause you to secrete a lot of saliva," he explains. That, in turn, will help restore the proper acid-base balance of the throat.

Actually, the ginger in the ginger ale may be helping, as well. Herbal experts have found that ginger helps kill flu viruses and may increase the immune system's ability to fight infection.

HE SAYS, "COME ON DOWN"

Finally we visit Robert, retired and resting comfortably, thank you very much, in Indiantown, Florida. He says he hasn't had a sore throat in years—a dramatic improvement over his days as a Long Island, New York, high school math teacher when students literally spread sore throats and other contagious maladies as they walked the halls.

"We'd hear what was going around, what the symptoms were, but there didn't seem like there was a whole lot you could do about it, with kids sneezing and coughing on you all the time," recalls the 61-year-old.

So, is his remedy to retire and join him in Florida? "Well, that's prevention, isn't it," he says, "treating the problem before it occurs?"

Indeed, it is. But you don't have to pack your bags just yet. A few commonsense steps can help keep you from catching someone else's sore throat, says Dr. Amedee. Tops on the list: wiping the telephone receiver and doorknobs with a paper towel sprayed with Lysol Disinfectant Spray after the sick person has used them. "These are the places that the germs of an upper respiratory infection—probably the true cause of the sore throat—tend to spread," he says.

Splinters

Popping Out Those Aggravating Slivers

Remember the folktale about the lion and the mouse and how a tiny thorn changed their entire relationship?

In that case, removing the thorn was a simple procedure—the mouse simply pulled the painful irritant from his grateful adversary's paw. (After that, the little guy didn't have to worry about becoming an hors d'oeuvre.)

The same rule of thumb applies to your own splinters. If you can see and grasp the splinter, pull it out. But poking and probing when you can't see what ails you is out of the question, says Gary Quick, M.D., chief of the Emergency Medicine and Trauma Care Department at the University of Oklahoma School of Medicine in Oklahoma City. "When you start searching for splinters, you are looking for the proverbial needle in a haystack," he says. "It seems like a simple process, but if the splinter goes beneath the deeper layers of skin, then it can migrate anyplace." Digging beneath the skin may yield nothing but an infection, says Dr. Quick.

Our survey takers don't rely on a lot of probing to remove their splinters. Instead, they have a number of strategies that they say help the splinter pop out. Here's what they do.

THEY'RE MAKIN' BACON WORK

Serious low-fat eating all but excludes bacon from the breakfast table. But according to our survey takers, the salty stuff has another purpose: treating splinters. In fact, bacon was the most commonly cited remedy for splinters.

For example, when Mabel's daughter Kathy came home with a swollen finger caused by a deeply embedded splinter, Mabel relied on bacon fat to treat the problem.

The 74-year-old New Haven, Indiana, resident, who learned about this remedy from her mother, trimmed a small slab of fat from some bacon and placed a piece on Kathy's finger. Next, she covered it with gauze and wrapped the finger with a bandage. Within just a few days, the splinter popped out, says Mabel. "You'd be surprised how well it works," she says. "You can just feel it draw the splinter out. The advantage is you don't have to keep digging."

Jan, a 44-year-old Cedar Rapids, Iowa, office manager, says the length of time she needs to wear a properly placed piece of bacon fat is directly proportional to the depth of the splinter. And checking the wound every so often just won't do. "You've got to let it work—that's what my mom told me," says Jan. "It's amazing how well it works."

Margaret never saw her son-in-law or his dad use bacon and a Band-Aid to help remove splinters, but she heard them talk about this remedy. "They worked with glass and wood all the time, and I think they used bacon for both," says the 74-year-old La Puente, California, resident. "I don't know if it's a Swedish thing or what—they were Swedish."

Although unsure whether bacon fat is truly effective on splinters, Dr. Quick says he's familiar with the theory. There is some thought that a substance with a high salt concentration—like bacon fat—would tend to draw moisture to the area. The extra moisture just might help the splinter pop out.

But Dr. Quick advises that if you do use bacon fat, you should first wash the area with soap and water.

OLD RUSSIAN REMEDY TAKES ON NEW LIFE

Once a farmer and still an avid gardener, Lois says she's been "stuck with all kinds of things" over the years. But her favorite treatment for splinters remains a remedy she learned from her Russian immigrant mother-in-law many years ago.

First she washes the area thoroughly and covers it with Vaseline petroleum jelly or some other lubricant. "They used to use lard," says the 71-year-old Sterling, Colorado, music teacher.

Then she covers the lubricant with aluminum foil. "They used to use the foil from a pack of cigarettes," Lois recalls. She covers the foil with a bandage or adhesive tape, and within 12 to 24 hours, the splinter comes to the surface of her skin so she can pull it out. If not, she repeats the procedure. "I didn't believe it either at first, but it works, and I've seen no adverse reaction in my family for years," she says.

Keeping the area moist—with or without foil—is actually a common tactic for treating wounds like splinters, says Dr. Quick. "If you have an opening in the skin, it tends to crust over with a scab. And if you keep a petroleum-based ointment such as one of the over-the-counter triple antibiotic ointments over that area, it tends to keep the skin surface soft and minimize scabbing. Skin healing occurs more quickly in such an environment," he explains. If the area is blocked with a scab, it will make it harder for the body to push a splinter back out again.

SLIVER-PULLING SALVE WORKS FOR THEM

Louise and her husband, residents of Lansing, New York, make frequent use of a homemade sliver-pulling salve.

"It contains beeswax and tallow," says Louise, who got the recipe from her grandfather. After heating the salve, Louise says she spreads some on a bandage. After allowing it to cool, she places the bandage over the splinter.

It's possible that these ingredients—homey as they sound—serve the same purpose as petroleum-based products, says Dr. Quick. "I have heard of that. It sounds like you have an emollient there in the beeswax and tallow that might tend to do the same thing," he says.

HE TAPES IT

Troubled occasionally by tiny splinters on the ends of his fingers—whether from work or chopping wood at home—Arthur resorts to a trick he learned from his grandmother, says his wife, Diane.

Arthur simply places a piece of adhesive tape over the splinter and by morning is usually able to pull out the offending piece of wood, says Diane, a resident of Geary, New Brunswick, Canada. "It seems like it has some kind of drawing power, like a poultice," she says.

"The tape probably creates an environment where the skin is kept more moist," explains Dr. Quick. That, in turn, softens the skin and probably helps the skin's natural tendency to push out a foreign object. "Have you ever noticed, if you put a Band-Aid on your finger overnight, how the skin looks white underneath and is soft? Same principle," he says.

SHE NUMBS IT

Erin, a 30-year-old resident of Redmond, Oregon, gets lots of opportunities to try her favorite splinter remedy, thanks to her nine-year-old son, Caleb.

When Caleb got a splinter in his thumb from playing on the deck of their new house, she sprayed the wound with Medi-Quik First Aid spray, an over-the-counter product used to treat minor cuts and scrapes. She waited a minute to let the area get numb. Then she pulled out the splinter with tweezers. "The kids can't feel it and it seems to make the splinter slip out easier," she says.

Medi-Quik contains a mild anesthetic and an antiseptic.

TEA SOAK HELPS HER SPLINTER

Mabel, from New Haven, Indiana, has one more splinter remedy to pass along: A friend of hers brews strong tea and sticks her finger in it whenever she has a splinter. While her etiquette might leave Miss Manners gasping, Mabel's friend is actually practicing a form of Dr. Quick's favorite treatment.

"If it's a minor splinter and it's not infected, I would simply recommend some warm soaks to see if it wouldn't pop out spontaneously," says Dr. Quick. "Use just salt water, five to ten minutes, four or five times a day. Most people won't do it that much. But soaking actually enhances the circulation in the area. That helps minimize the risk of infection."

Stress

Tranquilizing Options

When it comes to stress, our survey takers are real experts. They've survived lengthy illnesses, the deaths of loved ones, farm forfeitures, bankruptcies, hurtful words and broken hearts. They all say pretty much the same thing—that, for all of us, stressful situations, big and small, are unavoidable. And that how we react to them can make all the difference in the world.

Praying is a popular antidote to anxiety for our survey participants. But they also rely on everything from milk and cookies to Mantovani to soothe their frazzled nerves. In fact, their combination of action and acceptance—a kind of individualized stress management package, if you will—is exactly what a therapist might suggest, says Allen Elkin, Ph.D., program director for the Stress Management and Counseling Center in New York City.

"I'm not saying real stressors aren't out there and that sometimes we need to make changes in our lives," he says. "But the fact is, we also create stress by how we look at the world. Lots of stress comes from emotional exaggeration."

THEY TAKE TIME FOR FUN

"Both my father-in-law and sister were dying, and we were terribly stressed," says Janis, 44, of Thomasboro, Illinois. "So my husband and I and our kids made a point of doing something together that was fun. We spent just about every Sunday afternoon tubing down a creek at a nearby state park. We'd spend four or five hours just drifting along and return rejuvenated and ready to provide the love and support our sick family members needed."

"Nothing is more restorative than things that give you pleasure and satisfaction," Dr. Elkin says. "I think of them as stress buffers—they help balance the scale, and they are particularly helpful if you can't deal with the stress directly."

She Walks to Decompress

"When our town got a beautiful new park about three years ago, I started walking an hour each night after work," says Juanita, 50, office manager for her family's plumbing business in Cleveland, Georgia.

She didn't initially start walking to relieve stress, but, she says, "I noticed that the more I walked, the better I felt. I didn't feel so edgy and out of control when I got home. The days I walked, I could go home and sit down and relax. Now, when I get stressed out, I put my sneakers on and go for a walk."

"Walking along the country roads by my mother's house got me through a stressful period of taking care of her while she was dying," says Carole, a Lexington, Kentucky, resident who works in a senior citizens' home. "Walking frees up my mind and makes me feel closer to God."

A number of studies over the last several years have supported the use of exercise as a natural stress reducer. Studies show that people who are physically fit have less of a physiological reaction to stress (their heart rate and blood pressure go up less, for instance).

People often experience an immediate positive response to exercise, Dr. Elkin says. "It's incredibly distracting, for one thing. It's hard to exercise and worry at the same time," he says. Huff-and-puff exercise also causes your body to kick in feel-good chemicals—endorphins. "Plus, most people enjoy exercising and feel better because they're doing something good for themselves," he adds.

She Has Furry Friends

We talk to them, we cuddle them, we confide in them. Some of us even kiss them and let them crawl under the bedcovers. Pets, our survey takers tell us, can be great stress reducers.

"My grandcat, Brewster, as I call him—he belongs to my daughter, but we now have him—will jump up in my lap when I'm upset or anxious. He almost seems to be reminding me to take some time to relax," says Carole from Kentucky. At the senior citizens' home where she works, pets are welcome visitors. "People who are normally quiet will talk to an animal," she says. "It's really hard to resist a dog's imploring head in your lap."

Pets, especially dogs and cats, bring out the nurturing instinct in us, says Dr. Elkin. "Studies show that pet owners are less likely to develop stress-related illnesses such as heart disease than are people living alone," he says. Simply having a dog in the room or looking at an aquarium of fish can reduce blood pressure and lower pulse rate.

SHE GETS BY WITH A LITTLE HELP

"If you have friends, that helps stress about as much as anything," says Clara, 66, of Table Grove, Illinois, and Bonita Springs, Florida. She should know. Her husband died of AIDS, the result of a contaminated blood transfusion. "We had about seven years of nonstop stress," she says.

She's now alone in her big farmhouse in Illinois, but her long-time neighbors made sure she didn't feel entirely alone. "They would call me in the evening and ask me if I would like to come and eat with them," she remembers. "This would happen three, sometimes four, times a week. When they first started inviting me, I said, 'Now, I've already been down there a couple of times this week.' And they said, 'We wouldn't ask you if we didn't want you to come.' So, I sure would go, and it did make me feel a lot better."

Friends—what mental health professionals call a social support system—can reduce the sense of isolation people often feel when they're anxious, Dr. Elkin says. They can help you look on the positive side of things, offer a laugh, a shoulder to cry on or a kind word about yourself.

"This woman is very lucky," he says. But don't expect friends like these to appear out of nowhere. "Making friends is work. You need to find places like church where you can go to make friends," he says. Try being a friend, too, to reduce stress. "Phone someone you haven't talked to in a while," advises Dr. Elkin.

SHE TAKES TIME TO BE ALONE

"It's just plain solitude I crave," says Allene, 71, of Clifton, Texas. Years of working in high-pressure, people-oriented jobs, including her current stint as "general flunky to my husband," make her yearn for an afternoon of fishing or a long, quiet walk. "With no telephone and no one around to bother me—just the flow of the river and the sun—I can calm down, cool down or whatever," she says.

EDITOR'S NOTE: While solitude may soothe an introvert, it could be stress producing to someone who needs to be around people, Dr. Elkin says. "Know your personality type and your needs, and realize that sometimes what you need is change," he says.

HER BUBBLE BATH BECOMES THE BEACH

Some people use their mind's eye to help dissolve stress. By seeing relaxing situations in their minds, they produce relaxing changes in their bodies—momentarily lowering blood pressure and slowing heart rate, for example.

"I'll take a bubble bath, which is relaxing in itself, but I'll also close my eyes and imagine I'm basking in the sun on a hot beach, and it relaxes me even more," says Edith, of Raleigh, North Carolina. She's most likely to do this in the evening, after a particularly jaw-clenching day.

"The use of imagery can be incredibly useful for stress reduction," Dr. Elkin agrees. He likes to use a form of imagery he calls the blow-up technique. "Imagine your worry becoming exaggerated to the point of absurdity, where you begin laughing," he says. Someone who might worry about leaving the tap running at home, for instance, might imagine the whole house filling up with water until the windows and doors burst open.

SHE CREATES BAKER'S BLISS

"I use an apple-cinnamon potpourri around my house, particularly around the Christmas holidays," says Helen, 52, an X-ray technician from Chicago. "It's really soothing to come home to a fragrant-smelling house, and it's easier than baking an apple pie!"

Baby powder, apple pie, the smell of lilacs on a warm spring breeze. Can these scents calm you down? A branch of herbal medicine—aromatherapy—says yes. It uses the essential oils of plants to help heal the body. These oils and their fragrances can apparently have an effect on the central nervous system, making them a perfect choice for stress reduction. So it's no wonder that some people rely on a good sniff of one thing or another to alter their mental state.

In fact, food odors, especially a spicy apple scent, can produce a calming effect, Yale University researchers have found.

SHE BREATHES AWAY TENSION

"I learned from a biofeedback therapist to pay more attention to my breathing, especially when I am anxious," says Amy, 43, an elementary school teacher from Madison, Wisconsin. "I was taking rapid, shallow breaths, and I learned to consciously take slower, deeper breaths and to exhale fully. It's simple to do and really does help calm me down. In fact, I did this recently when someone ran into my car from the rear. It helped me to get out of the car calmly and get the information I needed without screaming or crying."

Slow, deep breaths can help relieve anxiety, Dr. Elkin agrees. "Such breathing sends a message to the rest of your body that all is well and helps to reverse other stress-related physiological reactions, such as rapid pulse, muscle tension and blood vessel constriction," he explains.

MUSIC SOOTHES HIS SAVAGE BREAST

Although some people try to get all the noise out of their lives when they're stressed, a few tune in to very specific wavelengths—whatever works to reduce stress for them. Most people say they prefer soft, quiet music—classical or what's called New Age. One woman prefers opera. "I don't understand the words, but that doesn't matter," she reports. "The music is what helps."

And one participant offers the kind of combination therapy an aging Baby Boomer can appreciate: "Dance by yourself to some fast music. You immediately feel better."

Few people would disagree that music can work soothing magic. Some experts theorize it's the rhythm; some say it's the "tonal atmospheres" created by music; others say it's just feeling comfortable with whatever you like. "It can be relaxing, distracting, energizing and evoke some beautiful memories," Dr. Elkin agrees.

Sunburn

Soothing the Scorch

You are, as they say, toast. A veritable crispy critter. Singe city. Our survey takers are all too familiar with that baked-to-a-crackly-crunch sunburned feeling. Located in hot spots across the country—Utah, California, Texas and Oklahoma, among others—they've had ample opportunity to discover a number of home remedies. Here are their favorites.

VINEGAR LOVERS SWEEP THE VOTING

Mary Ann, a 62-year-old Pittsburgh resident, captured the essence of those who swear by vinegar for treating a sunburn when she said, "Of course, you may smell like a pickle, but it takes the burn out."

In fact, nearly half of those who responded with remedies for this problem said nothing beats vinegar for soothing even the worst burns.

Pat's another example. A few years older than her two brothers, the Starkville, Mississippi, resident spent a lot of time as a kid taking care of them. Part of that care involved dousing one brother with vinegar after he spent too much time at the lake. "Even his armpits were blistered," she recalls. "I put vinegar on him every hour for eight or ten hours, and it never did even peel. It takes the heat right out."

You can almost count on Joy getting her first burn of the summer around May while participating in a bike- or walk-a-thon or working in her garden. It gets hot in Clinton, Oklahoma! When the inevitable happens, this motel manager mixes up a basin of three parts water for every part vinegar and dabs the solution on her burning shoulders. "It relieves the burning, that hot feeling, very quickly," she says. "You know how you feel hot in the middle of the night? I've used it then and been able to go right back to sleep."

Is this seemingly indispensable liquid good for yet another use? The experts say yes. "Vinegar is acetic acid and in low concentrations can be recommended medically for a number of situations where the skin is very irritated," says John E. Wolf, Jr., M.D., professor and chairman of the Department of Dermatology at Baylor College of Medicine in Houston, Texas. "I would think if people pour just plain vinegar on irritated skin, it would sting. But if they took the vinegar and diluted it significantly with cool or tepid water, then they'd have a soothing bath or compress."

EDITOR'S NOTE: Of course, severe sunburns, like those causing blisters, should be seen by a doctor. Extreme cases may need treatment with a powerful prescription topical steroid to heal properly.

THEY REACH FOR ALOE VERA

Carol, of Howell, Michigan, says aloe vera works so well she lathers the gel on with her sunscreen before tackling her lawn—a four-hour job. "Because of the healing properties, I figure it would be good to put on beforehand, too," says the fair-skinned 43-year-old massage therapist.

Of course, in those rare instances when she does get too much sun, Carol's quick to pour on the aloe vera gel she's purchased at a local health-food store.

Connie, a Palm Springs, California, resident who swears by aloe vera straight from the plant, wrote us with this testimonial: "My neighbor had a very bad sunburn. I suggested that she use aloe vera plants for relief. She broke a leaf in two and spread the substance over her sunburn. It gave her much relief, and I swear by it ever since."

Studies have shown that aloe vera gel hastens the healing of burns, frostbite and even surgical wounds. Among other substances, aloe vera has been found to contain salicylates, the painkilling and anti-inflammatory component in aspirin.

THEY MAKE TEA

Freshly brewed tea and even tea bags rated with our crew as another top sunburn stopper. Indeed, both aloe vera and apple cider vinegar users, like Carol, of New Jersey, recommend cool, wet tea bags for sunburned eyelids.

"Use four tea bags to a quart of water and cool it to lukewarm," advises Edith, a 53-year-old Taylorsville, Kentucky, resident. "Then you bring out a washrag or a towel, soak it in the tea and place it over your sunburn, and keep applying till the pain goes away, about 30 minutes."

Edith says she's used this remedy since she was a child. While on vacation with her parents in Florida, she got a severe sunburn, and a druggist told her mom about tea for sunburn. "We tried it and I didn't even blister," she recalls.

Joanne, a 53-year-old New York resident, opts for really strong tea. "Steep four tea bags in about a cup of water, cool and apply the liquid to the burn. The tea acid will soothe and cool immediately," she says.

Employing tea as a sunburn treatment isn't as far-fetched as it might sound, says Dr. Wolf. "Tea contains tannic acid. I don't know right offhand how the tannic acid would help, but it may be, in very dilute concentrations, soothing, just as acetic acid would be if it was diluted considerably," he says.

VITAMIN E HAS SOME FANS

John swears by vitamin E for leg cramps, and his wife found them effective during menopause. So it's no surprise the 76-year-old Forestville, Maryland, resident breaks open a few 400 IU (international units) capsules when he has a sunburn—or suggests the same for a pal.

Such was the case at work one day. "Someone spilled hot coffee on this fella's hand, and I told him to get some vitamin E," John recalls. "He said something like, 'Oh that stuff is voodoo medicine,' or something like that."

John didn't have any vitamin E handy to prove his theory, but a colleague did, and he was more than willing to share. The man reluctantly spread vitamin E oil from the capsules on his hand and, within a few minutes, said he was no longer in pain. The treatment made such an impression that a few months later the gentleman told John he successfully treated his wife with vitamin E after she suffered a sunburn while vacationing in Ocean City, Maryland. "I wouldn't use butter or ice or anything else for a sunburn. I would use vitamin E," says John. "It stops the burning and takes care of the blisters and peeling."

Daphne, a 63-year-old Dallas resident, can't stand those spray bottle sunburn remedies. "I always hated that stuff you get commercially," she says. "It comes out with such force against my parched skin, it hurts!"

Vitamin E oil, on the other hand, works so well that she even uses it on her pets (not for sunburn, but other skin problems). "I've always turned red and cooked," she says. "I like the vitamin E oil you can buy in a bottle. An oil lubricates the skin. It's soothing."

EDITOR'S NOTE: Although there's little research into vitamin E's use for sunburn, animal studies have documented improved wound healing of bedsores, diabetic ulcers and surgical wounds with vitamin E used topically. Be careful, though; vitamin E used on the skin can cause rashes in some.

BAKING SODA ENDS HER SORENESS

Karen doesn't get too many sunburns, but when she does, the 44-year-old Shelby, Ohio, resident has a two-step plan for relieving the pain.

First she draws a tepid bath, sprinkles in a cup of baking soda and soaks for 20 minutes. "That takes out some of the burn," she says. After patting dry—"you can't do much rubbing, you've got a sunburn"—she applies white vinegar with a cotton ball.

If the sunburn's bad enough, she'll repeat the procedure a couple times before bed.

Baking soda has a long folk history of use for sunburns, insect bites and poison ivy, says Dr. Wolf. Is there any reason why it might work? Could be. Bicarbonates—baking soda is 100 percent sodium bicarbonate—are sometimes mixed with local anesthetics to reduce the pain that follows injection, he says.

OATMEAL EASES HER PAIN

Aware of the damage excess sun can do to her skin, Catherine doesn't spend nearly as much time under those harsh rays as she used to. But when she does get too much, the 61-year-old Aldan, Pennsylvania, resident soaks in a soothing oatmeal bath a lot like her granny used to prepare.

"It was my grandmother's method—swirling two cups of oatmeal in some tepid bathwater until it almost had the consistency of gravy," she says. It's a lot easier these days, says Catherine. She uses a commercial brand manufactured for the bath (not for breakfast) called Aveeno colloidal oatmeal as directed.

Colloidal oatmeal with oil is one of Dr. Wolf's favorite sunburn remedies. "Theoretically, the colloidal oatmeal products should kind of coat the skin and the oil should give you a layer of oil and the two should help you retain water in the skin," he says. "And hydrated skin is going to feel better than skin that's all dried out from the sunburn effect."

THEY PREFER MOO

After her children spent a tough day in the sun picking corn and tobacco, Betty's mom would carefully spread the residue of freshly churned, homemade buttermilk on their sunburns. "It's the fat content that made it so good," remembers the 61-year-old Walbridge, Ohio, resident.

Instead of using buttermilk today—she says you can't find it like that anymore—Betty chills a can of evaporated milk for her kids and grandkids.

"It's rich enough," she says. "You put a little on your fingers and pat it on where it's sunburned. A washcloth or something like that is too rough. It will scrape the skin."

While there's not much science behind milk as a suitable sunburn remedy, there is some history, says Dr. Wolf. "It may be a little messy, but milk has fat in it, it's a liquid, and any kind of a liquid at a cool or tepid temperature does seem to make inflamed skin feel better. Milk baths have been used over the years for beautification, and some people do find them soothing, so milk would probably be soothing."

Swimmer's Ear

Stop the Waterlogged Pain

Every summer you splash in the pool. Every summer you complain about earache.

Do long hours in the water have to mean swimmer's ear? No, say our survey takers. They've come up with a number of ways to prevent or treat swimmer's ear—a painful bacterial infection associated with waterlogged ears. In fact, several participants say they had to deal with swimmer's ear for a few summers in a row until they discovered a sure cure. Here's what they say works to keep ears dry and healthy.

THEY DRY OUT WITH ALCOHOL AND VINEGAR

"My son, who is an avid swimmer, was in the doctor's office several times with swimmer's ear, until he started putting a solution of rubbing alcohol and vinegar in his ears," says Connie, 48, of Palm Springs, California. It was her pharmacist who suggested this solution. "He said it was similar to over-the-counter swimmer's ear products," Connie says.

"This solution can be very helpful because the vinegar is a mild acid that kills germs in the ear canal that cause swimmer's ear," says Edwin Monsell, M.D., Ph.D., head of the Division of Otology and Neurotology at the Henry Ford Hospital in Detroit. The alcohol helps by drying out the ear, he explains. It breaks up the surface tension of the water, allowing it to easily run out of the ear. It also washes out earwax.

Get an eyedropper-style bottle from the pharmacy and fill it with a mixture of half white vinegar and half rubbing alcohol, he suggests. After swimming or showering, tilt your head and put in enough drops to fill the ear canal. Then tilt your head the other way to let the solution pour out.

EDITOR'S NOTE: If your ears tend to be dry, or if the ear canal is irritated, use water instead of alcohol. "I tell people, especially diabetics, to use distilled vinegar and distilled, sterile water, not tap water, in their ears," says Dr. Monsell. "They can get a very serious type of ear infection if they aren't careful."

OIL PROTECTS HER EARS

"I used camphorated oil to treat any kind of earache, including swimmer's ear, in all six of my children—the same stuff my mother used for me," says Helen, 62, of Clearwater, Florida. She simply places the bottle of oil in hot water to warm it up a bit, then rubs the oil on the outer ear canal and applies just a bit inside the ear canal, using the tip of her finger. "Then, it's best to lie down for a while, using a heating pad on the ear," she says.

"Oil can help any sort of dry, flaky, irritated ear canal condition," Dr. Monsell agrees. He recommends using a few drops of mineral oil in each ear. There's even a prescription eardrop that incorporates acetic acid (vinegar) and oil. "Its advantage is that it tends to coat the ear canal and stay in there longer," he says. "It also helps to make up for skin oil production, which is impaired in swimmer's ear."

If you have dry ears, and also get swimmer's ear, Dr. Monsell suggests using a solution of water and vinegar first, followed by a few drops of mineral oil.

SHE TAKES AIM WITH HER BLOW-DRYER

"I've used a blow-dryer to dry my children's ears after a bath, and we also use this to dry ears after swimming, especially during the wintertime, when we swim at the Y," says Vivian, 46, a shipping clerk from Columbia, South Carolina. "It's easy, it gets their ears dry as well as anything, and we have no problems with swimmer's ear."

EDITOR'S NOTE: Doctors say it's fine to use a blow-dryer on your ears. Just set the dryer on warm or cool (not hot), and hold it about 18 inches away for a minute or so.

Teeth Grinding

Putting an End to the Same Old Grind

If you work for a living, no one has to tell you about the punishing effects of the daily grind. But did you know the stress you're carrying home from work in your briefcase or lunch bucket may also be causing your nightly teeth grinding?

Also called bruxism, teeth grinding seems to come naturally for those who have crooked teeth or suffer from too much stress, according to Dan L. Watt, D.D.S., a dentist in Reston, Virginia, and chairman of the International Dental Health Foundation, also in Reston.

A tiny but vocal group of people who responded to our survey know from experience that bruxism is more than just an annoying, unconscious habit. And they've had the sore jaws, headaches, stiff necks and broken teeth to prove it. Here's how they handle their gnashing.

SHE CHOOSES CHEWING

With bruxism so bad that it wore down one side of her teeth, Bonnie was searching for answers. Finally, she read one day that a combination of treatments, including gum chewing, calcium supplementation and simple jaw exercises, could ease her bruxism.

Nearly five years later, the 66-year-old Boulder, Colorado, resident says her nighttime grinding is under control.

Bonnie's regimen starts with an hour of gum chewing while she takes her afternoon walk. Next, she opens her mouth as wide as possible several times a day, stretching her jaw muscles. And just before she goes to bed, Bonnie says she takes two calcium tablets, which help relax her jaw muscles.

"It doesn't seem like much, but these things have really worked well for me," she says.

Based on what doctors know about bruxism, several of Bonnie's remedies could be contributing to her success, says Dr. Watt. Among the most important: stretching and contracting her jaw muscles.

"When you contract a muscle, the brain sends out two signals: one to contract the muscle and the other to relax the opposing muscle," explains Dr. Watt. "And that's what you're doing when you're stretching and yawning." Dr. Watt says he even recommends resting your jaw on your chin with your mouth open slightly while you watch television to help stengthen those muscles.

On the other hand, chewing gum would only be helpful if you keep your mouth open while chewing and don't bite too hard, he says.

Although Bonnie's contention that calcium helps relax her jaw muscles has not been documented by research, experts say her experience is consistent with a growing body of anecdotal evidence. There are a lot of people out there claiming that calcium seems to banish their bruxism. Since most folks need more calcium anyway, it wouldn't hurt to check with your doctor about taking supplements of this important mineral to see if it helps.

THEY SCORE WITH FOOTBALL MOUTHPIECES

Two of our survey participants say they tackled their bruxism by purchasing moldable football mouthpieces at their neighborhood sporting goods store and putting them in before bed.

Football mouthguards will stop you from grinding your teeth, says Dr. Watt. But if you continue to have jaw pain, that can be a sign that your teeth are out of alignment, and you may need a more elaborate mouthpiece that only a dentist can provide, he says.

"I'd say that in 30 to 40 percent of the cases, a tooth that's hitting too high when you bite down is triggering the problem. The next step, then, is to see if we need to keep from having the teeth hit together. And that's something you'd have to talk to your dentist about," he says.

SHE DELETES HER DENTURES

A 75-year-old woman who answered our survey says she simply removes her lower denture before bed to stop her nighttime gnashing.

While there's no doubt that taking out your dentures will stop your teeth from grinding, it's still a good idea to make sure your teeth are aligned properly, says Dr. Watt.

"If you can imagine your teeth hitting a couple millimeters before they do right now, then your tendency would be to clench. This woman probably just needs to have her dentures refitted," he says. In fact, it's a good idea to have dentures examined for fit on a yearly basis, he says.

STRETCHING, MASSAGE, EXERCISE EASE HER PAIN

After years of grinding her teeth, Helen took matters into her own hands.

Each morning and night, the 72-year-old Olympia, Washington, resident carefully massages her jawline, cheeks and neck with her fingertips in a bid to improve circulation and beat the stress and tension that's been linked to bruxism.

"When I was recuperating from an accident a few years ago, I became convinced of the value of improved circulation," says Helen. "And since I've been doing these things, I've noticed some improvement—and so has my dentist."

Helen has also developed a stretch for her jaw that she says has been of benefit. Bending her head back until her chin jaw is pointed toward the ceiling, Helen then extends her lower jaw until it reaches just beyond her top teeth for 30 seconds.

And as if that's not enough tension reduction, Helen says she tries to get regular exercise by walking as many as four miles a day or by swimming.

While her jaw-stretching program is certainly beneficial, Helen's overall exercise program may be providing the biggest benefit, says Dr. Watt.

"The first thing I try to talk to patients about is the stress in their lives," he says. "And, of course, we know daily cardiovascular exercise is great at helping relieve stress."

Because you're just as likely to grind during the day as you are at night, awareness can also go a long way in helping relieve the problem, says Dr. Watt. "Try to catch yourself clenching your teeth, and then deal with it," he says.

Tendinitis

Easing the Ache

Repetitive movements—things like painting your ceiling or tossing a baseball—can irritate and inflame your tendons—the tough, ropy structures that attach your muscles to your bones.

"The tendon floats back and forth smoothly. But once injured, you get a buildup of fluid or other irritative substances and pain," explains Ronald Lawrence, M.D., president of the American Medical Athletic Association and author of *Goodbye Pain*. That painful irritation is known as tendinitis.

Several of our survey takers suffer the ache of tendinitis from time to time. In addition to the ever-popular aspirin, they've discovered a number of techniques for managing the pain.

HEAT HELPS THEM

Moist heat is the favorite remedy for treating this stubborn problem.

"My way is placing a folded wet face towel in a clean saucer in a microwave for about 15 seconds to heat, then placing it on my sore tendon. Repeat a couple of times," says a North Carolina woman.

Either hot or cold packs should do the job, says Dr. Lawrence. "For more recent injuries, cold may be the best idea," he says. "For longer-term problems, moist heat is probably better. It increases blood flow, washing out the irritating substances. Twenty minutes, a half-hour—the amount of time you apply it doesn't mean anything as long as you are comfortable. If you've got the time, you can do more."

No microwave? You can take a moist towel or cloth and cover it with plastic wrap and put a heating pad over the top, he says.

SHE GIVES THIS PLANT AN A

The pain started in her elbow. And within a few months, Ruth's tendinitis was so bad she could barely raise her arm to comb her hair. Even weekly therapy at a local hospital didn't seem to help. In fact, not until the

North Tazewell, Virginia, resident started taking alfalfa tablets did she begin to feel relief.

As it turns out, two of Ruth's sisters—a Nashville nurse and an Atlanta psychologist—recommended alfalfa. But her Atlanta sister did one better: She actually gave Ruth a large bottle of alfalfa tablets. Ruth says she took two or three a day faithfully, and a week later the pain was gone. And as a result she didn't stop taking them until she polished off the bottle. "To this day, four or five years later, I haven't had any problem with it at all," she says.

Although there are few studies demonstrating alfalfa's effectiveness for tendinitis (or other "itis" aches like arthritis or bursitis), some believe chemicals in the plant have an aspirin-like effect, says Dr. Lawrence. "With some of these remedies, like alfalfa, the theory is that animals in attempting to heal themselves would seek out these things and eat them, and, lo and behold, they would be feeling better. So the assumption is, because they did this, or ate that, it must be good for us," says Dr. Lawrence. "It's safe to say it may have some benefit because of its aspirin-like effect, but it may not be strong enough for most people. I tried it many years ago and did not get great results."

She Swigs from the Jug

To this day, there's some question about whether Pat was suffering from tendinitis. After a battery of tests, her doctors were never sure just what was causing her severe knee pain. But the 58-year-old Starkville, Mississippi, resident has no doubt what took her pain away—two ounces a day of a vinegar-and-juice mixture called Jogging in a Jug. "My knee would barely bend enough for me to sit down," she says. "Within a week of taking this stuff, the pain went away. It works."

How'd she hear about it? A little Southern hospitality: A cousin who took Jogging in a Jug for leg cramps made the suggestion, she says.

Sold in grocery stores in 17 states, Jogging in a Jug is an apple/grape juice and apple cider vinegar drink created by Jack McWilliams, of Muscle Shoals, Alabama. A former cotton and dairy farmer, McWilliams says he once suffered from debilitating arthritis in his left shoulder. "I was being sustained on medication, but I wasn't enjoying the quality of life I wanted," he says.

Then he discovered the merits of drinking apple cider vinegar. In addition to experimenting on himself with good results, McWilliams encouraged his family to try his elixir. They gave it good marks, as well.

Today, McWilliams says people who buy Jogging in a Jug report the best results when they drink two ounces every 24 hours. A six-bottle case costs $34 and will last six months, he says.

As strange as it may sound, apple cider vinegar may tip the balance of your body's complex acid/alkaline level, says Dr. Lawrence. "When you're having inflammation, the tissue tends to have a slightly more alkaline base," he says. "When you use apple cider vinegar, you've got acetic acid in the vinegar, and it moves your body more toward the acid side, which I believe helps in the healing process. That's widely used by many people and with good results."

TMD

Coping with Temporomandibular Joint Disorder

Headaches, clicking sounds, neck pain, ringing in the ears, cheeks made sore from the simple act of chewing a meal . . . you wouldn't think all those things could result from a misaligned or dislocated jaw joint. But they can, and they do.

The jaw hinge that enables you to open and close your mouth and chew your food is known as the temporomandibular joint. And doctors call problems with this joint temporomandibular joint disorder, or simply, TMD.

How does the jaw hinge become dislocated? In some cases, a blow to the face may do the job. And if you haven't been sparring at the corner gym? Some experts believe that many small assaults on your jaw—like crunching ice, chewing pencils or gnawing a pipe stem—can add up to big problems over the years. Experts don't really have the last word on what causes TMD, and there's no single cure for everyone who has this problem.

If you suspect that you may have TMD, you should see your dentist. This condition requires professional evaluation and treatment. In some cases, TMD proves resistant to treatment, and unpleasant symptoms linger on while a number of treatments are tried.

Many of our survey takers tried several things before finding relief. Here's what they suggest.

HE SCORES RELIEF WITH A FOOTBALL MOUTHPIECE

When John's uncomfortably hard, professionally fitted tooth guard failed to deliver relief, the 35-year-old Rutherford, New Jersey, resident picked up a moldable football mouthpiece at a local sporting goods store to see if that would get the job done.

"It seemed logical to me that the softer, pliable mouthpiece would be a much more effective cushion for grinding teeth while sleeping," says John. "When I went into the store to buy it, a customer and the store clerk were there. The clerk asked what I needed it for, and after I explained, they both nodded knowingly. Maybe I'm not the only one doing this."

John wears the mouthpiece nearly every night and seems to have less pain than before, reports his wife, Cheryl, who is a nurse and suffers from TMD herself.

Although most TMD sufferers probably wouldn't benefit from using a football mouthpiece, some might, says Brendan Stack, D.D.S., in private practice in Vienna, Virginia, and past president of the American Academy of Head, Neck and Face Pain and TMD Orthopedics. "If you are dentally overclosed—meaning that when you bite down, your chin is too close to your nose—the soft mouthpiece would increase the space between your upper and lower jaws. In other words, it increases the distance between your chin and jaw. That would give you some relief if that were your problem."

SHE SWITCHED HER SLEEPING HABITS

Marion, a resident of River Edge, New Jersey, did everything she could think of to eliminate TMD pain. Searching for relief, she saw a dentist, a physician and a chiropractor. Finally, Marion's husband made a discovery that has kept her pain-free for over a decade.

He pointed out that Marion always slept on her left side—the same side where she was experiencing jaw pain. Marion says she simply forced herself to sleep on her right side—and within a few days the pain was gone. "I was amazed that it brought me almost immediate relief," she says. "I've never been bothered since."

In fact, studies show that most TMD sufferers are women who suffer pain in their left jaw and sleep on their left side, says Dr. Stack. "When you're sleeping, the muscle reflexes that keep everything aligned are asleep, so the muscle sags. And of course, it doesn't just sag down toward the mattress, but it also sags back toward the ear and pivots a little bit." As a result, changing sleeping positions has helped plenty of people, he says.

One way to prevent yourself from sleeping on a particular side is to sew a golf ball into the shoulder of your pajamas on the side you want to avoid, says Dr. Stack. "Every time you roll over to the left, you roll onto this golf ball and automatically correct to the other side," he explains. "That's one little trick that people do."

Your dentist can also make you a mouthpiece that will hold your jaw in place while you sleep, no matter what position you're in. "You could sleep upside down on your head if you want, and it will hold your jaw in place," says Dr. Stack.

SHE QUIT CRUNCHING

Kim, a 20-year-old Macungie, Pennsylvania, resident, wore a special retainer and braces in an attempt to end her TMD pain. She also went through physical therapy and surgery. Each treatment seemed to help for a time, she says, but in the end it was simple things like avoiding chewy foods that provided the most relief. "I honestly don't think you can cure it," she says.

Kim now nixes things like hoagies, apples, caramel, large hamburgers, gum—anything that forces her mouth open too wide or makes her chew too much. "You've got to take small bites," she says. "You can't just pack it in there."

Avoiding chewy foods can provide some relief, agrees Dr. Stack. Improper chewing technique can also play a role in TMD, he says. "There is a proper way to chew," he explains. "You should chew straight up and down in a hinge motion, not milling side to side like a cow chews cud. You want a vertical stroke as opposed to a milling type action. That's why we take patients off of peanuts—you mill peanuts as opposed to chewing something like red meat up and down."

THEY LIKE IT HOT OR COLD

Volia, of Glassboro, New Jersey, reports that she uses hot packs—hot water and a washcloth—every morning on her neck and jaw. Kim, our friend from Pennsylvania, says she heats a wet washcloth briefly in her microwave to place on her jaws when they begin pulsating with pain. And she applies ice when they feel achy. "I can't leave the ice on long, or it starts tensing up," she says.

Alternating cold and hot treatments may provide the most relief, says Dr. Stack. He suggests using a hot water bottle for 15 minutes followed by an ice pack for 15 minutes. "What I think you're doing is fooling the nerve that sends the painful impulses to the brain," he says. "That's called shutting down the gate in the central nervous system."

Toothache

Pre-dentist Pain Relievers

When talking toothaches, our survey takers offer a mouthful of choices. A majority prefer to dab on oil of clove or take an aspirin. And a couple even recommend a swig of whiskey (applied topically, of course).

Whatever you choose to temporarily ease the ache, make certain to see your dentist as soon as possible, says Elaine Kuracina, D.M.D., a member of the Academy of General Dentistry in private practice in Endicott, New York. Most things that cause toothache require professional care, she says.

THEY GET NUMB WITH CLOVES

Count Virginia among the many who favor cloves. Just like her mom years before, the retired 65-year-old Ramsey, Illinois, resident says she uses cloves and clove oil for toothaches. "We've used it all our lives," she says.

Virginia says she squirts a few drops of oil of clove on a cotton ball and then dabs that on the sore tooth. That's usually good for an hour's worth of relief, she says. She repeats the procedure until she can get to a dentist. The same technique also works after an extraction, she says. Virginia's careful not to use too much, though. "You have to be careful, because it will burn the gum."

Karen doesn't normally keep oil of clove around the house. But when suffering from a bad molar several years ago, she went straight to the health-food store to pick some up. Somewhere along the line, probably from her parents, the 44-year-old Shelby, Ohio, resident says she learned about cloves' pain-numbing properties. "I think you can get it in drops, or you can wet your finger and put a little on the tooth itself," she says.

Although oil of clove can burn the gums, it's the ingredient of choice for dentists treating a toothache, says Dr. Kuracina. "There's a chemical in clove that actually soothes the nerves," she says. Dentists use a product called Eugenol, which is the active ingredient in oil of cloves, she says.

"To soothe a toothache caused by a lost filling, you can soak a tiny piece of cotton (about the size of the tip of a cotton swab) in oil of clove, place it in the hole and then cover the hole with temporary dental filling material available in most drugstores," says Dr. Kuracina. "If you cannot find it in a drugstore, then a piece of chewed sugarless gum will do until you can see a dentist."

EDITOR'S NOTE: Because Eugenol can actually harm teeth, it should be used only as a short-term, stopgap measure before you see your dentist.

THEY CALL FOR WHISKEY

Whiskey—not down the hatch but dabbed on the sore tooth—is another toothache treatment our survey takers favor. "Don't drink it, just hold it on the affected area," says Lauri, 47, of Hinsdale, Illinois. "Rub whiskey over gum and tooth until you get to the dentist," says Bonnie, 43, of Cincinnati.

EDITOR'S NOTE: An antiseptic and disinfectant when applied topically, whiskey also works as an anesthetic, says Dr. Kuracina. Just don't use the hard stuff on children. "I don't believe in rubbing whiskey on children's teeth or gums," she says.

SOME LIKE IT COLD

One woman recommends rubbing an ice cube on the webbed area between the thumb and forefinger. "This worked one weekend when the dentist's office was closed," she reports. As unlikely as this remedy sounds, there's a reason ice may be nice for a toothache.

"There is supposed to be some kind of acupressure point in that spot," says Dr. Kuracina. "I had one patient come in to see me wearing a clothespin there. I've also heard of placing a clothespin on the earlobe, that there's an acupressure spot there, too."

In fact, a Canadian pain researcher says this ice treatment eases tooth pain by sending impulses along the same pathways toothache pain travels. The result: The impulses close the gate on incoming pain.

Ice can also be used inside your mouth for treating a toothache, says Dr. Kuracina. When a nerve inside your tooth is dying, gases are created that put pressure on the inside of the tooth, causing pain. Ice or cold water on the tooth can cause the gases to condense, relieving the pressure and pain, she says. "I've had people bring a glass of cold water into the office with them that they are sipping constantly to help ease the pain," she says.

FLAVORS KEEP THEM SMILING

If someone told you to take vanilla flavoring for a sore tooth, you might think they were trying to make you forget about your toothache by keeping your taste buds busy. Not so, according to several of our survey takers.

With 11 brothers and sisters, Joan's husband's family had enough folks to field a baseball team—and keep a dentist very, very busy. Mom, too, was busy dispensing vanilla extract to ease toothache. "It was their family remedy," says the 57-year-old San Jose, California, resident. "I learned it from his mom."

And learned it well. When her husband broke a tooth recently munching popcorn, one guess what they used until he could see the dentist. "You just put it on a cotton swab and dab it on the affected area," she says. "It dulls the pain."

Dr. Kuracina has a theory why it could work. "All flavorings like that have high alcohol content, which would help," says Dr. Kuracina.

THEY USE ASPIRIN

Unfortunately, several of our survey takers are still using the old trick of dissolving an aspirin on a sore tooth.

EDITOR'S NOTE: While there's no disputing aspirin's pain-relieving power, it also damages your gums when applied topically, says Dr. Kuracina. "Swallowing an aspirin for a toothache is fine," she says, "but you shouldn't leave it lying against your gums like a lozenge. Aspirin can cause an acidlike burn on your gums. You may not experience pain, but when I see it, the gum looks like an open ulcer, and it will take a while to heal."

Ulcers

Strategies for Ending the Pain

Doctors feel like they've finally got the goods on one of the leading causes of ulcers. The prime suspect: *Helicobacter pylori*, bacteria that set up shop in your stomach and either create or take advantage of weaknesses in your stomach's lining to produce those painful sores.

In most cases these days, shutting down the pain created by this gut-level bad guy is as easy as taking the right doctor-recommended antibiotics. "We think now if you eliminate the bacteria, you've gone a long way in curing the disease, so it's worth a shot," says Howard Mertz, M.D., a member of UCLA's Center for Ulcer Research and Education and an assistant professor of medicine and gastroenterology.

That we received relatively few suggestions for this condition may be a tribute to science's recent success. Many of our survey takers have taken antibiotics to treat their ulcers. But they've also come up with several other methods for banishing ulcer pain.

THEY HEAD FOR THE HEAD

We're not sure just how cabbage (raw or juiced) became folk remedy number one for ulcers, but our survey proved its popularity. In fact, no other suggestion for this condition had as many fans.

Linda Mae, 44, of East Canton, Ohio, and Austin, of Wichita Falls, Texas, were two such endorsers. "It's good for an ulcer in no time," says Austin.

In fact, there seems to be a real history to cabbage as a cure for ulcers. Roman doctors used cabbage to treat ulcers, as well as such diverse conditions as headache, colic and insomnia. The first "modern" reports successfully using cabbage juice against ulcers surfaced in 1953 at Stanford University in Stanford, California. Research there showed drinking a liter of fresh cabbage juice over the course of a day healed seven patients of peptic ulcers in an average of only ten days!

The key ingredient in cabbage's success? Research points to a component of the juice known as glutamine. In a study of 57 people, in which 24 took glutamine every day while the rest used conventional therapy (antacids, antispasmodics, diet, milk and bland diet), glutamine proved to be the more effective treatment. Half of the people using glutamine showed complete healing within two weeks, and 22 of the 24 showed complete relief and healing within four weeks.

SHE AVOIDS FRIED FOODS AND SPICES

Helen says she first started to suffer from ulcer pain when her eldest son was a baby—a stress reaction she thinks was associated with his birth. And when the pain really flares, to this day she takes a doctor-prescribed drug called Zantac.

But she believes she's successfully avoided some episodes by eliminating from her diet most fried foods like bacon as well as those spiked with spice. "I'd rather not eat them than to have a flare-up," says the Hendrum, Minnesota, resident.

While spicy, fatty or acidic foods don't cause ulcers, they have been found to make an already angry ulcer feel worse. You don't have to stick to bland food, but stay away from foods that turn on the burn, experts say.

Then again, if foods like these are bothersome, you may not have an ulcer at all, but heartburn, says Dr. Mertz. "Fatty foods and spicy foods are known to promote acid and reflux, which in some people is experienced as heartburn," he says. (Reflux happens when the stomach's contents move up into the lower part of the esophagus.)

SHE AVOIDS MOO

Roberta, 30, of Gardner, Kansas, says skipping milk is a smart ulcer avoidance tactic.

Many people who have ulcers seem to suffer after drinking milk, says Dr. Mertz. "It used to be thought that milk would neutralize acid, but that's an outdated principle," he says. "Milk protein in the stomach stimulates acid. So drinking milk is not a good treatment for ulcers."

HE TAKES GINGER AND LICORICE

An old hand at home remedies, Austin says gingerroot and licorice also work well for treating ulcers.

"I take the gingerroot first and then wait about 10 to 15 minutes and take the licorice and let it dissolve in my mouth," he says. "I let them work together."

Ginger, proven effective in preventing nausea and motion sickness, has a calming effect on the stomach. Doctors who favor natural healing therapies sometimes recommend deglycyrrhized licorice (or DGL) for people with ulcers to help protect the stomach's lining.

(DGL is simply licorice with the glycyrrhizin removed. Glycyrrhizin can cause high blood pressure in some people.) You can find DGL at many health-food stores.

SHE SIPS CHAMOMILE TEA

Barbara, a 47-year-old resident of San Francisco, says she's allergic to all but one of the various prescription ulcer medications. She's learned to cope with the recurring pain by drinking chamomile tea and eating bland food like mashed potatoes until the pain passes.

"It seems to ease the symptoms, not overnight, but within a few days," she says. "The other secret to this treatment is to recognize the signs of stomach problems during their onset and to start treatment immediately, instead of pretending that the pain will go away."

In fact, chamomile tea is taken throughout Europe to help aid digestion and fight infection. Tea made from German chamomile is available in many health-food stores. (German chamomile has the best reputation as a digestive aid.)

EDITOR'S NOTE: Chamomile is a member of the daisy family and can trigger an allergic reaction in people sensitive to ragweed, aster or chrysanthemums.

STRESS MANAGEMENT SPEAKS TO HIM

One 23-year-old man suggests keeping emotional stress to a minimum as a key for keeping an ulcer under control: "Stay calm. Don't get excited. Think briefly before speaking to keep you from getting upset. Speak without harsh words, and most importantly, say what's on your mind and don't keep it bottled up."

In fact, keeping stress to a minimum could play a substantial role in avoiding ulcers, says Dr. Mertz. "There is some scientific evidence that people under a lot of stress will secrete more stomach acid," he explains. "You can't get an ulcer without acid, so the acid and the *H. pylori* together allow you to get an ulcer. If you have a lot of stress, it's conceivable that you would generate a lot more stomach acid and then develop an ulcer."

Vaginal Problems

Banishing Troublesome Infections

Vaginal problems are certainly common enough. Three out of four women have had at least one run-in with some form of vulvovaginitis. That's medicalese for the gamut of vaginal ailments—from yeast infections to menopause-related dryness.

Different vaginal problems can have similar symptoms—itching, burning, discharge and, sometimes, abdominal pain—so it's important to know exactly what you are dealing with before you start any kind of home treatment, experts say.

"You want to make sure you don't have a serious infection that can move into the uterus and fallopian tubes and cause infertility," says Paul Reilly, N.D., a naturopathic doctor from Tacoma, Washington, and an instructor at Bastyr University in Seattle.

"Most women who have repeated yeast infections can tell when they have another one and don't necessarily need to go to the doctor each time they get one," Dr. Reilly says. "However, recurrent infections could mean you have a problem such as diabetes, a hormonal imbalance or an overgrowth of yeast in the intestines, which needs to be treated."

It's also wise to see a doctor for the first episode of an infection or if your infection is associated with a new sexual partner, with a change in menstrual patterns, with severe discomfort or with any kind of bodywide symptom, such as fever, Dr. Reilly adds.

With that in mind, there is a place for home remedies, Dr. Reilly says, especially when it comes to preventing recurring vaginal yeast infections. Here's what our participants say helps them.

THEY REACH FOR ACIDOPHILUS

By far, yeast infections are among the most common vaginal problems. While over-the-counter creams such as Monistat 7 (miconazole nitrate) are fairly effective, some women find they don't go far enough. "I'd use it, but the infection would come back," says Marcia, 52, a day care home operator from Midland, Michigan. In fact, for one reason or another, recurrence occurs in about 60 percent of women who use such creams, Dr. Reilly says.

Many of our survey takers rely on yogurt, or supplements containing the same beneficial bacteria often found in yogurt—*Lactobacillus acidophilus*—to control vaginal yeast infections.

They use acidophilus in several ways—eating yogurt or taking acidophilus tablets on a daily basis to prevent recurrence of infection; during an infection, inserting yogurt into the vagina; mixing yogurt or powdered acidophilus with water and using it as a douche; even using yogurt as a sexual lubricant.

"I used acidophilus tablets continually for a year or two, when I was having a lot of yeast infections, probably because of hormonal changes," Marcia says. "It definitely did help to prevent a recurrence." She took four to six capsules a day.

"If I need to take antibiotics, I'll automatically get a bad vaginal yeast infection unless I also take acidophilus tablets or eat lots of yogurt," says Karen, 42, a hair stylist from Shelby, Ohio. "I start taking them as soon as I can after I start the antibiotic, and I always continue for at least a few weeks after I stop taking the antibiotic. Most times, the tablets help prevent the infection."

In fact, after many years as a classic old wives' remedy, yogurt has won a vindication of sorts. In a scientific study, a doctor at Long Island Jewish Medical Center found that women who ate a cup of live-culture yogurt a day had fewer recurring yeast infections than they did when they did not eat yogurt. All the women had had a minimum of five yeast infections in the year prior to the study. The number of infections fell from an average of three during the first six months of the study to less than one while the women were eating yogurt.

"Eating yogurt rebalances the bacterial flora in the colon, which may help prevent vaginal infections by boosting immunity or by preventing recolonization of the vagina with yeast from the colon. However, if you want to take supplements, I recommend taking acidophilus capsules or powders instead of tablets, which are not as potent," says Dr. Reilly.

EDITOR'S NOTE: Don't use yogurt vaginally unless you know for sure that you are battling a yeast infection, not some sort of bacterial infection, says Dr. Reilly. Yogurt provides an ideal growth medium for some types of bacteria, so using it inside your vagina can actually make a bacterial vaginal infection much worse.

Powdered acidophilus has a higher concentration of beneficial bacteria than yogurt, Dr. Reilly adds, but a recent study showed that many brands of powdered acidophilus didn't live up to their claims for amounts or types of microorganisms. How can you be sure you have potent enough acidophilus? "Ask at your health-food store if the brand you are purchasing has regular assays done by an outside laboratory, or write to the manufacturer to verify this," he says.

A good acidophilus brand should contain at least one billion viable organisms per gram. An assay may also tell you whether or not that particular strain of acidophilus can inhibit yeast growth.

GARLIC GUARDS AGAINST INFECTIONS

Several women suggest using a douche that contains garlic oil or crushed garlic cloves for vaginal infections, yeast or otherwise. And some also include garlic in their diets to prevent recurrent vaginal infections.

"I've used a douche that contained two crushed cloves of garlic and two tablespoons of apple cider vinegar, and it always seemed to help," says Roberta, 32, of Wichita, Kansas. "I'd use it once a day for two or three days, and the infection would be gone."

"I like garlic, and I'll eat two or three cloves a day if I am taking antibiotics for something like a bladder infection, or if I develop a vaginal yeast infection," says Lynn, 34, a lab technician from Amherst, New York. "It's hard to tell what's doing what, but I do seem to get better faster if I take garlic." Her favorite way of indulging: garlic-laced tabbouleh or hummus, Caesar salad with sliced raw garlic, or simply a sliced garlic and salami sandwich. No, she's not a complete social outcast. "I work alone pretty much, and my husband and friends like garlic as much as I do."

It's true that garlic does have antibacterial and antifungal properties, experts say. In fact, it has been used therapeutically for thousands of years. More recent research has demonstrated that garlic juice and its constituents can slow or kill more than 60 kinds of fungi and more than 20 types of bacteria, including some of the most virulent.

"Raw garlic is excellent to eat, especially for chronic yeast infections," Dr. Reilly agrees. "I suggest people include it regularly in their diet."

EDITOR'S NOTE: Garlic oil used in a douche or even a clove of garlic wrapped in cheesecloth and inserted into the vagina will also help knock out yeast infections, and, in fact, several of our survey takers say they do this. But Dr. Reilly does not recommend this use of garlic. "It can be too irritating," he says.

BAGGY CLOTHES MAKE A DIFFERENCE

Lycra, Spandex, leather, tight jeans, pantyhose—they may show off your figure, but women say these constricting, airtight clothes create the kind of warm, moist environment yeasts love. So they opt instead for a loose fit that allows air to circulate.

"I've found that switching from pantyhose to thigh-high stockings instead has made a big difference," says Heidi, 23, an Environmental Protection Agency information writer from Baltimore, Ohio. She'd suffered for a few years from monthly yeast infections until she started following this advice from a book her mother gave her. In fact, doctors recommend exactly the same sort of clothes for vaginal yeast infections, especially cotton-crotch panties.

BLOW-DRYER DRIES UP HER ITCH

"I'd tried lots of things, including cotton underpants and vinegar douches, but nothing worked for me until I started drying my pubic hair with a blow-dryer after every shower or swim," says Alexa, 37, an environmental survey director from Washington, D.C. "It is embarrassing to do this in the ladies' health club dressing room five days a week," she admits. "But it's been absolutely miraculous. I have gone from chronic yeast infections so bad I had to quit swimming to daily swims and an infection only every few years."

Here again, eliminating moisture helps to deter the growth of yeast, Dr. Reilly says.

SHE WATCHES HER SWEET TOOTH

Some women find that overindulgence in sweets seems to precipitate vaginal yeast infections. That's certainly the case for Dorothy, 67, of Aberdeen, Washington, who's had adult-onset diabetes for many years. "If my blood sugar gets out of control because I am not watching my diet, I'm sure to develop a vaginal yeast infection," she says. By eating nothing sweeter than a daily piece of fruit or two, she's able to control her blood sugar and reduce her tendency for infections.

"For women prone to infections, reducing sweets and improving diet in general is very important. It tackles an important cause of reinfection—yeast growth in the colon," Dr. Reilly agrees. (Yeast thrives on sugars.)

In addition to waving aside the dessert cart, he suggests adding vitamin- and mineral-rich vegetables and grains, more fiber, aromatic spices like thyme and sage (which fight yeast overgrowth in the intestines) and copious amounts of garlic and yogurt, along with a good multivitamin/mineral supplement. "This sort of diet is the foundation of treatment for chronic yeast infections," he explains.

Varicose Veins

Keeping the Flow Going

I f your throbbing, aching legs look like a map of the interstate high-way system, your problem is a matter of flow—blood flow. Standing or sitting all day can stress the gates or valves in the veins in your legs. These gates help move your blood back up to your heart.

When the gates struggle or fail, blood pools in your legs, squeezing your veins out of shape and bulging them toward the surface of your skin, explains Walter de Groot, M.D., FASC, past president of the North American Society of Phlebology and a Seattle surgeon.

"Gravity is our enemy," he says. "I always say varicose veins are the price we pay for walking upright."

Our survey takers claim they've found the fast lane for relief. Here's what they do.

THEY STOCK UP ON STOCKINGS

There are, no doubt, flashier home remedies than support hose. Still, our survey takers agree that few work as well for varicose veins.

Standing on a concrete floor for hours on end while working at a print shop, Joyce developed throbbing, aching varicose veins. The Spokane, Washington, resident began wearing elastic stockings.

"When I told the doctor that I was wearing elastic stockings, he said, 'Great,'" recalls the retired 62-year-old. "If you get the stockings before the varicose veins are too bad, you can prevent them from getting any worse."

Evelyn, 66, of Buffalo, New York, and Sammie, 68, of Ralls, Texas, also found support hose helpful for their varicose veins. And one 76-year-old woman took the time to share her dos and don'ts for proper relief: "Wear support hose. Do not wear midcalf hose."

Wearing quality stockings is the equivalent of having friendly hands gently squeezing your legs, says Dr. de Groot. "Stockings treat varicose veins at the cause," he says. "The important thing about support hose is that they be graduated. If you have moderate pressure at the ankle and heavy pressure above the knee, your stockings act like a tourniquet, which is exactly the wrong thing to do."

Instead, Dr. de Groot says, your stockings should provide the most pressure at the ankle and gradually decrease in pressure as they get higher on your leg. Medically prescribed support hose do just that. Good over-the-counter brands include J.C. Penney, Givenchy and Nordstrom Total Support Hose. "Always the words to look for are 'total support hose,' " he says.

EXERCISE EASES HIS PAIN

Ed, 65, already has the best body at the local health club—or so says his wife, Arlene. But when varicose veins caused increasing pain and numbness in his legs, the Columbia Station, Ohio, resident added another exercise to his training routine: calf raises.

Ed simply places a barbell over his shoulders, steps onto a block of wood and then raises and lowers his heels 20 times, rests for a few minutes and then repeats the exercise. "He's pain-free now, and he's got great-looking legs, I'll tell you that," says Arlene.

Any exercise like weight training, bicycling or walking is a natural pump pushing the blood back up to the heart, says Dr. de Groot. "Realistically speaking, a ten-minute walk in the morning and the evening would be a good way to do it," he says. Consistent exercise can reduce symptoms like throbbing and aching within several months, he says.

SHE TAKES A LOAD OFF

Yvonne's doctor suggested elastic stockings to help treat her varicose veins. And she might have taken his advice but for two things: It's too hot in Austin, Texas, to wear them, and frankly, she felt like they would make her look old.

Instead, Yvonne had her varicose veins removed by a doctor several years ago. And to keep them from coming back, she's figured out how to use gravity to her advantage.

Yvonne structures her workday to include a project every hour that allows her to get off her feet for 15 minutes. "You know, chores that you can do while you are sitting," she says. She also puts her feet up whenever she can.

Yvonne's technique is great for relieving gravity's grip on her legs, says Dr. de Groot. "Normally, your feet hang down, so gravity is against you. When you lie down, gravity is working for you. If I am sitting and I put my legs out horizontally in front of me, this treats the cause: gravity."

HE OPTS FOR ASPIRIN

Anthony wore surgical stockings he hated and covered his legs with warm compresses to treat both his varicose veins and phlebitis (another leg circulation disorder). "Those stockings are like having ants crawling up and down your leg," he says.

But it wasn't until he suffered from a heart attack during a winter hunting trip that the Norristown, Pennsylvania, resident learned aspirin was the key for his treatment. "My doctor told me I've got the thickest blood he's ever seen," he says.

Since he started taking an aspirin a day, his varicose veins have virtually vanished.

In fact, aspirin does prevent one of the complications of varicose veins, says Dr. de Groot. "Clotting of the superficial veins is not a threat to your life at all, but it's very painful," he says. "They call that phlebitis. Theoretically, aspirin could help prevent it by thinning the blood."

DIET DOES IT FOR HER

When Patricia got serious about dropping meat and as much fat as possible from her diet, she thought she'd probably lose a few pounds and improve her overall health. Little did she know the varicose veins on one leg and a "hot spot" on the other would virtually disappear, too.

"When I was off my feet, that hot spot—a lot of little broken blood vessels—was fine. Then I would be on my feet and it would turn bright red. The varicose veins are much, much less in evidence now," says the 53-year-old Toronto day-care worker.

Some experts say carrying extra body weight, especially in the form of abdominal fat, actually slows the flow of blood back to the heart. Losing weight can help prevent and ease varicose veins.

SHE RUBS AWAY THE PAIN

When pain threatened to knock her off her feet, Patricia says she would rub on an oil-based lotion made from the herb arnica. "Rubbing would stop the pain," she says.

Massaging the legs with arnica—or any other lotion, for that matter—is a well-known way to force blood out of the legs and back up into the heart. "A lot of people sit here and tell me their complaints, and they say, 'At the end of the day, I have to grab my leg and squeeze it,' " says Dr. de Groot. "And, of course, they are sending blood back up to the heart. If you put your foot up on your desk, you decrease gravity, but if you grab your leg and squeeze, you will squeeze blood back up to the heart and out of that vein."

Tincture of arnica, which can be purchased at most health-food stores, is recommended by some experts for bruises, sore muscles and sprains. It helps reduce pain and inflammation.

EDITOR'S NOTE: Do not apply arnica to broken skin or take it internally. This plant is toxic when ingested.

VITAMIN C WORKS FOR HIM

Sam, 61, of Marietta, Pennsylvania, encourages the use of vitamin C.

Indeed, vitamin C may be of some benefit for varicose veins. "Vitamin C theoretically reduces the fragility of blood vessels, so that might help," says Dr. de Groot.

HE GETS AN E

Remember Ed with the great legs? His wife, Arlene, convinced him to take 400 IU (international units) of vitamin E a day after she read that this nutrient is good for varicose veins and phlebitis.

Arlene may be onto something. Some experts believe vitamin E can reduce the symptoms of intermittent claudication—calf pain that seems to be caused by narrowing leg arteries. In one study, patients who took 300 to 800 IU daily for at least three months walked with less pain than those who received a blank pill. Blood flow through their legs also apparently improved.

EDITOR'S NOTE: Although the Daily Value for vitamin E is only 30 IU, 400 IU a day is safe for most people. If you suffer from moderate coagulation factor deficiency, however, don't take this much vitamin E. It can cause dangerous bleeding in people who have this condition.

CONNIE VOTES FOR VINEGAR

Connie says credit for her apple cider vinegar and sugar remedy goes to her Aunt Maude, an 89-year-old Ohio woman "with legs like a 35-year-old."

"All her life she has taken two ounces of this stuff every day, and she just has beautiful legs," says the Camden, Arkansas, flower shop owner. Even more remarkable, both of Aunt Maude's parents suffered from terrible varicose veins, Connie says. (The problem is hereditary.)

Aunt Maude insisted Connie begin drinking the tart mixture—one pint of warm water, three tablespoons of sugar and two tablespoons of apple cider vinegar—to avoid having another painful varicose vein operation.

And she did comply for several years with a daily dose—although recently she hasn't had any. Still the veins have not returned. "I probably need to get back on it, though," she says.

Mahlon, 62, is another vinegar fan. He not only rubs his legs with full-strength vinegar, but he also mixes two tablespoons of vinegar with honey and then drinks it for his varicose veins.

Although he's never heard of drinking apple cider vinegar for varicose veins, it can't hurt, says Dr. de Groot. "I am an open-minded doctor, and I say listen to your patients. I'm not aware of it, but I'm not laughing at it, either," he says. "If the patient derives comfort from it, even if it's from the placebo effect, there's nothing wrong with the placebo effect. And drinking vinegar can't hurt."

Warts

Banishing Those Unsightly Sprouts

When it comes to home remedies for warts, people get weird. Even the most rational among us attack warts with potions and incantations worthy of the Middle Ages.

Our survey takers offer their share of wonderfully wacky treatments . . . along with a number of suggestions that are downright down-homey.

WISHING MAKES IT SO

"When I was a little girl," one survey taker wrote, "my grandfather rubbed the warts on my hands and my cousin's hands with a bean and buried the bean we didn't know where. Both of us had our warts disappear in a week or so."

Ordinarily such treatments would seem like they wouldn't amount to much more than a hill of bean sprouts. But there's some evidence that, in the case of warts, at least, believing you're using the right treatment may be as important as the treatment itself.

"Warts are caused by a viral infection that is not really curable," says Libby Edwards, M.D., chief of dermatology, Carolinas Medical Center, Charlotte, North Carolina. "But they are very responsive to your immune system. So anything you can do to increase your immune response will help to get rid of warts. And that means injuring the wart in any way that brings it to your immune system's attention and believing that it works. When people believe something will work, it often does. The body will take care of it."

CASTOR OIL GREASES THEIR WART REMOVAL

Barbara, a resident of Dryden, Ontario, has lots of reasons to believe that castor oil removes warts—almost 100 reasons, actually. Barbara says she successfully treated that many warts with castor oil after she had them burned off and they grew back! "I had a terrible time with them. I was ashamed to let anyone see my hands. They were a mess," says the 82-year-old former nurse. "And after I had the warts burned off, they came back bigger than ever."

Then Barbara says she remembered that an elderly patient told her to rub castor oil once a day on her hands like cream to get rid of warts. "I did, and within three months they had all disappeared," she recalls.

Vic and his son James, residents of Flemington, New Jersey, are also among those who swear by the wart-removing properties of castor oil. James, 8, was visiting the family doctor for another ailment when he showed the doctor two warts that had sprouted on his fingers.

Rather than burning them off in his office, the doctor simply instructed the family to buy some castor oil. "He said castor oil is the main ingredient in some over-the-counter wart remedies," says Vic.

James applied the castor oil faithfully. "Within several days we saw a marked difference," says Vic. "They were probably gone in a week or two weeks' time."

Eleanor, 59, of Sun City, Arizona, remembers well treating a wart with castor oil as a child. The reason: Her mother made a fuss over her applying the gooey stuff herself like a big girl. "I applied it every night, and it just sort of fell off after a week or so," she recalls.

"Kept on long enough, it would soften a wart, so it might be easier to dig off the top and gradually remove it," says Dr. Edwards. "When the top cells of your skin stay wet long enough, they lose their cohesiveness. Rather than lying flat, they become round and plump and soft. Especially if they are covered with a Band-Aid."

THEY USE VITAMIN E OIL

Vitamin E oil is another top-rated wart treatment among our survey takers.

Whenever he has a wart, Claude, a 67-year-old Springfield, Louisiana, resident smears on some vitamin E oil he purchased at a local health-food store. "It makes them dry up, and the tops fall off," he says. For warts that appear on his body, Claude says he applies vitamin E when he bathes. For those that show up on his hands, face or neck, he'll spread on some vitamin E several times a day.

Connie, of West Linn, Oregon, says she helped her husband successfully battle no fewer than 23 warts on his hands by faithfully applying the contents of vitamin E capsules for several weeks. For good measure, he also swallowed one 400 IU (international units) capsule a day.

Although unaware of any properties vitamin E might have for fighting the virus that causes warts, continuous coverage with vitamin E oil could, just like castor oil, cause warts to crumble, says Dr. Edwards. "As far as vitamin E itself going in and rooting out that virus and clobbering it and making the virus go away, there is no evidence of that. Only by its lubricating or softening properties could vitamin E be of benefit," she says.

THEY STIFLE THEIR WARTS

Allene, a resident of Valley Mills, Texas, smothers warts with clear fingernail polish. "It cuts off the air, and they just go away," says the retired 70-year-old.

The goal, she says, is to create an airtight seal over the wart. It's not necessary to add more fingernail polish unless the seal is broken, she says. Depending on the wart's size, it should wash off with soap and water within a few days, she says.

Other survey takers suggest smothering the warts with adhesive tape or Elmer's Glue.

Could such wart abuse serve a medicinal purpose? In fact, it may be one of the most effective treatments, says Dr. Edwards. "Tape, glue, fingernail polish—they are all the same concept and, according to some doctors I've talked to, do seem to work. Maybe that's because if you cover the wart, it will get soft, just like if you wear rubber gloves your skin will get soft and moist. The same thing happens with warts."

DANDELION DOES IT FOR THEM

A dandelion lover from way back—she often picks dandelions for her salads—Nicole says her favorite green also works wonders on warts. "I had one just below my fingers, near my palm, and it was really bugging me," says the 55-year-old Fountain, Colorado, resident. "You just break off the dandelion stem, and it has that white milk in there. You put it on several times a day, and within a week or so the wart just shrivels."

One survey taker who identified himself only as a 40-year-old Native American also suggests dandelion milk.

Dandelion roots, stems and leaves have a long history as healing agents. Since the nineteenth century, the plant has been used as a diuretic to flush excess water from the body. And there's evidence that ancient Chinese physicians used chopped dandelion to treat breast cancer. But could it really work as a wart remedy?

"I have no idea what's in dandelion, but anything that's irritating that you put on a wart is likely to cause an immune system reaction," says Dr. Edwards.

EDITOR'S NOTE: If your skin is sensitive, be careful. Dandelion can cause skin rashes.

IODINE IS DIVINE, THEY SAY

"When I was growing up, I had a lot of warts and did everything to get rid of them. I was very ashamed of them," says Diana, an 83-year-old resident of Pensacola, Florida. A few weeks after applying iodine several times a day, however, Dorothy says her warts vanished. "It didn't seem to take long. It softens up, and pretty soon it falls off," she says.

While messy and and not her favorite treatment, iodine may theoretically be of some benefit, says Dr. Edwards. "Iodine can be irritating, and if it's an irritant, it might help get rid of some warts," she says.

ASPIRIN WORKS FOR HER

"The warts on my hands were so bad I could no longer grip a tennis racket. My doctor suggested I have them burned off," recalls Carol, a resident of Abilene, Texas.

After reading how aspirin can eliminate warts, she soaked her hands in warm water and then taped a slightly damp aspirin tablet on one of the warts. "One overnight application and within days the wart turned black and fell off," she says.

Carol has apparently stumbled upon a wart-buster of professional proportions. "Salicylic acid, which is closely related to aspirin, is a standard treatment for warts," says Dr. Edwards. A typical over-the-counter remedy has salicylic acid imbedded in a patch that delivers the acid gradually.

EDITOR'S NOTE: If you are allergic or sensitive to aspirin, do not try either of these remedies. Rubbing aspirin into the skin could cause a reaction. And people who are sensitive to aspirin can have an allergic reaction just from coming in contact with salicylic acid.

HE SINGLES OUT SALT

"My wart disappeared in about a month when I kept it covered with moist table salt and a Band-Aid," says Edward, 64, a retired manufacturing engineering manager from Centerville, Ohio. "I learned from my grandmother that in Norway they covered warts with salted fish. I didn't want to go around with salted fish on my forehead, so I tried the salt without the fish, and it worked for me."

Nothing fishy about this remedy. The salt is a mild skin irritant, and the Band-Aid serves to keep the skin covered and moist.

Water Retention

Ways to Wring Out the Water

Our bodies are composed mostly of water, a holdover from our aquatic origins. Sometimes, like sponges, our bodies hold more water than is normal—or comfortable. That condition, known as edema, can show up as a puffy face and eyes, swollen hands and ankles, a throbbing headache, stiff joints, tender breasts or a bloated belly.

"I know I have it when my ankles get swollen, especially at the end of the day," says Marilyn, 64, a retired nursing home worker from Oneida, New York. "I can definitely see it in my face, which is puffy and fat-looking, and I hate it," says Melanie, 38, a nurse's aide from Troy, New York.

Most causes of fluid retention are fairly innocuous—premenstrual hormone changes in the body, for example, or eating too much salt. Fluid retention can also be the first sign of potentially life-threatening disorders such as heart or kidney disease. That's why it's important to see your doctor right away if you have a sudden weight gain, swollen ankles or difficulty breathing, or if you find that an indentation remains when you press your skin. That's a sign of pitting edema—a type of fluid buildup that needs a doctor's attention.

Here, then, is what people do to dry up when they're feeling waterlogged.

THEY SHAKE THE SALT HABIT

"More times than not, I retain fluid when I've eaten too much of something that's particularly salty," says Linda, 39, a school food service preparer from Columbus, Indiana. Among the worst of her personal culprits: Chinese foods, hot dogs or other lunch meats, movie theater popcorn, pickles and her favorite—preserved fish such as kippers, herring or lox. "I can really pack that stuff in, and I pay the price later," she says.

It's true that too much salt makes your body retain fluid, agrees Norman C. Staub, M.D., a professor in the Department of Physiology at the University of California, San Francisco. That fluid stays with you until your kidneys have a chance to excrete the excess salt, which can take about 24 hours. So if you avoid salty foods, you are less likely to have noticeable fluid retention, Dr. Staub says.

SHE SWEARS BY JUICES

"Cabbage juice, mixed with raw pineapple juice, is the one thing that keeps my feet from swelling during the summertime," says Glenna, 74, of Spokane, Washington. She juices a whole cabbage and a whole pineapple and drinks the results over the course of a day. "You've got to be near a bathroom if you do this," she cautions.

Cabbage, like most leafy vegetables, contains a hefty amount of potassium. Potassium, along with magnesium, acts to chemically counterbalance sodium in the body and so helps to reduce fluid retention, says Patrick Donovan, N.D., a naturopathic doctor in practice in Seattle and Tacoma, Washington, and a faculty member at Bastyr University in Seattle.

"For sodium to be released from a cell, there must be potassium available for the cell to pick up," Dr. Donovan explains. Water normally follows sodium from a cell, traveling from an area of lower to higher salt concentration. This helps drain fluid from tissues.

"In fact, I encourage people to get more potassium by eating lots of fruits and vegetables, particularly green leafy vegetables," Dr. Donovan says. Grape and orange juice are also good sources, as are many vegetable juices.

WATERMELON SEED DRAINS HER

"Watermelon seed tea is better than anything!" That enthusiastic endorsement comes from Janie, 45, a massage therapist from Pottsville, Pennsylvania, who says that sipping two or three cups of this tea throughout the day helps relieve her fluid retention.

Watermelon, its seeds, and its relatives—cucumbers and other melons—contain a chemical called cucurbocitrin that apparently increases the permeability (leakiness) of capillaries in the kidneys, allowing more water than usual to escape into the urine.

"Watermelon is used in Chinese medicine for this reason," Dr. Donovan says.

Watermelon seed kernels are also a good source of both potassium and magnesium, minerals that offset sodium's fluid-retaining properties.

If you want to try watermelon seeds, use dried seeds for best results, Dr. Donovan says. Grind them into a powder and use about one heaping teaspoon per cup of boiling water.

THEY GO FOR THE GREENS

Several people say they take a natural diuretic to relieve fluid retention. Asparagus spears and parsley are among the foods they say have a draining effect.

"Just one serving—three or four spears—of asparagus usually works for me if my fingers are puffy," says Kathleen, a retired schoolteacher from Wichita, Kansas. It doesn't matter how you cook it, she says.

"I've used parsley tea several times to relieve premenstrual swelling, and it does seem to help," says Pattie, 27, a Durham, North Carolina, textiles worker. "I read about this in an herb book and decided to try it, just out of curiosity." She steeps one heaping teaspoon of dried parsley flakes per cup of boiling water.

"Asparagus has a very weak diuretic effect. Parsley is stronger, as are dandelion leaves and celery and celery leaves," Dr. Donovan says. (A diuretic is a substance that causes the body to lose excess water.)

MORE WATER EQUALS LESS FOR THEM

Want to get rid of excess water? Then drink up, several of our survey takers say.

"Whenever I notice that my body is retaining water, my remedy is to start drinking at least 16 eight-ounce glasses of liquid a day. Drinking this much water has always taken care of the problem. I put a couple of drops of lemon juice in the water or drink herbal teas," says Anna, of Wichita, Kansas.

"I retain fluid when I eat salty foods, such as Chinese food, and I can reduce the swelling by drinking three or four glasses of water," says Bonnie, 46, a freelance writer from Epping, New Hampshire.

Drinking more water can indeed draw water out of your tissues and out of your body via urine, Dr. Staub agrees. "It works by removing salt from your body," he explains. Salt causes fluid retention, but all body fluids, including urine, contain some salt. So the more you drink, the more you urinate; and the more salt you remove from your body, the less fluid you retain.

EDITOR'S NOTE: Plain water is definitely the best, because just about every other drink—juices, soda, milk—has a little sodium in it.

IT'S FEET UP FOR THEM

Several women say they'll stop whatever they're doing and prop their feet up on a chair for a few minutes when their ankles start to swell. "And if you can lie down and put your feet up, that works best," says Janie, from Pottsville, Pennsylvania. A massage therapist, she spends most of her day on her feet, making other people feel better.

Sometimes getting off your feet is the simplest and best thing to do, Dr. Staub says. If you recline with your feet in a raised position, you allow fluid that has pooled in your legs to make its way into the circulatory system and then to your kidneys, where it can be excreted.

VITAMIN B₆ STOPS HER SWELLING

Several people say they take vitamin B_6 to prevent or reduce fluid retention associated with circulation problems or premenstrual symptoms.

"I take it every day, and have for years, for the slight swelling I have in my ankles as a result of heart trouble," says Marilyn, of New York. Her ankles swell up by the end of the day and are especially bad during the hot days of summer. She says she takes a 100-milligram tablet twice a day, along with a B-complex vitamin and a multitude of other vitamins and minerals. "My doctor didn't recommend this, but he knows I do this and doesn't have a problem with it," she says.

Vitamin B_6 is sometimes recommended for fluid retention, especially when it's associated with premenstrual hormone fluctuations, Dr. Donovan says. "B_6 is involved in the body's manufacture of certain hormones associated with fluid balance and so may be helpful," he says. He prescribes 50 to 100 milligrams a day of the most biologically active form of B_6—pyridoxal 5-phosphate.

EDITOR'S NOTE: Most doctors recommend that you take no more than 50 milligrams a day of vitamin B_6 without medical supervision. That's because nerve damage has been associated with long-term use of high doses of vitamin B_6.

Weight Loss

No Diets Here, Just Dedication

We've all heard of some pretty wacko weight-loss plans and maybe even tried a few. (I was particularly disappointed when the Foot-Long Italian Hoagie Diet failed to generate washboard abdominals as advertised.)

We shouldn't be surprised when they fail, though. For one thing, few are based on sound nutritional principles. And for another, research shows the best way to trim down and tone up is by developing your own sensible eating and exercise plan and sticking to it, says Susan Olson, Ph.D., coauthor of *Keeping It Off: Winning at Weight Loss* and director of psychological services at the Southwest Bariatric Nutrition Center in Scottsdale, Arizona. "A diet is not something that you can do for the rest of your life. Psychologically, it just won't happen," she says. "But when you do it yourself, you're not following someone else's diet. Until it becomes your own, it really isn't going to last."

Which may be why our survey takers claim such tremendous slimming success. Devoid of dopey diets, their stories stress homegrown consistency and common sense. And in most cases, they rely on several techniques simultaneously.

CUTTING FAT IS THEIR FOCUS

Originally, Regina started cutting fat from her family's diet to help improve her husband's high cholesterol. Peter's cholesterol isn't the only thing that's gone down: In just a few months, he's also lost about ten pounds.

It's not hard to understand why. Until her health awakening, the 49-year-old St. Augustine, Florida, mom served the same "standard American diet"—things like pork chops, ham and hamburgers—she was fed as a kid. Now only lean cuts of beef—like marinated, grilled flank steak—make it to her family's plates. And then it's just once a week. Most other days, she feeds them chicken, fish or pasta.

She's also recruited her kids, Noah, Luke and Skylar, into her low-fat eating campaign. At the supermarket, they scour food labels looking for the lowest-fat choices. Regina doesn't even have to coax them at restaurants; the kids often order a salad or a McLean Deluxe at McDonald's.

Pat wasn't fat—at least nobody said she was. But, while eating cafeteria food during the years she worked as a Baltimore middle school librarian, the 45-year-old could feel herself packing on the extra pounds. Convinced she needed to lose weight, Pat cut much of the fat and sweets out of her diet and began walking and working out on a NordicTrack ski machine. Within six months, she lost 30 pounds and her dress size dropped from a 12 to a 4. "I had to buy all new clothes," she says. "That is a good problem."

Instead of eating high-fat school cafeteria food ("they'd give you french fries with a lasagna if you're not careful"), Pat says she now brings a lean turkey sandwich from home for lunch. "And I haven't had a french fry in almost a year," she says.

Dorothy's no lightweight, and she's the first to admit it. But the 82-year-old Pensacola, Florida, resident has lost and kept off at least ten pounds over the past year by cutting back on fat.

Of course, Dorothy splurges once in a while. The day we talked, she had just been to lunch with some girlfriends and had chicken fingers!

But the bad, old high-fat days of coating her baked potato in butter and sour cream or dining on lobster soaked in butter or steak once a week are behind her. Instead, you'll find Dorothy trimming the skin from her chicken breasts and skimming the fat off her chicken soup. She eats low-fat cheese only and enjoys plenty of oatmeal, orange juice and apples.

Eating less fat is a proven weight-loss strategy—and not just because fat has over twice the calories of carbohydrates, says Dr. Olson. "You know why I think watching your fat helps? It's because it gives you more freedom," she says. "I think when people are counting calories, they can feel restricted. But counting fat grams makes you feel like you have more say in what you eat."

Many nutritionists today suggest that no more than 25 percent of the calories in your diet come from fat. For a woman who weighs 160 pounds and eats 1,900 calories a day, that means no more than 53 grams of fat. And how much fat is that? To give you an idea, a single cup of gourmet vanilla ice cream can have as much as 24 grams of fat; a glazed doughnut weighs in at about 10 fat grams.

EXERCISE DOES IT FOR THEM

A retired schoolteacher, Nina has learned well that exercise is an important factor in weight loss. The 68-year-old Gonzalez, Florida, resident has lost 80 pounds since tipping the scales at 250.

Every day, Nina walks for at least 35 minutes—a trip that usually takes her past a nearby high school. (She's also learned how to pass on sweets—until recently her biggest weakness.)

Carole calls her walking program more "a saunter, really," but, between that and trimming the fat from her diet, she's dropped 30 pounds in just a few months.

Nearly every day, the 59-year-old Lexington, Kentucky, resident walks with her husband two to three miles, "checking out the neighborhood, seeing if everyone is doing his repair work," she says, laughing. Before she began walking at her doctor's suggestion, Carole weighed 138 pounds "and wasn't exercising at all," she says.

Jim, a 51-year-old Rochester, New York, resident, loves to ski. Before he started his exercise regime, you'd find him on the slopes every winter. But that's the only time he was active.

Jim now participates in a 75-minute step class twice weekly, uses the StairMaster at the gym and lifts weights. After six months on this program, he lost 20 pounds. What lay behind all this activity? "I just got sick and tired of being out of shape," he says. "I haven't felt this good since, probably, I was 20 years old."

Walking, aerobics and weight training are among the best techniques to trim your weight, says Dr. Olson. "Walking is really the number one aerobic exercise for losing fat, and 30 to 35 minutes a day would probably be just perfect, because it's something that you can keep up with for the rest of your life," she says. It can make a big difference in your metabolism, helping to keep it efficient, she adds.

Weight training actually enhances an aerobic fitness routine by building muscle mass that burns fat even while you sleep, says Dr. Olson.

She Overcame an Emotional Problem

Bobby remembers herself as a chubby kid and teen who ate for the wrong reasons. "I'd put food in my mouth not out of hunger but nervousness or whatever," says the 51-year-old Manhattan resident.

When she got to college and discovered she disliked the taste of the cafeteria food, she developed a sweet tooth that had her eating more than ever. Ice cream was one of her favorites—a snack that helped push her weight to 167.

A short time later, Bobby began experimenting with the effect of certain foods on her metabolism and weight. She dropped sugar and most meats, because they made her feel sluggish. She stopped smoking. And she started jogging, although she now prefers to walk. In fact, she doesn't even own a car. And she consciously worked at finding nonfood ways to satisfy her emotional needs and deal with stress.

"I've realized that prevention is the best thing, and I'm very devoted to my health," she says. "I discovered this a long time ago."

For the record, Bobby now weighs 120 pounds, but she's less concerned about what the scale says than how she feels. "Weight for me is not a problem," she says. "I can tell from my clothes if I'm getting heavier."

Putting on weight is a protective mechanism for many people, says Dr. Olson. "Eating carbohydrates is like taking a drug," she explains. "It produces a chemical in the brain called serotonin that not only gives you a feeling of well-being but helps you relax. So people are getting a 'numbing-out' when they binge or when they overeat, and it's an escape. And the weight itself can put distance between you and someone else. Some people eat when they are stressed or when they are bored or if they are angry at somebody or if they want to reward themselves."

Wrinkles

Face-Saving Tactics

Maybe we should have asked for photographic proof. Our survey participants who suggest home remedies for wrinkles seem almost too smooth to be true. "I can just watch someone's mouth drop open when I tell him how old I am," says Amelie, 53, an airline reservations agent from Aurora, Colorado. "People are always telling me how good my skin looks for my age," adds Anne, 64, of Hagerstown, Maryland.

Invariably, the conversation gets around to the little secrets these apparently ageless beauties employ to create such breathtaking effects.

And here's where our survey takers break into two categories. There's the "good genes and cold cream" group—those who do very little to their skin but nevertheless remain youthful looking. Then there's the "I'll do anything to look good" group—those with a long list of wrinkle minimizers, from exercise and diet to a medicine cabinet full of moisturizers, scrubs, sunscreens, and hemorrhoid creams. (No mistake. More later.)

So what works? Here's what our smooth-faced friends recommend.

SUNSCREEN'S THEIR BEST FRIEND

"I started using sunscreen every day about five years ago, and I noticed an improvement within a few months," says Laura, 45, a doctor's assistant from El Paso, Texas. That difference is especially apparent to her in the autumn. "I do still get a bit of a tan. But it used to be, when my tan faded, the wrinkles and dark spots would really stand out during the winter months," she says. "Now, those lines aren't so pronounced. I feel like my skin is holding its own against time, maybe even improving a little."

She usually uses a water-resistant discount store brand with a sun protection factor (SPF) of 32. "I also sometimes use a makeup that contains zinc oxide on my nose and around my eyes, and a lip moisturizer that contains sunscreen," she says. (Zinc oxide is the opaque sun-blocking paste life-guards use on their noses.)

Skin experts agree: Short of holing up in a cave, sunscreens are the best way to prevent wrinkles, not to mention skin cancer. The sun's ultraviolet rays damage the deep skin cell layers that generate the connective tissues that hold skin together, providing strength and elasticity.

Your best bet: Use a sunscreen that offers protection from all the sun's potentially damaging wavelengths, suggests Vincent DeLeo, M.D., associate professor of dermatology and director of Environmental Dermatology at New York City's Columbia-Presbyterian Medical Center. Look for sun-screens that include oxybenzone; dioxybenzone; 2-ethylhexyl, 2-cyano-3, 3-diphenylacrylate (also known as octocrylene); or titanium dioxide. And use one that offers a sun protection factor of at least 15.

To be most effective, apply it to the skin at least a half-hour before going out—the ingredients need to be absorbed by the skin before they work. And reapply after swimming or heavy sweating.

THEY WEAR WIDE-BRIMMED HATS

"I have several hats that I use for gardening or walking," says Lenora, 51, of Manhassett, New York. Her favorite is a long-brimmed baseball cap designed for fishermen. ("It's cool and it definitely shades my eyes.") She also finds that a tightly woven straw hat with a four-inch brim provides the most sun-blocking protection, especially when the rays are coming in at an angle. "That's my gardening hat," she says.

Hats, like sunscreens, block harmful ultraviolet rays. And because they shield your eyes from the sun's rays, they help you avoid squinting, which deepens the lines around your eyes.

Do note, though, that hats are useless for protecting you from sunlight coming from below as it bounces off reflective surfaces such as snow, sand or water. For that, only a sunscreen works, Dr. DeLeo says.

EGG MASK HELPS HER STAY SMOOTH

You can't turn back the clock, but for a special occasion, would you set-tle for about two hours of smoother-looking skin, especially if it costs only about ten cents—the price of one ordinary egg?

Here's the recipe from Eleanor, 58, a hospital issuance clerk from Soddy-Daisy, Tennessee, who got it from her mother-in-law.

Whisk an egg white until it's a little frothy. Then, with your fingertips or a cotton ball, dab it on your face. Let it dry. During this time, don't move your face at all, Eleanor warns, or the egg won't do its magic. Rinse your face with cool water and apply moisturizer and makeup. Alternatively, dab the whisked egg white on problem areas, such as under your eyes, and apply your makeup over the dried egg white.

"The egg white dries tight and shiny and tightens your skin to flatten out wrinkles," she says. Unfortunately, the effects only last a few hours.

"This works as well as a $100-an-ounce wrinkle cream," confirms Cleveland dermatologist Jerome Z. Litt, M.D., author of *Your Skin: From Acne to Zits.*

She Grabs the Moisturizer

"I have been using a good moisturizer for years, and it certainly seems to make my face look smoother," says Irma, 56, a housewife from Frederick, Maryland. She wears it at night and under her makeup during the day.

Moisturizers can help your skin look smoother by holding moisture in the outer layers of your skin, Dr. Litt explains. Look for a moisturizer that contains liposomes, he recommends. These are fatty acids, similar to those found in the membranes of skin cells, that attract, hold and then redistribute the moisture in your skin. Better yet, use a moisturizer-sunscreen combination. In one study, this mix, meant to be the placebo—inert treatment—fared well, with 48 percent of those using it for six months showing improvement in brown spots, wrinkling and roughness.

She Opts for Hemorrhoid Healer

Leave it to someone from Texas—a state that's produced more Miss Americas than most—to clue us in on an old beauty pageant skin secret: Preparation H. Some women maintain that this ointment known for soothing throbbing hemorrhoids can reduce fine lines and wrinkles.

"I've used this over the years, and so have some of my friends," says Carolyn, 54, of Houston, Texas. "I do other things as well, so it's hard to tell exactly what's doing what, but Preparation H works at least as well as many moisturizers I've used."

Any scientific backing to this claim? Perhaps, in a roundabout way. A component of Preparation H—live yeast cell derivative—which supplies something called skin respiratory factor, apparently helps to speed healing, at least when it comes to burns.

But when it comes to wrinkles, "Preparation H is not worth a darn," Dr. Litt says. "Not everything with grease in it makes a good face cream." Also, there is the possibility of developing a rash on your face if you become allergic to it, he says.

SHE PUTS ON A HAPPY FACE

"I know that tension shows up on my face, so when I have the time, I simply lie down and imagine all the tension draining out of my face like melting ice," says Connie, 44, a junior high school English teacher from Chicago. Taking a hot bath, or better still, relaxing in the steam room at her health club, helps her relax even more, she says. "Even just cupping my hands over my eyes for a few minutes helps," she says.

Experts agree that some wrinkles are caused primarily by facial expressions, not aging. (Vertical frown lines between the brows are a good example of this.) These wrinkles are caused by muscle contractions, often unconscious. You can, by conscious effort, help to minimize these kinds of lines.

THEY STAY YOUNG WITH VITAMIN E

Here's the youthful skin secret from the woman we mentioned earlier, the one who leaves people agape when they learn her age. Amelie, 53, an airline reservations agent from Aurora, Colorado, credits her smooth skin, at least in part, to her daily use of vitamin E, both topically and orally, for the past three years.

"The air is very dry out here, and the moisturizer I was using didn't work well enough," she says. "I had some vitamin E on hand and started using that at night. Now I say, 'Never underestimate the power of vitamin E.'" She simply opens a capsule of oil with a pin and rubs it on her face.

Vitamin E oil or creams are popular with several other survey takers, too.

Little research has been done to determine if, indeed, vitamin E can help wrinkle-proof skin. Most of that work has involved the vitamin's potential to prevent sun- or aging-related damage, including precancerous skin cell changes.

One study, by researcher Helen Gensler, Ph.D., of the University of Arizona College of Medicine, Tucson, found that only one type of vitamin E, alpha tocopherol, helped prevent sun-related skin cancer, but this form of vitamin E is next to impossible to find. (*Note:* Alpha tocopherol acetate, the form of vitamin E found in sunscreens and most supplements, was not helpful when used topically and, in fact, may even enhance your risk of skin cancer.)

Your best bet for now is to improve your skin from the inside by taking vitamin E orally. Either form will do, says Dr. Gensler, since alpha tocopherol acetate is converted to alpha tocopherol in the body.

SHE MOVES AWAY FROM WRINKLES

"I do know I look better than a lot of my friends my same age, and that lots of aerobic exercise is one thing that distinguishes me from them," says Karen, 47, of Beaverton, Oregon.

Karen may well be onto something. Know how a good brisk walk brings a healthy glow to your cheeks? Well, that blush isn't just pretty. It's a sign that exercise is flushing your skin with blood. The result: denser, thicker skin that springs back to its original shape after being stretched. That translates into fewer wrinkles and not-so-baggy eyes, says James White, Ph.D., an exercise physiologist and author of *Jump for Joy*, a book of exercise programs for people concerned about their skin or recovering from plastic surgery.

Index